Psychosocial Strategies for Athletic Training

Psychosocial Strategies for Athletic Training

Megan D. Granquist, PhD, ATC
Assistant Professor
Department of Kinesiology
University of La Verne
La Verne, California

Jennifer Jordan Hamson-Utley, PhD, ATC, LAT
Director of Teaching & Learning
Assistant Professor of Athletic Training
Department of Health Promotion and Human Performance
Weber State University
Ogden, Utah
Doctoral Faculty
School for Advanced Studies
University of Phoenix

Laura J. Kenow, MS, ATC
Associate Professor, Athletic Training Program Director,
and Athletic Trainer
Department of Health, Human Performance and Athletics
Linfield College
McMinnville, Oregon

Jennifer Stiller-Ostrowski, PhD, ATC, LAT
Assistant Professor of Athletic Training and Undergraduate
Athletic Training Program Director
Department of Health Promotion and Human Performance
Weber State University
Ogden, Utah

F.A. Davis Company • Philadelphia

F.A. Davis Company
1915 Arch Street
Philadelphia, PA 19103
www.fadavis.com

Printed in the United States of America

Last digit indicates print number: 10 9 8 7 6 5 4 3 2 1

Publisher: T. Quincy McDonald
Director of Content Development: George W. Lang
Developmental Editor: Joanna Cain
Art and Design Manager: Carolyn O'Brien

As new scientific information becomes available through basic and clinical research, recommended treatments and drug therapies undergo changes. The author(s) and publisher have done everything possible to make this book accurate, up to date, and in accord with accepted standards at the time of publication. The author(s), editors, and publisher are not responsible for errors or omissions or for consequences from application of the book and make no warranty, expressed or implied, in regard to the contents of the book. Any practice described in this book should be applied by the reader in accordance with Director of Content Developmentprofessional standards of care used in regard to the unique circumstances that may apply in each situation. The reader is advised always to check product information (package inserts) for changes and new information regarding dose and contraindications before administering any drug. Caution is especially urged when using new or infrequently ordered drugs.

Library of Congress Cataloging-in-Publication Data

Granquist, Megan D.

Psychosocial strategies for athletic training / Megan D. Granquist, PhD, ATC, Assistant Professor, Department of Kinesiology, University of La Verne, La Verne, CA, Jennifer Jordan Hamson-Utley, PhD, ATC, LAT, Assistant Professor of Athletic Training, Department of Health Promotion and Human Performance, Weber State University, Ogden, UT, Doctoral Faculty, School for Advanced Studies, University of Phoenix, Laura J. Kenow, MS, ATC, Associate Professor, Athletic Training Program Director, and Athletic Trainer, Department of Health, Human Performance and Athletics, Linfield College, McMinnville, OR, Jennifer Stiller-Ostrowski, PhD, ATC, LAT, Assistant Professor of Athletic Training and Undergraduate Athletic Training Program Director, Department of Health Promotion and Human Performance, Weber State University, Ogden, UT.

p. cm.

ISBN 978-0-8036-3817-4

1. Athletes—Mental health. 2. Athletes—Psychology. 3. Athletic trainers. 4. Medical referral. 5. Sports—Psychological aspects. 6. Sports—Social aspects. 7. Physical education and training. I. Title.

RC451.4.A83G73 2014

617.1'027—dc23

2014005676

To my mentors and teachers, my colleagues and students, my family and friends—for your guidance and encouragement.
To Dad—for your model of work ethic.
To Mom—for your example and for always being there for me.
To Doug—for your support and immense love.
—Megan

For my family, Michael and Seth, whose patience, love, and support allow me to move mountains. And for my parents, whose encouragement and guidance has led me down this path; "keep it on the high side of the road and out of the ditch."
—Jennifer Jordan "Casey"

To Mom and Dad (and Buddy),
My success stems from the unconditional love and support you so readily provide. Thank you and I love you.

To the injured athletes with whom I work,
You inspire me daily to strive to understand how to better facilitate the healing of body, mind, and spirit.
It is a privilege to work with you.
—Laura

To John, Mike, and Maryn—in all of the hours that went into this book, you were always on my mind, and so you have become a part of it. With you beside me, all things are possible.
—Jenn

Preface

Prompted by the recent revision of the Psychosocial Strategies and Referral (PS) content area within the fifth edition of the Athletic Training Education Competencies, this collaborative textbook came into existence because of our commitment to educating athletic trainers and athletic training students so that they may provide the best possible care by treating the *whole* person in a *holistic approach* to patient care.

The purpose of this textbook is to provide a theoretically sound basis for the integration of psychosocial aspects related to athletic training. Our aim is to provide a user-friendly introduction to the practical use of psychosocial strategies as they relate specifically to the field of athletic training and to offer athletic training students and certified athletic trainers an applied reference that will provide useful tools with which to enhance their clinical practice. As such, each chapter provides an overview of the research literature in each area to introduce major concepts and theories that are reinforced by evidence-based practice examples that illustrate clinical integration.

The structure of each chapter is similar and begins and closes with a case-study–type narrative, referred to as the Athlete Insider. Each chapter also contains Key Terms, Chapter Objectives, and End-of-Chapter Exercises to guide the reader to relevant concepts and to encourage critical thinking on associated topics. In addition, the discussion of Strategies and Competencies and Board of Certification (BOC) Style questions presented at the end of each chapter aim to provide the reader with a study tool for the BOC Examination.

SPECIAL FEATURES

The following special features are contained within this textbook and supplement the text:

- **Evidence-Based Practice:** This feature summarizes peer-reviewed research and provides the reader with applications to athletic training practice. This feature is consistent with the profession's emphasis on an evidence-based approach to care of the athlete.
- **Clinical Tips:** This feature provides examples that the authors or contributors have used within their own clinical practice to integrate psychosocial strategies into athletic training.
- **Special Considerations:** This feature may address gender considerations, cultural considerations, and/or special populations related to psychosocial aspects of athletic training.
- **Red Flag:** This feature highlights issues related to the physical and psychological well-being and/or safety of athletes.
- **Virtual Field Trips:** This feature provides links to resources and learning activities that can be found on the Internet to supplement the text.

Throughout this textbook, we made an effort to use consistent terminology and would like the reader to recognize that terminology varies across the literature, as well as nationally and internationally. The term *psychosocial* (i.e., the integration of psychological and social factors) related to injury, rehabilitation, and return to play is used throughout this textbook and is consistent with the terminology used within the fifth edition of the Athletic Training Education Competencies. Although we recognize the terms *client* and *patient* are preferred by the National Athletic Trainers' Association, we have chosen to use the term *athlete* throughout this textbook in reference to an active population. We have also focused on the traditional athletic settings but acknowledge that many athletic trainers work with participants in a range of competition levels (e.g., recreation to professional), with participants of all ages (e.g., youth to masters), and with active participants in settings outside of the sport domain (e.g., military personnel, industrial workers, performing artists).

To our readers: thank you for your consideration of integrating psychosocial strategies within your athletic training practice. Your dedication to those with whom you work will make all the difference in their recovery and return to participation.

Contributors

Monna Arvinen-Barrow, PhD (C. Psychol.)
Assistant Professor
Department of Kinesiology
University of Wisconsin-Milwaukee
Milwaukee, Wisconsin

Britton W. Brewer, PhD
Professor of Psychology
Springfield College
Springfield, Massachusetts

Cindra S. Kamphoff, PhD
Director, Center for Sport and Performance Psychology
Associate Professor of Sport and Exercise Psychology
Minnesota State University, Mankato
Mankato, Minnesota

Leslie Podlog, PhD
Assistant Professor of Exercise and Sport Science
University of Utah
Salt Lake City, Utah

Stephanie A. Stadden, PhD, LAT, ATC, CSCS
Associate Professor in the School of Health, Exercise, and Sport Science
Assistant Athletic Trainer
Lenoir-Rhyne University
Hickory, North Carolina

Jill Tracey, PhD
Associate Professor of Kinesiology and Physical Education
Wilfrid Laurier University
Waterloo, Ontario, Canada

Reviewers

Adam Annaccone, MEd, ATC, PES
Instructor/Assistant Athletic Trainer, Health Science
California University of Pennsylvania
California, Pennsylvania

Jennifer Austin, PhD, ATC
Associate Professor and Director, Exercise and Sport Sciences
Colby-Sawyer College
New London, New Hampshire

Joseph A. Beckett, EdD, ATC
Professor and Director, Athletic Training
Concord University
Athens, West Virginia

Theresa Bianco, PhD
Lecturer and Acting Undergraduate Program Director, Psychology
Concordia University, Montreal
Montreal, Quebec

Kirk W. Brown, PhD, LAT, ATC
Director, Associate Professor of Athletic Training Education
University of North Carolina–Wilmington
Wilmington, North Carolina

Laura E. Clark, MS, ATC
Clinical Instructor, Clinical Coordinator
Colorado State University–Pueblo
Pueblo, Colorado

Christopher C. Dake, Athletic Trainer
Head Athletic Trainer/Clinical Coordinator, Athletics/Health and Leisure Services
University of West Florida
Pensacola, Florida

Linda G. Diaz, EdD, ATC, CMT
Associate Professor and ATEP Program Director, Kinesiology
William Paterson University
Wayne, New Jersey

Elizabeth A. Drake, MS, ATC, ATR
Adjunct Faculty/Doctoral Assistant, Human Performance
Minnesota State University, Mankato
Mankato, Minnesota

Shandra Dawn Esparza, EdD, ATC, LAT
Assistant Professor/Clinical Coordinator, Athletic Training Education
University of the Incarnate Word
San Antonio, Texas

Cordial M. Gillette, PhD, ATC, LAT
Sr. Lecturer/Clinical Coordinator/Assistant Athletic Trainer, Exercise and Sport Science/Athletics
University of Wisconsin, La Crosse
La Crosse, Wisconsin

Margo Greicar, EdD, ATC
Assistant Professor, Department of Kinesiology
Temple University
Philadelphia, Pennsylvania

Makayla Lynn Merritt, MPH, ATC, LAT
Clinical Coordinator, Visiting Instructor, Human Performance and Recreation
University of Southern Mississippi
Hattiesburg, Mississippi

Marguerite Theresa Moore, PhD, AT, ATC
Assistant Professor, Health, Physical Education and Recreation
Northern Michigan University
Marquette, Michigan

Jason Porter, MS, ATC
Assistant Athletics Director of Sports Medicine & Adjunct Professor ATEP, Athletics
Liberty University
Lynchburg, Virginia

Robb S. Rehberg, PhD, ATC, NREMT
Associate Professor, Kinesiology
William Patterson University
Wayne, New Jersey

Daniel Tarara, MS, ATC, LAT
Director, Athletic Training Education
High Point University
High Point, North Carolina

Susan P. Wehring, MS, ATC, LAT
Director/ATEP, Health, Human Performance and Recreation
Southeast Missouri State University
Cape Girardeau, Missouri

Jennifer Zuberbier, MS, LAT
Assistant Athletic Trainer, Athletic Training
University of Wisconsin–Oshkosh
Oshkosh, Wisconsin

Acknowledgments

This textbook was truly a collaborative effort. We sincerely thank our coauthors and contributors for their expertise and the time and care that they dedicated to this project. Thank you also to those whose research served as our foundation; we hope that our extension of your work makes you proud.

Thank you to Quincy McDonald from F.A. Davis for seeing the value in our project. With great gratitude we thank Joanna Cain, Pamela Speh, and Gayle Crist of Auctorial Pursuits, Inc. for their guidance and patience with us throughout this endeavor.

Contents

Chapter 1

Introduction to Psychosocial Aspects of Athletic Training

Jennifer Jordan Hamson-Utley and Jennifer Stiller-Ostrowski

CHAPTER OUTLINE

KEY TERMS

Athletic identity The degree to which a person identifies the self as an athlete.

Burnout Psychological, emotional, and physical withdrawal from an activity that was previously enjoyable; a response to excessive stress and dissatisfaction with sports participation.

Coping skills Mechanisms that promote the ability to cope with a stressor or situation; built from experience or learned.

Demographic variables Factors that explain or provide context for data being gathered.

Extrinsic motivation Behavior that is driven by a desire to attain a specific outcome; motivation from an outside source.

Hardiness Stable personality trait composed of three components: perceived control over the situation, view of the situation as a challenge as opposed to a threat, and commitment to changing the situation.

Holistic Related to healing; a holistic approach includes all parts of the healing system—the mind and the body—in the healing process.

Injury severity Grading of an injury that includes the amount of deformity, disability, and lack of strength to complete daily living activities; typically includes strength, range of motion, and functional deficit.

Injury type Kind of injury; soft tissue or bony; relates to severity.

Intrinsic motivation Behavior that is driven by an interest or enjoyment in the task itself (e.g., personal best).

Mood state Transitory, fluctuating state of mind of the athlete.

Motivational orientation An individual propensity to be driven by internal or external factors.

Nonpharmacological pain management Strategies designed to increase an individual's perception of control over pain that he or she experiences.

Pain tolerance The ability of the patient to withstand pain or painful stimuli for a period of time.

Personality A stable trait of an individual's general emotional, behavioral, and attitudinal response patterns.

Positive affirmation A positive declaration of truth; used in rehabilitation and healing to improve mind-set and to motivate.

Psychological skills Mental skills, techniques by which the individual can use the mind to control the body or to create an outcome.

Psychosocial Integration of psychology and sociology within injury and healing processes; interplay between the two fields best captures individual and situational factors.

Recovery status The percentage toward recovery; can be seen as varying on a continuum from 10% to 100% or reported as "not fully recovered" or "fully recovered".

Relaxation Release of tension in the body; return to equilibrium.

Self-talk Internal and/or external statements to the self, multidimensional in nature, that have interpretive elements associated with their content; it is dynamic and serves at least two functions (instructional and motivational).

Subjective report What athletes or patients tell the practitioner about their injury or condition.

Thought stopping A psychological strategy that allows the athlete to gain control over the thought process, changing negative thoughts to more productive positive thoughts.

CHAPTER OBJECTIVES

After reading this chapter, you will be able to:

1. Recall basic research findings related to the psychosocial aspects of athletic injury and recovery, from injury prevention to return to play.
2. Recognize the role of stress and other psychosocial antecedents to injury.
3. Identify the psychosocial aspects of athletic injury and what athletes expect from their health-care providers.
4. Identify typical postinjury emotions and the role athletic trainers can play in facilitating a positive coping response.
5. Describe the important role of communication throughout the injury process—from initial injury and throughout rehabilitation and recovery.
6. Explain the importance of educating injured athletes on interpreting the meaning of pain and its implications for training and rehabilitation.
7. Recognize the role of the athletic trainer both as a source of social support for injured athletes and as a facilitator to identify other sources of social support in the athlete's life.
8. Describe the integration of the psychosocial approach into injury recovery, and identify useful tools for the athletic trainer to implement with the athlete including positive self-talk, motivation, and pain-management strategies.
9. Identify the basic elements of response to sports injuries and how athletic trainers can play a role in athlete recovery and referral.
10. Identify the psychosocial role of the athletic trainer as outlined by the Role Delineation Study (Sixth Edition) and the Commission on Accreditation of Athletic Training Education guidelines, as well as *Psychosocial Strategies and Referral Competencies and Clinical Integration Proficiencies* (Fifth Edition).

ATHLETE INSIDER

Seth is a freshman on the football team of a large Division I university. He was a standout as a high school athlete and was aggressively recruited for his athletic talents. Now, feeling like a small fish in a big pond at college, he begins to doubt whether he has the ability to make the plays he did in high school and is apprehensive about being hit by some of the larger players on the defenses of opposing teams. During the first week of practice, he is tackled awkwardly and tears his anterior cruciate ligament (ACL); he sees his college career crumbling in an instant and feels frustrated and anxious. He is worried about letting his father, his coaches, and his teammates down. An athletic training student waits with Seth as he is prepared for surgery. Seth can't stop thinking about his injury and wonders if he will ever return to play. The next day, he meets with his team's athletic trainer and begins his rehabilitation.

INTRODUCTION

This introductory chapter answers the question "Why should athletic trainers be concerned about psychosocial aspects of injury?" by tackling head-on the misconception that injury mechanisms and rehabilitation techniques should center on the physical nature of injury. The chapter provides an overview of the primary areas of the psychology of injury research, highlighting the essential role of

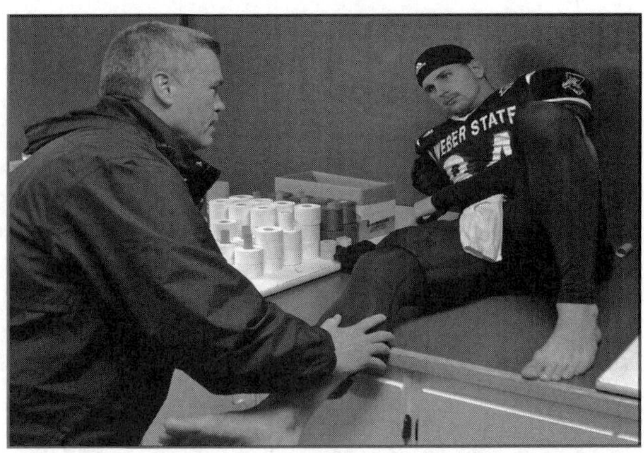

Figure 1-1 | Athlete Insider

psychosocial strategies from injury prevention through the return to sport. By the end of the chapter, you will recognize the important role of the use of psychosocial strategies. Beginning *before* injury occurs and infiltrating every facet of both physical and mental recovery processes, presenting an applied and integrated approach to the care of the injured athlete, illustrates current evidence-based care. This chapter serves as an introduction to the entire psychosocial content area and acts as a road map to the rest of this textbook. Major topics will be introduced, and you will be directed to subsequent chapters for additional information.

IMPORTANCE OF PSYCHOSOCIAL ASPECTS OF INJURY

Until the 1990s, rehabilitative interventions primarily addressed the physical dimensions of sport injury, focusing on helping athletes return to a preinjury level of function by treating the obvious physical symptoms. However, pain is both physical and psychological, and often overlooked in the injury treatment and rehabilitation processes are the emotional and cognitive components. Pain does not occur in the body without the mind reacting and contributing to the experience; therefore, treatment of the physical symptoms is only half of the solution. Because of their frequent contact with injured athletes during recovery and rehabilitation, athletic trainers are in a position to provide psychosocial skills training and emotional support to their athletes. ***Holistically*** educated and skilled athletic trainers are in an excellent position to provide care for the entire athlete, not just his or her injured body part.

The Psychosocial Strategies and Referral content area consists of topics that many athletic training students often struggle with because they are not as concrete as other topics (e.g., orthopedic evaluation, therapeutic exercise). Similar to rehabilitation, modalities, and other more traditional athletic training techniques, athletic trainers need to evaluate athletes' receptivity and educate them on the technique to increase it. The psychosocial approach to injury prevention, injury rehabilitation, and return to play of the injured athlete has many facets. These factors or components can best be described as personal/individual and environmental/situational factors, and they are summarized in Table 1-1. Psychology of injury research is typically divided into three areas: psychosocial antecedents to injury, emotional and behavioral responses to injury, and psychosocial factors that influence the rehabilitation and recovery process. These three areas are summarized in the following sections.

What Are Psychosocial Aspects and How Do They Play Into Injury Prevention?

Stress is a psychosomatic phenomenon, which means that it has both psychological and physical components. Stress can be either positive or negative; in fact, there would be little constructive activity without positive stress. For example, without the stress of a deadline, would you be motivated to get that term paper done? Even many things that we view as positive can be stressful, such as planning a vacation, renting an apartment, or planning a wedding. Negative stress, however, is stress that produces fear and anxiety. There are two general categories of negative

TABLE 1-1 Personal and Situational Factors: Psychosocial Approach to Care of the Athlete

Personal/Individual Factors	Environmental/ Situational Factors
Injury history	Sport type
Injury severity and type	Level of competition
Injury cause	Time in season
Recovery status	Scholarship status
Personality	Playing status
Self-motivation, self-esteem	Coach and teammate influences
Motivational orientation	Family dynamics
Athletic identity	Athletic trainer influences
Pain tolerance	Social support networks
Coping skills, psychological skills	Sport ethics
Mood states	Rehabilitation environment
Gender, age, and ethnicity	Accessibility of services
Prior sports experiences	
Socioeconomic status	
Physical and nutritional health	

stress: life events and daily hassles (you will learn more about negative stress in Chapter 3).

Stress forces can disrupt the body's equilibrium, and these negative effects can lead to injury in sports. In these situations, stress has the effect of decreasing attentional focus, creating excessive muscle tension, and hindering skills and motor coordination. Research has established a clear relationship among life stress, competitive anxiety, coping resources, and injury. Athletes who are injured tend to have greater levels of competitive anxiety and stress, to appraise difficult situations as being threatening (vs. challenging), and to have low levels of coping resources. Research has shown that athletes with high stress or high anxiety are more likely to be injured or severely injured, whereas those with very low stress and anxiety are more likely to remain uninjured or receive a less severe injury. In addition, athletes with few coping resources are more likely to be severely injured. Consider the scenario with Seth in the Athlete Insider section at the beginning of this chapter. Can you identify sources of stress that may have served as psychosocial antecedents to his injury?

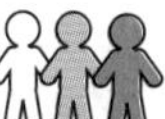

SPECIAL CONSIDERATIONS

Watching big-time college football on television one Saturday, an athletic trainer sees his favorite team's quarterback being blitzed, avoiding the sack, and throwing—right into the hands of the other team. Interception! As the network shows the replay repeatedly, it is clear that a defender closely covered the receiver. How did the quarterback not see the defender? Consider the physical effects of stress. The quarterback was clearly in a high-stress situation as he dodged the onslaught of defenders. As his stress level increased, muscle tension likely increased, and his attentional field narrowed. When he looked downfield, all he saw was his receiver; he never saw the defender just a few feet away. In rehabilitation and return to sport, stress becomes an important management issue to avoid reinjury.

Application and Integration

So, how can athletic trainers use psychosocial strategies to help prevent athletic injury? Athletic trainers can educate coaches and support staff about the stress–injury relationship by explaining how and why being in a stress state may predispose an athlete to injury (you will learn more about psychological antecedents to injury in Chapter 3). Athletic trainers can also monitor an athlete's stress levels and seek education about signs that may indicate that the athlete is stressed (such as deviations from athlete stress profiles). They can also help athletes learn to cope with stress by providing social support and by assisting them in finding additional sources of support. Athletes receive social support from a variety of people, so an athletic trainer's role may include both providing appropriate social support and evaluating whether the athlete is receiving enough social support from important others (the role of social support is discussed in depth in Chapter 9).

CLINICAL TIP

Athletes with a history of many stressors, ***personality*** characteristics that exacerbate the stress response, and few coping resources will be (when placed in a stressful situation) more likely to appraise the situation as stressful and to exhibit greater psychological activation and attentional disruptions. ***Mood state*** refers to an individual's transient, fluctuating internal state. For example, mood is collected via ***subjective report*** by the athlete and can include emotions such as happy and energized or sad and down. Research shows that mood state has an impact on an athlete's motivation to perform, rehabilitate, and return to play. One can assess an athlete's mood state using the Profile of Mood States Questionnaire (POMS; McNair, Lorr, & Droppleman, 1971), which examines six identifiable mood states including the athlete's level of tension-anxiety, depression-dejection, anger-hostility, fatigue-inertia, vigor-activity, and confusion-bewilderment. The graphic display of the results of POMS screening is the iceberg profile (Morgan, 1980) (Fig. 1-2).

Emotional Response and Coping With Injury

Many factors influence an athlete's emotional response to injury. In fact, many of the same factors that serve as antecedents to injury may also play a role in how the athlete interprets the injury. Personal or individual factors are those that describe the athlete and what that person individually brings to the preinjury, healing, or return-to-play situation. Factors such as injury history, ***injury type***, and ***injury severity***, as well as ***recovery status***, are individual characteristics that play into the athlete's psychosocial reaction. One key factor that demands particular attention on the part of athletic trainers is the influence of ***athletic identity*** on emotional response. Individuals with a strong athletic identity may have more difficulty coping with forced time away from their sport. Many theories surround emotional response to athletic injury (these theories are discussed in depth in Chapter 4). In general, athletes' emotions often form a U-shaped pattern, with periods of the greatest emotional disturbance occurring immediately after injury and just before returning to play, when anxiety may be high and confidence in the involved body part may be low (Fig. 1-3). As the athlete makes visible progress throughout the course of rehabilitation, emotions tend to become more positive. Overall, emotional responses progress from negative to positive; however, there is large

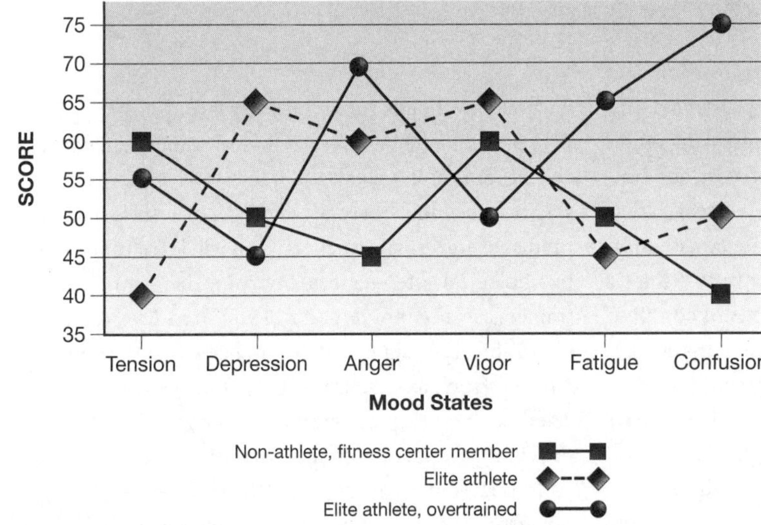

Figure 1-2 | Profile of mood states: Profile of Mood States Questionnaire

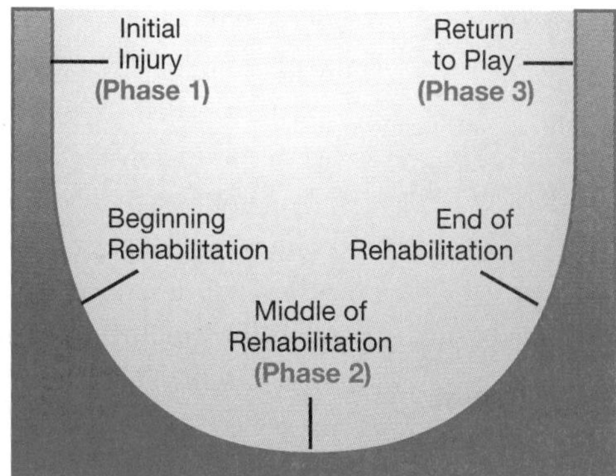

Figure 1-3 | Emotional response to injury.

individual variation, and some athletes may need psychosocial intervention to help them cope with injury. The negative psychological impact of sports injuries has been well documented in the literature. It is important for athletic trainers to develop an understanding of common emotional reactions so that they can identify when an athlete's emotional state is such that he or she potentially requires referral for treatment.

History of injury, including the type and severity of injury, has an impact on recovery status. According to the 2008 report, "Go Out and Play: Participation in Team or Organized Sports," conducted by the Women's Sports Foundation, 69% of girls and 75% of boys in the United States participate in organized and team sports. With sports participation on the rise, injuries are occurring now more than ever before, and athletic trainers should consider the personal/individual factors of the athlete to provide the best care. Compare the following two high school basketball athletes:

- Athlete 1 is a female basketball player who sustained a grade 1 ankle injury 3 weeks ago. She never fully rehabilitated the injury; as a result, she has had a series of recurrent ankle sprains.
- Athlete 2 is a female basketball player who has sustained a grade 2 ankle injury, an ACL rupture, and a fractured radius, all three of which were rehabilitated to 100%.

How does the injury history of athlete 1 position her to respond to the next injury occurrence? It is possible that, because of a lack of experience suffering through more severe injuries and a history of recurrent injuries related to incomplete rehabilitation, this athlete is at risk for having a negative perception of the rehabilitation and recovery process. Athlete 1 may tend to perceive any subsequent injury as being more severe and more threatening because of her history of not overcoming a fairly insignificant injury. Contrast this with athlete 2, who has extensive injury experience but has built confidence in her ability to return to sports based on multiple successful rehabilitation situations. Compared with athlete 1, athlete 2 is likely to respond to injury in a very different manner; athlete 2 will likely face even a severe injury with a positive outlook in relation to her ability to return to a preinjury level of participation. Injury history allows the athlete to create expectations about the injury experience and to prepare for what follows the injury event. Having this experience, as well as other personality traits (e.g., ***hardiness***) and states, will likely have a positive impact on the initial response to the injury and spill over into the injury rehabilitation and return-to-sport phases (Fig. 1-4). You will learn more about psychosocial antecedents to injury and how an athlete's injury history can influence his or her emotional responses in Chapters 3 and 4.

CLINICAL TIP

The personality trait of *hardiness* has been shown to moderate the stress–injury relationship. Individuals with this trait tend to view a new situation as a challenge (vs. being threatened by it) and have a sense of control over their lives and situations. Research indicates that "tough-minded" athletes are less likely to be injured than "tender-minded" athletes. Athletic trainers should be mindful of the level of hardiness that the athlete brings to the injury and recovery situations to best situate the athlete for success.

Overview of Emotional Response Models

Initial models of emotional response to injury attempted to predict how an athlete would respond following injury, suggesting athletes should progress linearly through various emotional stages. Recently, however, experts have developed cognitive appraisal models, which focus on developing an

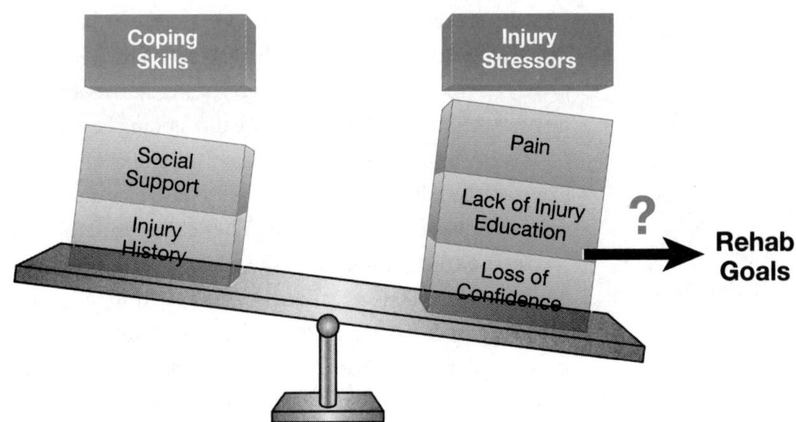

Figure 1-4 | Importance of psychosocial strategies.

understanding of how the individual's perception of the injury shapes the emotional response and subsequent behaviors. These models take into account individual variations (e.g., personality traits, coping resources), injury severity, and characteristics of the injury scenario (contact vs. noncontact, senior year vs. freshman year, preseason vs. playoffs, starter vs. nonstarter; see more factors in Table 1-1). These models propose that the athlete's appraisal, or perception, of the injury is more important in determining the emotional response than the injury itself. An athlete who views the injury as threatening, perhaps resulting in the loss of a starting position or the loss of a potential scholarship, will likely have a negative emotional response to injury and may not be motivated during rehabilitation. Conversely, an athlete with the same injury who views the injury as having positive consequences (possibly as a much-needed break from his or her sport) will likely have a positive emotional response. The evolution of emotional response theories and cognitive appraisal models is discussed in depth in Chapter 4. Based on what we know about Seth, what factors are likely to influence his emotional response to injury and the rehabilitation process?

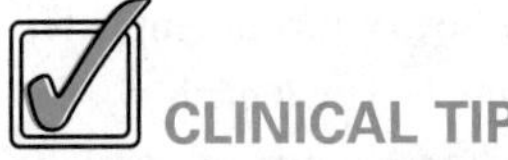

CLINICAL TIP

Research has shown that anxiety, pessimism, and confusion regarding what to expect from the rehabilitation process result in decreased adherence to the rehabilitation program. Negative emotions are common and should be expected following an injury that is perceived by athletes to be severe or threatening to their place on the team. Many athletes are surprised when they are injured, and they must develop an entirely new skill set to aid them in coping with the injury and its physical and emotional effects. Learning to communicate effectively with injured athletes is key in identifying these troublesome mood states and areas of uncertainty, as well as in helping athletes navigate their way through the often difficult process ahead. Establishing open lines of communication is also an important component of identifying athletes in need of psychosocial referral and in approaching athletes about it.

Application and Integration

Athletic trainers need to recognize that emotions can create anxiety and tension, which can result in increased physical discomfort following injury. Athletic trainers can help relieve some of this anxiety by answering athletes' questions and helping them to arrive at a realistic appraisal of the severity of the injury and its consequences. Athletic trainers should encourage athletes to openly and honestly express their feelings following injury and acknowledge that injury results in the loss of some sense of the self (you will learn more about facilitating positive emotional responses in Chapter 4). Athletic trainers must develop their own communication skills, because communication is essential both before and after injury (communication skills are addressed in depth in Chapter 5). Finally, athletic trainers must learn to facilitate adherence to rehabilitation and motivation by using psychosocial strategies, such as goal setting, stress management, imagery, and ***self-talk*** (and much more, as discussed in Chapter 10).

Environmental and Situational Factors That Influence Response to Injury

Personal/individual factors are not the only concern for the athletic trainer; environmental and situational factors also play into the psychosocial aspect of care of the athlete. Categories of situational factors are sport, social, and environmental. Situational sport factors include level of competition, time in season, playing status, scholarship status, sport type (contact vs. noncontact), and sport dynamic (team vs. individual). Examples of social situational factors include, but are not limited to, teammate and coach influences, family dynamics, athletic trainer influences, and the athlete's sport ethical alignment. The last category of situational factors is environmental and includes things such as the rehabilitation environment and accessibility to that environment (you will learn more about the rehabilitation process in Chapter 8).

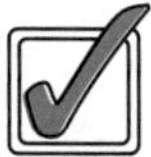

CLINICAL TIP

Injured athletes often worry that once injured they will gain weight. It is a common misconception that injured athletes should eat less or take in fewer calories during the recovery process. Actually, during the first 1 to 2 weeks of healing (depending on severity), the metabolic rate rises, meaning that the athlete burns more calories at rest than he or she did preinjury. Restricting calories during the early healing phase (phase 1) has a direct impact on the healing process by prolonging the inflammatory response and decreasing immune function. Athletic trainers need to educate injured athletes on the importance of nutrition during injury rehabilitation and suggest healthy ways to fuel the body.

VIRTUAL FIELD TRIP

Education is a psychosocial strategy that can assist the injured athlete with the healing process. The athlete should be encouraged to continue to eat healthy during injury rehabilitation. To help guide the injured athlete on what and how much to eat during a phase of recovery, explore the resources at http://davisplus.fadavis.com, which includes a link to ChooseMyPlate.gov.

Sport factors are those that are specific to the sport in which the athlete competes. For instance:

- A college freshman has different sport experiences than a college senior in the same sport.
- A scholarship athlete may have a different interpretation of an injury as compared with a nonscholarship athlete.
- An elite athlete may have a different mind-set than a high school athlete.
- An athlete who is a starter versus an athlete who is not may perceive his or her involvement in the team's success differently.
- Athletes participating in a team sport versus athletes in an individual sport are likely to have vastly different social support networks and ***motivational orientations*** or climates.

How each of these factors might come into play will become evident in the following scenario:

> *Matt is a Division I college soccer athlete who starts for his team. It is the end of the season going into playoffs of his senior year of eligibility. He sustains an injury in the game, and his team is down by two goals. They must win to advance into the playoffs.*

Soccer is a team contact sport where injury often occurs and is expected at some point in a college career. Because Matt is a "starter" and a scholarship athlete, he is likely to feel that he has let his team down by becoming injured. He is being "paid to play" this sport by the school. The situational factor of being a team sport carries with it a commitment to perform for the good of the team. Even though Matt had no control over his injury situation, he may no longer see himself as an asset to the team. Another situational factor of great importance is time in season. The level of competition and timing of this match, with the team going into the playoffs resting on this win, increases the weight of the injury occurrence on Matt. All of these factors may affect how Matt will perceive his injury. It is best for the athletic trainer to appreciate these factors. Athletic trainers are better able to assist when they understand athletes' cognitive, behavioral, and emotional responses as they progress through the injury recovery phase.

Of social importance, the athlete's relationships with the coach, teammates, family, significant others, and an athletic trainer may have a large influence on how the athlete responds to stressors and sport injury. Relationships with these individuals can be functional and productive, or they could be the exact opposite and impede progress for the athlete in terms of resolving stress or facilitating injury rehabilitation. Coaches can play a vital role in the support of the athlete. For example, the athletic trainer communicating with the coach about the athlete's progress in rehabilitation allows for that coach to ask informed questions and seem up to date, increasing that athlete's feelings of self-worth and connectedness.

Athletic trainers stand to play a vital role in the support and care of the athlete. Athletes look to their athletic trainers as a source of information about their injury, and research shows they expect education and quality time with the athletic trainer. The athletic trainer can influence the athlete's perception of the injury by being present, by providing the support and education that improves the athlete's awareness, and by offering comfort regarding the upcoming surgery and rehabilitation process. The athletic trainer can also function as a source of information about other stressors, such as sexually transmitted diseases, drug addiction, and eating disorders. See Chapter 9 for more information on social support.

The athletic trainer also faces the challenge of providing an environment conducive to healing and recovery for the injured or otherwise stressed athlete. Environmental factors include the athletic training facility and rehabilitation area, the athletic trainer's office, and the team training facility, to name a few. Specifically, if these places are too busy, too loud, or too overrun by teammates or other athletes, it is likely that the athlete will not feel comfortable. In this case, activities or tasks to be completed will be limited in that location. Athletes may even avoid going to the athletic training room because they may see certain teammates and feel ashamed by their injury. This category also includes the accessibility to the earlier mentioned personnel and facilities. If the athletic trainer is too busy all the time to ask about certain signs and symptoms of a likely disease or injury, the athlete may avoid seeking education or care altogether. Understanding how both personal/individual and situational/environmental factors affect how the athlete responds cognitively, behaviorally, and emotionally to stress and injury events will undoubtedly improve the care provided by the athletic trainer.

Factors That Influence the Rehabilitation and Recovery Process

Injured athletes will experience different levels of ***intrinsic motivation*** at various points during the rehabilitation process. For example, an athlete with a minor injury who will return to sport this season will likely be highly intrinsically motivated (desire to compete in upcoming games/matches will provide that). However, athletes who sustain an injury and will not return to sports this season or who sustain an injury during the off-season may need additional ***extrinsic motivation*** strategies to keep them motivated at a time when the ability to compete is not within the short-term realm. Individual factors also play a role in athlete motivation and adherence to rehabilitation. For example, factors including mood state, ***pain tolerance***, ***coping skills***, and ***psychological skills*** help to describe the preparation of an athlete to handle challenging sports injury situations. We have already discussed the impact of mood state on both preinjury and postinjury factors. Pain tolerance is a personal/individual trait that describes the athlete's ability to withstand painful situations, such as chronic and acute injuries. For example, some athletes can play through a ruptured spleen, whereas others cannot play through a sprained ankle. Although athletic trainers do not recommend continuing participation through pain, having a high pain tolerance can be a positive attribute within sports injury rehabilitation. Consider the case of Seth in the Athlete Insider section at the start of this chapter. Seth has recently undergone reconstruction of his ACL and is beginning to work on achieving 90° of knee flexion range of motion (ROM). Even though the athletic trainer has educated the athlete that it is safe to attempt to achieve the set goal of 90°, the athlete is experiencing pain and cannot continue as a result. In this scenario, having a higher pain tolerance can allow the athlete to push through this pain and make progress toward the goal of 90° of knee flexion. It has been suggested that those athletes who are perceived to have a higher pain tolerance may actually have better developed nonpharmacological pain-management strategies. These strategies are not necessarily inherent to the athlete; rather, the athletic trainer can facilitate them through educational interventions (you will learn more about helping athletes interpret and manage their pain in Chapter 7).

Coping skills include tools that athletes bring to the situation that assist in promoting a positive outcome. These tools can include social support networks, ***relaxation*** and imagery exercises, positive self-talk (***thought stopping***) or ***positive affirmation*** statements, goal setting, and pain-management exercises. It is common for athletes to enter the college sport setting without knowledge or experience using such skills. It is also highly probable that high school athletes have limited experience with learned coping skills and may also have limited social support networks (i.e., teammates, friends, significant others, family, coaches, athletic trainers). It is important for the athletic trainer to be mindful of the usefulness of coping skills in injury prevention, injury education, rehabilitation, and return to sport, and to be prepared to teach athletes how to use coping skills in diverse settings to facilitate specific outcomes. In addition, athletic trainers should learn to identify unhealthy or "negative" coping strategies as well (Table 1-2) and be prepared to intervene and suggest replacement positive coping behaviors (Table 1-3). As a reminder, see Chapter 9 for an overview of the role of social support and Chapter 10 for further discussion of coping skills and psychosocial strategies.

Gender can also play a significant role in both injury prevention and the appraisal of injury, rehabilitation, and return to sport. There are many theories as to why and how male and female individuals differ when it comes to athletic participation; however, what is important in this textbook is how it relates to injury and recovery. Research shows that male and female athletes expect different types of skills from their athletic trainers during injury care and rehabilitation. It is important for athletic trainers to pay attention to the clinical implications of research or best practices provided by research regarding gender differences in clinical care. For example, female athletes tend to covet more hands-on, companionship-like traits in the rehabilitation setting, whereas male athletes desire education and open communication to facilitate injury prevention and recovery. In addition, male athletes are often less forthcoming about their pain when the athletic trainer is a woman. However, both male and female individuals want education and open communication. An effective athletic trainer acts accordingly based on gender to provide the best prevention and care possible. Another personal/individual factor worth examining is ethnicity, which can provide layers of insight for the athletic trainer about an athlete's injury and rehabilitation behaviors. See Chapter 2 for more information about sociocultural influences on delivery of effective athletic injury care.

TABLE 1-2 **Identifying Healthy and Unhealthy Coping Strategies**

Healthy Coping Strategies	Unhealthy Coping Strategies
Practicing relaxation	Using alcohol, binge drinking
Practicing behavior modification	Using marijuana
Utilizing social support networks	Binge eating/purging
Journaling	Consuming too much caffeine
Exercising	Smoking
Deep breathing	Compulsive spending
Meditating	Isolation
Listening to music	Violent behavior
Eating right	Denial
Laughing	Disassociation
Sleeping	Overtraining

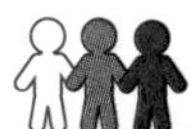

SPECIAL CONSIDERATIONS

The athletic trainer should be aware that the female athlete might be at a heightened risk for injury because of maladaptive eating patterns. The "female athlete triad" has three components: (1) energy availability, (2) bone health, and (3) menstrual status. Low energy availability is the principal element, impairing both the menstrual cycle and bone health. However, named after the female because of common occurrence, the triad also pertains to male

Continued

athletes, particularly in weight-class sports, distance running, and military training. Because athletic trainers work with all of the above, they should remain open to considering stress fractures caused by low energy availability in the male athlete.

Finally, personal/individual factors such as socioeconomic status and prior sports experience can also play into the evaluation of injury and return to sport. Consider the high school athlete whose parents cannot afford to send her to rehabilitation for her torn ACL and the athletic trainer who does not have the time to spend with her daily or weekly on rehabilitation exercises and treatments. What disadvantage does this pose to the athlete? The athlete in this situation has nowhere to turn for help; she is out of options and is likely discouraged because of her injury. This athlete may quit her sport or experience depression that is also likely to go untreated, placing her at risk for suicide. Also consider the athlete who is just beginning participation in sports and becomes injured. How can this factor alone—that is, lack of prior sports experience—predispose the athlete to a negative injury and rehabilitation outcome? It is likely that this athlete has little invested in sports and will quit altogether. Such athletes are apt to have low motivation to work hard in rehabilitation and may experience more pain and lack of progress as a result. See Chapter 11 for an in-depth discussion of psychosocial aspects of returning to athletic participation.

ATHLETES' EXPECTATIONS OF THEIR HEALTH-CARE PROVIDERS

Types of Psychosocial Strategies Athletic Trainers Should Use

Creating and maintaining an open, motivational, and supportive environment in the athletic training facility is an important step in ensuring a healthy recovery. The more we know about how athletic trainers and athletes best interact, the more efficient, effective, and mutually beneficial this relationship can be. Research has identified

TABLE 1-3 Stress and Positive Coping Strategies

Common Athlete Stressors	Positive Coping Strategies
Academic examinations	*Organize* the class materials, set aside *time* for studying each subject/class, make study guides, study in groups, *communicate* with professors if comprehension is low, and be *positive* with self-talk
Chronic or severe injury	*Communicate* to establish roadblocks, set goals for recovery, *act* with behaviors to achieve those goals, *reward* daily achievements, and stay *positive*
Personal relationships	Use *communication* skills, use "I feel" vs. "you make me feel" statements, ask close friends and family for *advice*, eat right, and get plenty of sleep
Teammate relationships	Clear the air, address the problem, open *communication* lines and alert the coaching staff if the issue involves violence or danger
Coach relationship	Meet with the coach to express concerns; *communicate* about possible ways to solve the problem to maintain a level of mutual respect and hard work
Financial concerns	*Communicate* with the financial aid office, seek help from a social worker, and establish a budget and act within the lines
Family planning	*Communicate* about roadblocks and emotions, visit medical care providers such as a family planning clinic, or seek guidance from health services on campus

several important psychosocial learning experiences that should be included as part of professional training. These experiences include:

- Having discussions and educating injured athletes
- Facilitating coping behaviors and positive responses to injury and subsequent rehabilitation
- Obtaining practical experience in dealing with dysfunctional behaviors related to rehabilitation
- Applying psychosocial intervention techniques during rehabilitation
- Recognizing professional limitations
- Understanding when to refer and to whom referrals should be made

These skills do not develop naturally as the result of "attending" classes and clinical placements; rather, they are experiences that must be carefully crafted and focused on to develop an appropriate skill set.

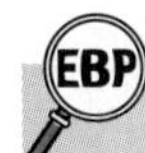

EVIDENCE-BASED PRACTICE

Stiller-Ostrowski, J. L., & Ostrowski, J. A. (2009). Recently certified athletic trainers' undergraduate educational preparation in psychosocial intervention and referral. *Journal of Athletic Training, 44*(1), 67–75.

Description of the Study

This study explored the educational preparation of recently certified athletic trainers within the psychosocial intervention and referral content area, with the purpose of identifying areas in which entry-level athletic trainers may be underprepared. Semistructured focus group interviews were conducted with 11 recently certified athletic trainers (certified an average of 2.7 years) who had graduated from accredited athletic training (AT) programs. Key open-ended questions focused on type of communication practice/training engaged in during undergraduate education; type of training received regarding ensuring rehabilitation adherence/motivating injured athletes; type of education received regarding stress-management and mental skills training; and type of education received concerning recognizing, intervening, and referring for psychosocial issues.

Results of the Study

Responses indicate that the participants were adequately prepared for handling common communication and interpersonal issues but were underprepared or unprepared to handle scenarios involving unmotivated athletes, counseling and social support, mental skills training, and psychosocial referral. Anecdotal experiences shared by participants established successful educational strategies in these areas.

Implications for Athletic Training Practice

Themes contained within the psychosocial intervention and referral content area have an impact on all aspects of the athletic training profession, including injury prevention, facilitating healthy emotional response to injury, motivating athletes during rehabilitation, and preparing athletes physically and psychologically to return to participation. To be prudent entry-level professionals, athletic training students must not only be educated in these areas but also must be given practical experience to engage in the practice of the field.

What Athletes Expect From Athletic Trainers

Injured athletes themselves are in the best position to tell athletic trainers what types of psychosocial support skills they need from caregivers. Research with injured athletes has indicated that the types of skills fall into three general categories: communication/education, motivation, and atmosphere/social support. Developing communication skills is essential to virtually every aspect of the injury process; in fact, the development of rapport with uninjured athletes has even been associated with earlier reporting of injuries. After athletes sustain an injury, communication becomes even more important as they now must be educated about their injury, their physical limitations, and what they can do to help speed their recovery. Additional research shows that gender and experience with athletic training services play a role in the number and type of expectations injured athletes have of their caregiver. Male athletes expect less overall from the athletic trainer; however, first-time injured males expect to be educated by their athletic trainer on elements related to their injury and recovery. Female athletes expect more overall from their athletic trainer, regardless of experience with athletic training services. For more on this research and athlete expectations, see Chapter 10. Clarifying expectations about what injured athletes should expect during the rehabilitation process is essential to decreasing their anxiety and facilitating adherence to the rehabilitation program. Finally, it is important to educate athletes on the risks of returning to participation too soon and to develop two-way communication regarding any fears or apprehensions they might have about returning to sport (you will learn more about developing communication skills in Chapter 5 and about facilitating psychosocial return to activity in Chapter 11).

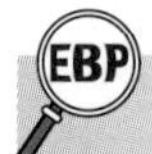

EVIDENCE-BASED PRACTICE

Clement, D., Hamson-Utley, J., Arvinen-Barrow, M., Kamphoff, C. S., Zakrajsek, R. A., & Martin, S. B. (2012). College athletes' expectations about injury rehabilitation with an athletic trainer. *International Journal of Athletic Therapy & Training, 17*(4), 18–27.

Description of the Study

Injured athletes typically enter injury rehabilitation with certain expectations of what the working relationships will be like with athletic trainers. This study determined whether male and female athletes differed in their expectations of athletic trainers' rehabilitation services and assessed the interaction between past athletic training experience, gender, and athletes' expectations about injury rehabilitation. Student–athletes were administered a self-report questionnaire that measured their expectations of athletic training and injury rehabilitation. A total of 759 questionnaires were distributed, and 679 (89.5%) student–athletes at 5 colleges and universities located in various regions across the United States returned completed questionnaires (65.2% males [n = 443] and 34.8% females [n = 236]). The Expectations About Athletic Training (EAAT) was used to measure athletes' expectations about athletic training and injury rehabilitation. The EAAT includes subscales assessing: (a) Personal Commitment, (b) Facilitative Conditions, (c) Athletic Training Expertise, and (d) Realism.

Results of the Study

The researchers found a significant interaction between past athletic training experience and gender for expectations. Results indicated that male athletes with no past athletic training experience had lower expectations of personal commitment to athletic training and injury rehabilitation and of athletic trainers providing them with a facilitative environment. They also found that female athletes with athletic training experience were less likely to have realistic expectations of athletic training and injury rehabilitation.

Implications for Athletic Training Practice

Female athletes expect athletic trainers to provide a rehabilitation environment that is accepting, nurturing, and based on trust that allows for self-disclosure and personal growth. This type of rehabilitation environment may facilitate adherence and injury recovery more quickly for this group. For injured male athletes, however, who expect less from the athletic trainer in the rehabilitation process, educating them about the process and how the athletic trainer can help within it (e.g., social support, communication/active listening, relaxation, and imagery strategies) helps to influence self-efficacy, self-motivation, and communication.

Motivation and rehabilitation adherence increase incrementally, from when athletic trainers are physically present, to when they provide personal attention and feedback, to when they elicit feedback from athletes (Fig. 1-5). Basically, whenever possible, the athlete should not be left to rehabilitate alone. Athletic trainers should engage in

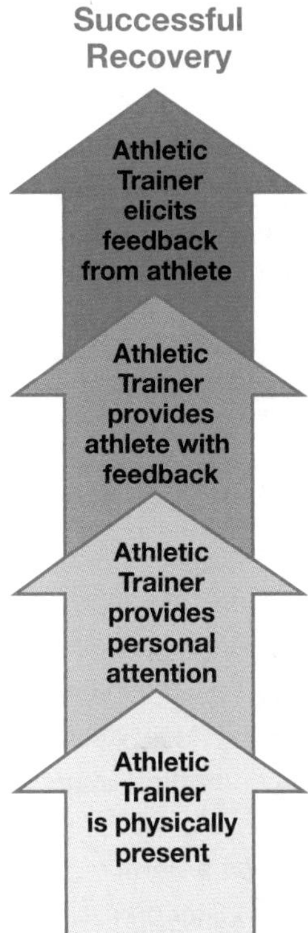

Figure 1-5 | Increasing athlete motivation and rehabilitation adherence.

conversation about the individual as well as the injury. Providing feedback and cues to improve the quality of the exercise being performed while also eliciting feedback from the athlete regarding his or her perception of the rehabilitation program and progress toward recovery are helpful to enhance rehabilitation adherence. Another strategy to improve athlete motivation is to engage in short-term goal setting; motivation increases by setting and meeting goals, as well as by the excitement athletic trainers demonstrate when goals are met. Reports also show that the willingness of the athletic trainer to perform rehabilitation exercises with the athlete increases athlete motivation and effort during rehabilitation. The key to keeping athletes motivated and adherent to rehabilitation is to develop creative, individual programs and to push them to reach their ultimate potential (you will learn more strategies to keep athletes motivated during rehabilitation in Chapter 8). Finally, the athletic trainer can demonstrate an understanding of the urgency of the situation from the athlete's perspective. Although a particular rehabilitation program may not be the athletic trainer's top priority, it *is* the top priority for the injured athlete. Athletes should perceive that their recovery is important to the athletic trainer (you will learn more about strategies to enhance adherence and motivation in Chapter 8).

Atmosphere and Social Support

Injured athletes tend to thrive in rehabilitation environments that are inviting, positive, and supportive. We have already discussed the importance of communicating with and educating injured athletes, but the perceived availability and approachability of the athletic trainer cannot be emphasized enough. Athletes must feel comfortable initiating conversation and asking questions (especially questions that they may feel are "dumb questions" or those that they have asked previously but are still unclear about). In addition, athletes should perceive the athletic training room as a positive place full of athletic trainers who can help them maintain a positive outlook on the rehabilitation process. Injured athletes expect athletic trainers to provide many levels of social support, with the primary focus being on support related to their athletic injury (specifically, listening and emotional support, emotional challenge, task appreciation, and task challenge). In addition, they expect athletic trainers to possess the ability to listen, display empathy, and counsel them as needed in situations unrelated to sport and injury. Athletic trainers should also help foster the development of support structures. This may include pairing athletes up with other injured athletes who may share common challenges, or it may involve helping the athlete identify sources of support within his or her personal life (such as parents, friends, and significant others; you will learn more about domains of social support and provision strategies in Chapter 9).

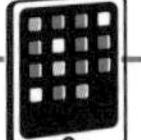

VIRTUAL FIELD TRIP

To learn more about some of the expectations an athlete may have of an athletic trainer following injury, visit http://davisplus.fadavis.com and complete the critical listening exercises associated with this chapter.

ROLE OF PSYCHOSOCIAL STRATEGIES IN FACILITATING RECOVERY FROM ATHLETIC INJURY

Research shows psychosocial strategies to be invaluable tools for athletic trainers leading the rehabilitation process. Strategies have been shown to be effective in the following ways:

- Reducing pain
- Improving positive outlook
- Increasing adherence/reducing recovery time
- Improving relaxation
- Increasing injured athletes' satisfaction with rehabilitation.

Other members of the sports medicine team (i.e., physicians) acknowledge that athletes struggle with psychological issues following injury and value psychosocial techniques. Orthopedics and family medicine physicians endorse the multifactorial approach to postinjury rehabilitation, including both mental and physical exercises. Research has shown that formal education in the Psychosocial Strategies and Referral content area can increase both knowledge about the importance of techniques and the frequency with which athletic trainers use psychosocial strategies.

Athletic trainers should recognize the value of encouraging athletes to transfer and use psychosocial strategies they utilize in their sport in the injury rehabilitation context as well. Athletic trainers' perceptions of the importance of psychosocial strategies have increased drastically over the past 20 years. In 1991, the majority of athletic trainers believed that focusing on short-term goals and encouraging positive self-thoughts were the only effective techniques for facilitating injured athletes' recovery. In 2000, physiotherapists (the most equivalent professional to athletic training in Europe) also rated practical strategies such as communication, social support, and reinforcement as most important. Physiotherapists ranked psychosocial strategies such as relaxation, mental imagery, and concentration development as less important. More recently, in 2008, both physical therapists and athletic trainers reported increasingly positive attitudes about the effectiveness and use of psychosocial strategies with injured athletes. Goal setting remains the top-rated skill; however, positive self-talk, relaxation, pain management, and imagery were rated positively overall. For more details on this recent research, see the following evidence-based practice feature. The recent positive ratings are encouraging and stand to influence the implementation of psychosocial strategies with injured and recovering athletes.

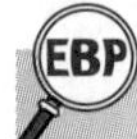

EVIDENCE-BASED PRACTICE

Hamson-Utley, J. J., Martin, S., & Walters, J. (2008). Athletic trainers' and physical therapists' perceptions of the effectiveness of psychological skills within sport-injury rehabilitation programs. *Journal of Athletic Training, 43*(3), 258–264.

Description of the Study

Psychological skills are alleged to augment the rehabilitation from sport injury; however, implementation of psychological skills within the rehabilitation programs of injured athletes is limited. The purpose of this study was to examine attitudes of both certified athletic trainers and physical therapists on the effectiveness of mental imagery, goal setting, and positive self-talk to improve adherence and recovery speed of injured athletes. Athletic trainers and physical therapists were contacted via electronic and physical mailings to survey their beliefs on the effectiveness of psychological skills for increasing adherence and recovery speed of injured athletes undergoing rehabilitation. Professional member databases of the National Athletic Trainers' Association and American Physical Therapy Association provided selected participant lists. Of the 1,000 athletic trainers and 1,000 physical therapists who were randomly selected, 309 certified athletic trainers (age: 34 ± 8.32 years, years in profession: 10.67 ± 7.34) and 356 physical therapists (age: 38.58 ± 7.51 years, years in profession: 13.18 ± 6.17) responded. The survey used in the study—Attitudes About Imagery (AAI)—measured attitudes about psychological skills for enhancing adherence and recovery speed of injured athletes. The AAI was developed based on athletic injury response models and feedback from four experts representing three areas of specialization (sport psychology, athletic training, and physical therapy). Test–retest reliability ranged from 0.60 to 0.84, and Cronbach's alphas ranged from 0.65 to 0.90. The measures of internal reliability and interitem reliability support the experts' guidance on content validity. One-way analyses of variance were calculated to determine whether significant differences existed in attitudes as a result of the professional's education, training experience, and interest. The AAI survey includes **demographic variables** and 15 items on a 7-point Likert scale that measure attitudes about the effectiveness of mental imagery, positive self-talk, goal setting, and pain control on adherence to rehabilitation and recovery speed of injured athletes.

Results of the Study

The researchers found significant mean differences on attitudes of effectiveness of psychological skills for those who reported formal training and those who reported interest in receiving formal training ($p < 0.05$). In addition, athletic trainers held significantly more positive attitudes than physical therapists on 9 of 15 AAI items ($p < 0.05$). Although only 24.6% of certified athletic trainers and 11% of physical therapists reported having formal training on mental imagery, 72.5% of certified athletic trainers and 53.7% of physical therapists reported they would seek formal training if it was available. Regarding the effectiveness of educational standards, 61.5% of certified athletic trainers reported graduating from an accredited program, yet only 24.6% reported receiving education on the use of mental imagery with injured athletes.

Implications for Athletic Training Practice

Overall, athletic trainers and physical therapists hold positive attitudes on the effectiveness of psychological skills to augment the rehabilitation process. Communicating with athletes to discover the issues and roadblocks they face is a first step in teaching and implementing effective skills that stand to improve the rehabilitation process for injured athletes. Athletic trainers who are unsure of how to use psychological strategies with athletes should seek continuing education.

Although early studies may have indicated that athletic trainers viewed psychosocial strategies as less important in injury rehabilitation, more recent studies have shown these skills to be important to successful recovery and rehabilitation. The Athletic Trainer and Sport Psychology Questionnaire (ATSPQ) was developed for use in this line of research (Larson, Starkey, & Zaichkowsky, 1996). Questions focus on behaviors associated with successful and unsuccessful coping with athletic injury, frequency of use of psychological skills with athletes during injury, rating of the importance of using and learning about psychological skills and techniques in relation to athletic injury, rating of the importance of the psychological aspect of athletic injury, and the importance of a course in sport psychology in the education of an athletic trainer. The ATSPQ has also been modified to be used with sport physiotherapists in the United Kingdom and restructured as the Physiotherapist and Sport Psychology Questionnaire (PSPQ) (Hemmings & Povey, 2002). Research has shown consistent findings across professions with regard to both the Likert scale and open-ended questions. Specifically, both types of professionals listed the same top five characteristics of athletes who cope successfully and four of the top five characteristics of athletes who cope unsuccessfully. Successful coping characteristics included adherence with the rehabilitation program, positive attitude, motivation to rehabilitate, patience with the injury program, and determination. This similarity between the two studies indicates that injury-relevant psychological issues are similar across athletes at multiple competitive levels and in multiple countries. Taken together, the results of these studies indicate the importance of incorporating mental skills and strategies into athletes' injury rehabilitation programs.

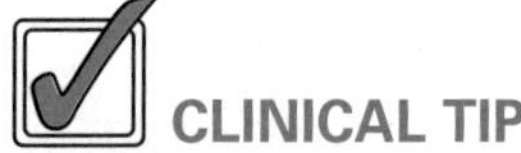

CLINICAL TIP

In a recent study, athletic trainers reported that the top three selected psychosocial strategies that are important when working with injured athletes are: (1) keeping the athlete involved with the team, (2) using short-term goals, and (3) creating variety in rehabilitation exercises (Clement, Granquist, & Arvinen-Barrow, 2013).

ROLE DELINEATION STUDY AND EDUCATIONAL PREPARATION OF ATHLETIC TRAINERS

The Role Delineation Study identifies essential knowledge and skills for the profession of athletic training. The certifying body for entry-level athletic training—the Board of Certification (BOC)—identified these essential skills via a Practice Analysis that also serves as a foundation for BOC examination development. Five domains were identified in the sixth edition of the Role Delineation Study (2011b):

1. Injury/illness prevention and wellness protection
2. Clinical evaluation and diagnosis
3. Immediate and emergency care
4. Treatment and rehabilitation
5. Organizational and professional health and well-being

The Role Delineation Study and Practice Analysis outline the essential knowledge and skills an entry-level professional should possess to perform athletic training job duties to the standards required for certification.

As the sixth edition Role Delineation Study outlines, athletic trainers are involved in the prevention and care of athletic injury (Domain 1), and it is imperative to recognize the important role that athletic trainers have in both physical and mental injury-prevention techniques. The athletic trainer must develop communication skills that help athletes recognize emotions, conflicts, and personal problems that may contribute to stress and serve as psychosocial antecedents to injury. It is also important to understand imbalances between physical load and emotional coping resources, such as overtraining and ***burnout***. Key roles of athletic trainers include immediate and emergency care (Domain 3) and clinical evaluation and diagnosis (Domain 2). During emergency situations, athletic trainers must be able to control both their own emotions and the emotions of the injured athlete. Mental skills such as relaxation and focused breathing may be essential to control the athlete's response to injury, as well as to aid the athletic trainer in maintaining control and focus. After an unfavorable diagnosis, athletic trainers must recognize and anticipate potential negative emotional responses and must have the skills necessary to facilitate more positive responses and behaviors. Athletic trainers are also involved in the treatment and rehabilitation of injuries (Domain 4), playing a vital role in athletes' motivation and rehabilitation adherence. Finally, a component of professional behavior (Domain 5) is an awareness of one's own professional limitations and willingness to identify professionals to whom they can refer athletes when needed.

The professional success of certified athletic trainers is influenced by more than the ability to provide effective physical interventions to injured athletes. Specifically, the importance of psychological recovery from athletic injury is receiving more attention. AT programs generally focus primarily on the physical nature of athletic injury, and for good reason. The primary roles of athletic trainers include physical injury prevention, evaluation and treatment, and rehabilitation. However, the BOC and the Professional Education Council (PEC) agree that knowledge regarding psychology and sociology (i.e., psychosocial aspects) of injury is also essential for the entry-level athletic trainer. This is evidenced by the inclusion of Psychosocial Strategies and Referral as one of eight content areas accredited AT programs must address. In addition, two of the nine clinical integration proficiencies (CIPs) require demonstration of proficiency in using various psychosocial interventions including verbal motivation and goal setting, imagery, pain-management techniques, self-talk and relaxation (CIP-7), and recognition and referral of patients for mental health issues (CIP-8). Graduating athletic training students must consider both physical and mental aspects of injury to fully care for the injured athlete, and both aspects must be emphasized in the athletic training curriculum.

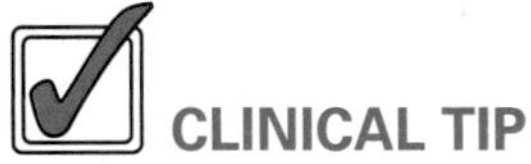

CLINICAL TIP

Stiller-Ostrowski and Hamson-Utley (2010) examined the effectiveness of AT programs in addressing psychosocial aspects of injury and recovery. They found that 61.5% of athletic trainers reported graduating from an accredited program, yet only 24.6% reported receiving education on the use of mental imagery and other psychosocial strategies with injured athletes. Even though students graduate from an accredited program, they need practice as certified professionals in the clinical setting. Those who feel less competent in selecting and implementing psychosocial strategies that facilitate athlete recovery should seek continuing education.

PSYCHOSOCIAL STRATEGIES

Many psychosocial strategies have been useful with the athlete population, both before injury and in returning to sport after injury. Many athletic trainers refer to the Phase of Rehabilitation theory for guidance on which skills may work best in certain situations across the recovery timeline (for more details on this theory, see Chapter 8). In the Athlete Insider section at the beginning of this chapter, Seth may have increased his risk for injury by worrying about the size of the opponent and the hits that he might incur while playing his position at the college level. Certain psychosocial strategies can assist the athlete with self-doubt and anxiety, and might even act as injury-prevention mechanisms by moderating the impact of stress on the risk for injury. For example, the first useful skill in Seth's scenario might be communication. Noticing that Seth seems somehow preoccupied in the athletic training room before practice and on the practice field, the athletic trainer should take the time to communicate with him regarding his apprehensions and gather information that might lead to identifying a tool that would calm his fear. Psychosocial antecedents to injury and communication skills are addressed in Chapters 3 and 5, respectively.

Positive Self-talk and Relaxation

One skill set that might benefit Seth and further decrease his risk for injury is a combination of relaxation and positive self-talk. He could use relaxation techniques to help decrease muscle tension that may be caused by his anxiety about playing against larger, stronger athletes. Learning to identify muscle tension and voluntarily regulate it would aid in maintaining the skills and coordination that are essential on the field. Adding in positive affirmations ("I am quick enough to miss the majority of the tackles.") may aid in building Seth's confidence in his ability to avoid injury. Chapter 10 will provide an evidence-based practice approach to psychological skills techniques.

Nonpharmacological Pain Management

The techniques of ***nonpharmacological pain management*** provide a method of controlling the pain associated with injury. Athletes like to be in control, but within the injury and rehabilitation scenario, they are rarely in the lead. Providing athletes with the skills that allow them to be in control of their pain will assist in improving motivation and overall healing. Such techniques could include either associative or dissociative techniques (e.g., focusing on deep, diaphragmatic breathing). In addition, athletes can learn forms of mental imagery (specifically, healing imagery) or self-talk techniques that help to reframe the meaning of pain. For example, rather than a negative experience, athletes could interpret pain as information that they are being too aggressive in rehabilitation and should back off before disturbing the healing cycle (or "setback"). Chapter 7 will provide further information on pain-management strategies.

Motivation

Motivation could be a combination of highlights from Seth's successful high school performances and the use of goal setting. Highlight reels focus on individual strengths and successes, which empower the athlete to return to play with confidence (motivational imagery). Goal setting could increase athlete motivation during rehabilitation by providing athletes with direction while improving their sense of control over the rehabilitation process. The process of setting and attaining goals builds confidence in both the injured athlete's abilities and in the success of the rehabilitation program. To enhance the value of goal setting, the athlete must connect achievement of short-term goals to a successful return to sport. Imagery techniques can be combined with goal setting to enhance the value of both. The use of "possible selves" imagery involves visualizing oneself achieving a goal that has been set (for examples, see Box 1-1). Psychosocial aspects of rehabilitation, including facilitating athlete motivation and adherence, will be discussed in Chapter 8.

Education

Knowledge reduces anxiety and improves confidence; it might involve injury or recovery education. Especially effective before or just after surgery, education about the injury and/or surgical process, including what to expect in the days and weeks to come, has been shown to reduce anxiety and improve overall healing. Education increases awareness and reduces anxiety about the injury or pain the athlete experiences. For instance, when athletes understand that the pain is no longer harmful but is a sign of progress (e.g., gaining ROM), they can exhale or relax. This reduces tension in the surrounding musculature, which results in vasodilatation and lessens pain. The vasodilatation increases the blood flow to the injured area, bringing more healing properties to the area and removing injury by-products. Athlete education techniques will be provided in Chapter 5.

ATHLETE INSIDER CONCLUSION

Seth met many challenges within rehabilitation, including understanding his injury and how to work effectively toward his goals. He spent many hours in rehabilitation and found himself asking the athletic trainer questions every day to understand his progress

BOX 1-1 | Possible Selves (Performance Imagery)

- Visualize a series of possible selves over the course of a rehabilitation program.
- Use in conjunction with a series of short-term goals.
- For example:
  - Get knee to 90° of flexion → imagine yourself accomplishing this, focusing on the kinesthetic feeling (tightness as knee nears 90°, sliding your heel back and back along a tabletop or flat surface...)
  - Perform straight-leg raise with knee fully extended → imagine yourself accomplishing this (sensation of knee locking out, feeling shaking of quad as you lift your leg off the table)
  - Single-leg balance → imagine yourself accomplishing this (feel foot wobble underneath you and see yourself putting your arms out to the side as you work to maintain balance)
  - Mini-squat → imagine yourself accomplishing this (see your knees bending until they are just over your toes, and feel the wall against your back as you slide down)
  - Beginning a running progression → imagine yourself accomplishing this (see yourself in good running form; feel yourself getting winded from the exertion; feel your heart begin to race from the excitement of being at this point in your rehabilitation)
  - Returning to sport → imagine yourself back to full participation (see yourself completing the same activity in which you were injured and feel the strength in your injured body part as you successfully complete the activity)

KEYS TO SUCCESS

1. Make it vivid (see and feel it).
2. Have a plan (want attention focused on developing the image for the athlete vs. creating it off the top of your head).
3. Create first-person perspective for athlete.
4. Educate the athlete (education is KEY for healing imagery to be effective).

and when he would be ready to return to play. He found that when he understood the next step and how short-term goals contributed to his ultimate goal, he was more focused and worried less about returning to play. He built a strong relationship with the athletic trainer by spending quality time in a positive environment that allowed for open communication and social support (Fig. 1-6).

Effective Psychosocial Strategies for the Athletic Trainer to Use With Seth

The following psychosocial strategies can be effectively applied by the athletic trainer in working with Seth throughout his recovery and return to competition:

1. Goal setting and possible self imagery (Box 1-1)
2. Performance imagery as Seth prepares to return to sport: Seth likely will engage in "injury replay imagery" (playing the "video" of his injury repeatedly in his mind). To assist Seth in forming positive images, the athletic trainer can prepare a script that leads him to avoid the injuring tackle and see himself running his route without pain (see sample imagery script at http://davisplus.fadavis.com).
3. Education about his injury to lessen his anxiety and keep him focused on rehabilitation goals
4. Teaching Seth to use positive self-talk in the rehabilitation setting when he meets a challenging exercise or something that causes pain; teaching him also to transfer this skill to the field as he readies to return to play (Fig. 1-7)

CONCLUSION

This chapter provides an overview of the role of the athletic trainer and the use of psychosocial strategies throughout the injury process, beginning with skills for identifying psychosocial antecedents that may predispose an athlete to injury and concluding with strategies designed to facilitate a psychosocially healthy return to participation. It is important for both athletic training students and certified athletic trainers to recognize the role that they play in "the mental side of injury" (Fig. 1-8).

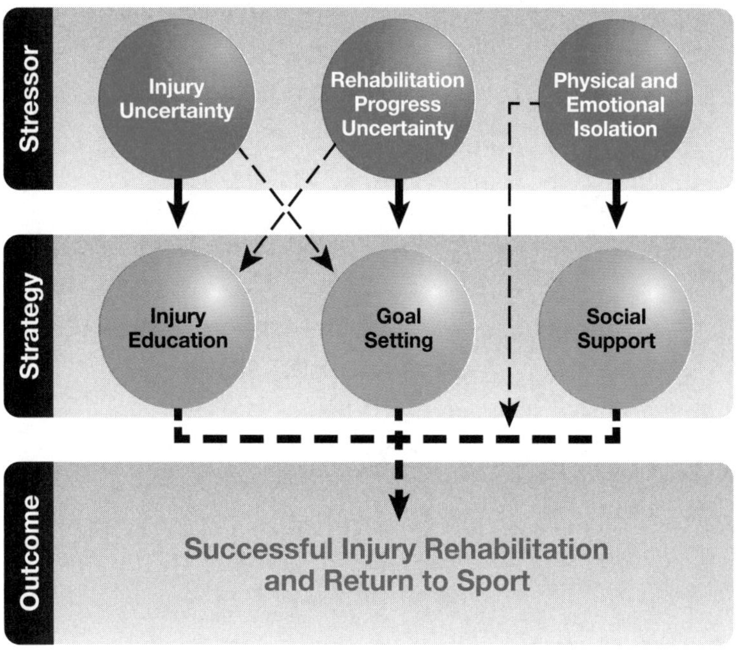

Figure 1-6 | Using psychosocial strategies with Seth.

Motivated
Humble
I know I can do this
I am strong enough
Positive
I am made stronger by this experience
Energetic
I am in control
Intelligent

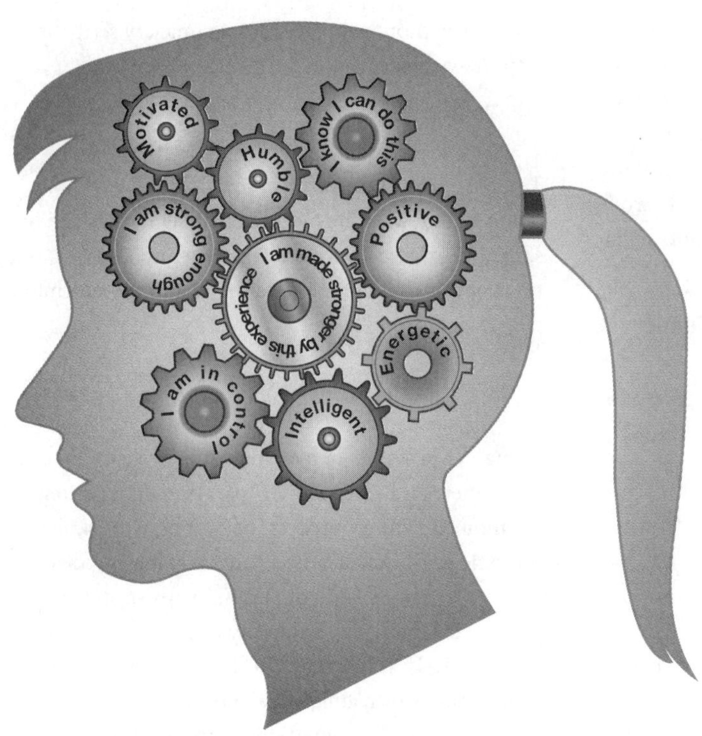

Figure 1-7 | Role of positive self-talk in injury rehabilitation.

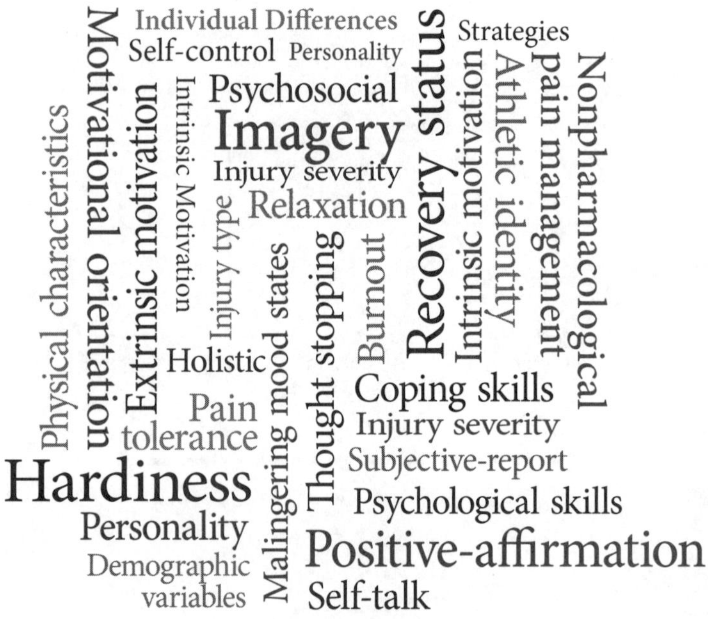

Individual Differences
Self-control Personality
Strategies
Motivational orientation
Physical characteristics
Extrinsic motivation
Intrinsic Motivation
Psychosocial
Imagery
Injury severity
Relaxation
Injury type
Holistic
Pain tolerance
Hardiness
Personality
Demographic variables
Malingering mood states
Thought stopping
Burnout
Recovery status
Intrinsic motivation
Athletic identity
pain management
Nonpharmacological
Coping skills
Injury severity
Subjective-report
Psychological skills
Positive-affirmation
Self-talk

Figure 1-8 | The psychology of injury.

REFERENCES

Andersen, M. B., & Williams, J. M. (1988). A model of stress and athletic injury: Prediction and prevention. *Journal of Sport & Exercise Psychology, 10*(3), 294–306.

Clement, D., Hamson-Utley, J., Arvinen-Barrow, M., Kamphoff, C. S., Zakrajsek, R. A., & Martin, S. B. (2012). College athletes' expectations about injury rehabilitation with an athletic trainer. *International Journal of Athletic Therapy & Training, 17*(4), 18–27.

Clement, D., Granquist, M. D., & Arvinen-Barrow, M. (2013). Psychosocial aspects of athletic injuries as perceived by athletic trainers. *Journal of Athletic Training, 48*(4), 512–521.

Hamson-Utley, J. J., Martin, S., & Walters, J. (2008). Athletic trainers' and physical therapists' perceptions of the effectiveness of psychological skills within sport-injury rehabilitation programs. *Journal of Athletic Training, 43*(3), 258–264.

Hemmings, B., & Povey, L. (2002). Views of chartered physiotherapists on the psychological content of their practice: A preliminary study in the United Kingdom. *British Journal of Sports Medicine, 36*(1), 61–64.

Larson, G. A., Starkey, C., & Zaichkowsky, L. D. (1996). Psychological aspects of athletic injuries as perceived by athletic trainers. *The Sport Psychologist, 10*(1), 37–47.

McNair, D., Lorr, M., & Droppleman, L. (1971). Manual for the Profile of Mood States. San Diego: Educational and Industrial Testing Service.

Morgan, W. P. (1980). Test of champions: The iceberg profile. *Psychology Today*, 92–99.

National Athletic Trainers' Association. (2011a). *Athletic training educational competencies* (5th ed.). Dallas, TX: National Athletic Trainers' Association.

National Athletic Trainers' Association. (2011b). *Role delineation study/practice analysis* (6th ed.). Dallas, TX: National Athletic Trainers' Association.

Stiller-Ostrowski, J. L., & Hamson-Utley, J. J. (2010). The ATEP educated athletic trainer: Educational satisfaction and technique use within the psychosocial intervention and referral content area. *Athletic Training Education Journal, 5*(1), 4–11.

Stiller-Ostrowski, J. L., & Ostrowski, J. A. (2009). Recently certified athletic trainers' undergraduate educational preparation in psychosocial intervention and referral. *Journal of Athletic Training, 44*(1), 67–75.

BOARD OF CERTIFICATION STRATEGIES AND COMPETENCIES

As the sixth edition of the BOC's Role Delineation Study outlines, athletic trainers are involved in both the prevention and the care of athletic injury. The PEC develops educational competencies that are required in all AT programs; implementation of these competencies is enforced by the Commission on Accreditation of Athletic Training Education (CAATE). The main focus of the Psychosocial Strategies and Referral content area is to recognize and assist (and potentially refer) the athlete who is struggling to cope with a stressor or injury situation. Furthermore, the CAATE educational guidelines acknowledge the importance of psychosocial strategies by requiring programs to include coursework on facilitating coping skills aimed at preventing injury and on assisting athletes in managing preinjury stressors and their emotions following injury. Psychosocial strategies such as verbal motivation, goal setting, imagery, pain management, self-talk, and relaxation are effective in injury prevention and rehabilitation. The athletic trainer is in a key position to implement strategies that have the potential to impact prevention, cognitive appraisal of an injury, and the return-to-play confidence of the athlete.

Each chapter throughout this textbook will address a variety of Psychosocial Strategies and Referral (PS) competencies and clinical integration proficiencies from the fifth edition of the Athletic Training Education Competencies and Clinical Integration Proficiencies (2011a). The PS competencies address three areas of knowledge: Theoretical Background (PS-1 through PS-5), Psychosocial Strategies (PS-6 through PS-10), and Mental Health and Referral (PS-11 through PS-18). The two CIPs address selecting and integrating psychosocial techniques into an athlete's treatment and rehabilitation (CIP-7) and recognizing the need for and referring athletes to mental health providers (CIP-8).

Board of Certification Style Questions

1. An athlete is getting ready to return to play and is experiencing anxiety. What psychosocial strategy might be used in the athletic training room just before practice? (Select all that apply.)
   a. Relaxation
   b. Motivation and positive self-talk
   c. Goal setting
   d. Pain management

2. What is an effective strategy for the athletic trainer to teach the athlete about his or her injury and recovery? (Select all that apply.)
   a. An environment with a feeling of open communication
   b. Positive self-talk
   c. A thought-stopping program
   d. Positive affirmations about return to play

3. What is the moderating variable to the stress response according to the Andersen and Williams (1988) model? (Select all that apply.)
   a. Personality
   b. Coping resources
   c. History of stressors
   d. All of the above
   e. a and b only

4. Anxiety is best described as a negative psychological and physical reaction to a(n):
   a. subjectively perceived threat.
   b. objectively perceived threat.
   c. well-known threat.
   d. fear.

END-OF-CHAPTER EXERCISES

1. Make a list of four characteristics that create a supportive environment in which to rehabilitate from athletic injury. Then describe how the athletic trainer can work to make those elements apparent/available to the injured athlete.

2. Illustrate how education can play a vital role in the injury recovery process. Think about the athletes or patients with whom you have worked this week and select an injury. Outline important aspects of that injury and the overall recovery process. Then consider how to implement this process with the injured athlete.

3. Research has shown that increased stress and anxiety coupled with decreased coping resources predispose an individual to injury. What explains this relationship? How could these antecedents be mediated?

4. List four expectations that athletes have of their athletic trainer in terms of psychosocial strategies. Then provide a practical example of how the athletic trainer can demonstrate each skill.

5. Using the following chart, list three behaviors that an athlete may display that potentially interfere with the progress of rehabilitation or healing. In the second column, pair the behavior with an effective psychosocial strategy to modify the behavior to facilitate rehabilitation or healing.

Problem Behavior	Effective Psychosocial Strategy

6. Consider the busy athletic training room. Develop a strategy that facilitates effective communication between the athlete and athletic trainer when one-on-one communication is needed and not available. How would the athletic trainer make this strategy known? What is needed to implement this strategy? For example, the head athletic trainer gives athletes at the beginning of the season (and posts on his or her office door) the cell phone numbers of all of the athletic trainers for texting purposes. Athletes who need something and feel they cannot get it at the time they arrive at the athletic training room can text the athletic trainer to set up communication for a later time. The purpose of this exercise is to highlight those situations when athletes in psychological or physical need are not served.

7. Think of a time this month when an athlete needed emotional support from the head athletic trainer but was unable to receive it. What can you do as an athletic training student to remedy this situation?

8. Consider an athlete with whom you are working right now to rehabilitate an athletic injury. What motivates that athlete? If he or she is lacking motivation at times, how can you assist in the motivation process?

9. Examine your athletic training room for resources available to athletes who need psychosocial strategies. Complete the following chart with examples of resources found in your athletic training room for common psychosocial needs of the athlete.

Psychosocial Needs of the Athlete	Resource(s) Available in the Athletic Training Room
Stress management	
Pain management	
Eating disorder	
Substance abuse issue	
Return-to-play anxiety (after rehabilitation)	

10. Have you worked with an athlete this semester who is physically but not psychologically ready to return to play? What techniques might be useful in this scenario?

11. Consider the comparison between the elite athlete who has 30 years of experience playing a sport and has received four severe injuries that were rehabilitated successfully and the high school athlete who has 4 years of participation and no severe injuries in his or her history. How do they differ?

Chapter 2

Sociocultural Aspects of Injury and Injury Response

Laura J. Kenow with Cindra S. Kamphoff

CHAPTER OUTLINE

KEY TERMS

Macrotrauma Injury resulting from a single impact or force that creates tissue damage (e.g., fracture, sprain, or dislocation).

Malingering Intentionally pretending to have or exaggerating physical or psychological symptoms, especially to avoid work or a return to participation.

Microtrauma Injury resulting from repeated smaller forces that gradually result in tissue damage over time (e.g., stress fracture, tendinitis).

Normative behavior Behavior that is expected by societal standards.

Overconformer Athlete who unconditionally accepts the norms of the sport ethic and follows them without reservation.

Secondary gain Favorable consequences, such as increased attention from significant others and escape from stressful situations, or medication use, that occur in conjunction with the generally undesirable injury.

Sport ethic Socially defined criteria for consideration as an athlete in competitive sports.

Sport norms Standards, beliefs, or models considered to be normal in sports settings.

Sport socioculture Social and cultural climates, contexts, and structures that surround sport and drive the way individuals act and relate to one another in the sport environment.

Underconformer Athlete who rejects or dismisses the norms of the sport ethic.

CHAPTER OBJECTIVES

After reading this chapter, you will be able to:

1. Describe what the dominant sports culture is in high-intensity sports today.
2. Describe how this culture contributes to injury risk and athlete behaviors following injury.
3. Define the sport ethic and the normative behavior it elicits.
4. Identify the athletic trainer's role in the sport culture.
5. Assess the degree to which athletic trainers and the athletes with whom they work conform to the sport ethic.
6. Identify strategies to mediate both overconformity and underconformity to the sport ethic norms.

ATHLETE INSIDER

Petra Majdic, an Olympic cross-country skier from the small country of Slovenia, arrived at the 2010 Vancouver Olympic Games as a medal favorite in multiple events. This wasn't Petra's first Olympic experience. Four years earlier, at the Turin games, a poor choice of skis—cold-weather skis on an unexpectedly warm day—contributed to her disappointing finish out of the medals. In Vancouver, 22 years of training and sacrifice brought her to what might likely be her last chance at an Olympic medal. No one from Slovenia had ever medaled in Olympic cross-country skiing, and Petra no doubt felt the excitement and anticipation of her entire country at the prospect of showing that this tiny nation could compete and even win against the world.

During her warm-up for her first event qualifier, the independent sprint, Petra slid off an icy curve and plunged 10 feet into a craggy creek bed, slamming her ribs into rocks. The impact of the fall snapped her ski poles and broke the tip of one ski. Despite feeling significant pain in her chest, Petra begged to be taken to the start line for her qualifying heat, which was to begin in 20 minutes. Her coaches told her to drop out if the pain was too great, but Petra was determined. She completed the 1.4-kilometer course, qualifying for the next round, and then collapsed, screaming in pain. With only 90 minutes before her quarterfinal heat, she was taken to an on-site medical tent for evaluation. An ultrasound suggested no fractures, and Petra was told she could continue to race if she could tolerate the pain. Despite being unable to stand or sit without significant pain, Petra continued through her quarterfinal and semifinal heats, qualifying for the finals. The pain worsened with each round, and prior to the finals, Petra heard an ominous clicking sound as her ribs moved in her chest. She realized something was significantly wrong. Her support team encouraged her with the story of Kerri Strug, the U.S. Olympic gymnast famous for her gold medal–clinching vault on a seriously injured ankle at the 1996 Olympics, and reminded Petra of the 22 years of sacrifice she made to reach this race. Petra pushed on into the finals and fended off a Swedish skier down the stretch to win the bronze medal, Slovenia's first Olympic medal in cross-country skiing (Epstein, 2011).

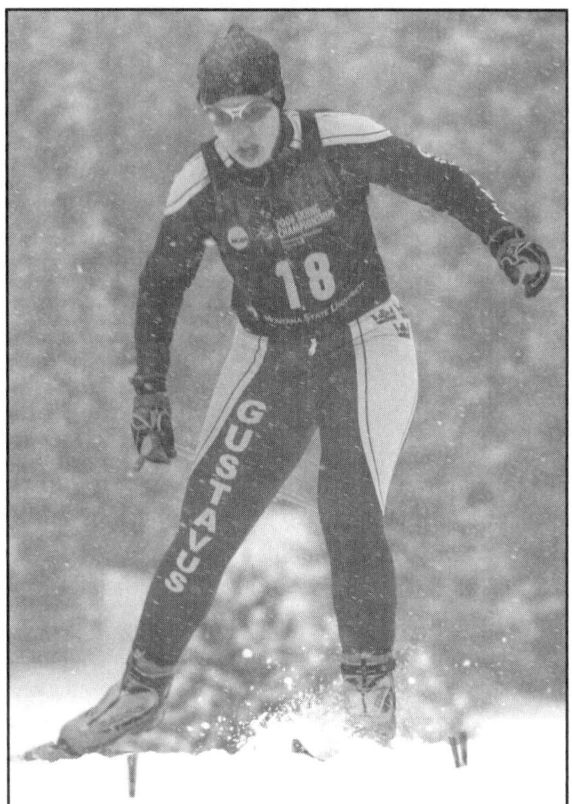

Figure 2-1 | Athlete Insider *(Courtesy of Gustavus Adolphus College, Sports Information)*

INTRODUCTION

Petra's story is not an isolated event; other tales of toughness stick in our minds. Recall Lindsey Vonn's 2010 Olympic gold-medal downhill ski run on a leg that she admittedly "numbed" up with lidocaine before the race to compete. Or Tiger Woods's 2008 U.S. Open performance, where he alternately used his golf clubs to hit shots and then to support himself as he limped through the final round, ultimately winning his 14th major on a leg diagnosed with double stress fractures and a knee that would later require ligament reconstruction. If you hear mention of "the bloody sock" in relation to baseball, does your mind immediately jump to Curt Schilling's 2004 gutsy pitching performance in the American League Championship Series as the pitcher for the Boston Red Sox? Or what about NBA star Alonzo Mourning's determination to continue playing basketball with the Miami Heat while he waited for a kidney transplant? And, as mentioned earlier, there is Kerri Strug's incredible second vault on a severely injured ankle in the 1996 Olympic Games that secured the gold medal for the U.S. women's gymnastics Olympic team.

Events such as these permeate the sports news headlines. Members of the media play these stories over and over again, reminding us of the pain and sacrifice athletes are willing to endure to obtain sports glory. But have you ever paused to ask, At what price? Will these athletes pay down the road in long-term health consequences as a result of their moment of glory? What messages are we sending to young children, who glue their eyes to the TV sets to watch their idols perform through pain and injury? Although these stories make for great news headlines, do they contribute to a societal acceptance of a win-at-all-costs mentality, and, if so, is that mentality healthy?

The social culture in high-intensity sports today expects athletes to "be tough" and play through pain and injury. The behavior is normalized, encouraged, and often glorified by those involved in sports (e.g., coaches, athletes, media, fans). This chapter discusses how this dominant sport culture contributes to risk for sport injury and influences athletes' behaviors following injury. The chapter encourages you to critically examine society's portrayal of sport injury, as well as your own personal views on "toughness" and playing through pain. This chapter concludes with strategies that athletic trainers can use to mediate the socially constructed "culture of risk" in sports and the behaviors this culture instills in athletes.

DEFINING THE SOCIOCULTURE OF SPORT

The ***sport socioculture*** refers to the social and cultural climates, contexts, and structures that surround sports and drive the way individuals act and relate to one another within the sport environment. In relation to sport injury, the sport socioculture influences sport injury risk, how individuals respond to and recover from injury, and how athletes determine when to return to sport following injury. For example, athletes are bombarded with common locker room slogans (Fig. 2-2) that send distinct messages about what is expected and what it takes to succeed in sports. These slogans clearly indicate that there will be some pain involved in achieving athletic success, but true athletes will not let that or anything else stand in the way of victory. Locker room slogans are great at creating intense focus and drive in athletes; however, they can become problematic when they are internalized and accepted without reservation. The sport culture emphasizes a "push-the-limits" mentality that constantly challenges athletes to put it all on the line for the good of the game; however, after injury, this mentality may be contradictory to efficient healing.

SOCIOCULTURAL FACTORS AND SPORT INJURY RISK

Sport participation involves risk. Each time athletes step on to the playing field, they risk many things, including falling short of their goals, losing a game, being critically

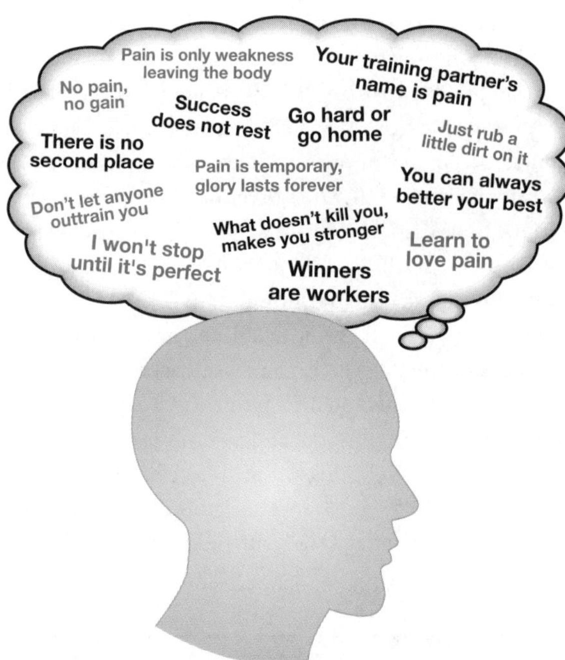

Figure 2-2 | Common locker room slogans that contribute to the sport culture.

evaluated by others, and possibly sustaining injury. As a result, some have gone so far as to label sports as a "culture of risk." The truth of this claim is debatable, but what is not under debate is that, each time athletes participate in sports, there is a chance they will get hurt. The risk for injury inherent in sports is a contributing factor to the sport culture.

A myriad of factors contribute to athletes' injury risks. Physical factors, such as athletes' strength, flexibility, and fitness, may be the first to come to mind, but they are far from the only factors that contribute to injury risk. Environmental, psychological, and sociocultural factors interact with physical factors to create unique injury risks for each athlete. Athletic trainers need to understand the complex interaction of these contributory influences to develop and devise effective injury prevention and intervention strategies. The following sections examine these influences in greater detail.

Physical Risk Factors

Multiple physical factors can make athletes more susceptible to injury. Athletes who are out of shape or lack appropriate strength and flexibility may be at greater risk for injury. Athletes' age and skeletal maturity can also contribute to injury risk. For instance, young athletes whose skeletons are still growing and developing may be at greater risk for growth plate injuries, or older athletes may encounter injury issues because of joint degeneration or decreasing flexibility. Prior injuries may make athletes more susceptible to reinjury, and training patterns that are excessive or lack variety can contribute to overuse injury issues.

Environmental Risk Factors

The environments in which athletes practice and compete also contribute to injury risk. The location of the field can become problematic when space issues force fields to be built in places that lack sufficient clearance between sidelines and potentially hazardous structures such as walls, benches, or fences. Athletes can easily sustain injury when they find they do not have enough time to stop before running into such structures. Consider the anxiety and anticipation experienced when you watch an NBA player fly into the first rows of the crowd while trying to chase down a loose ball. You can almost hear the collective sigh of relief when the athlete rises from the toppled chairs and spilled popcorn and beverages to return safely to the court. In addition, improperly padded goalposts or volleyball standards can increase injury risk if athletes collide with them. Old or improperly fitted equipment, sometimes used out of necessity in youth sports, cannot properly provide the intended protection, thus increasing the likelihood of injury. Weather conditions, such as rain or ice, can make playing surfaces slippery or frozen, increasing the likelihood of injury, as can uneven playing surfaces (Fig. 2-3). Fortunately, many of these environmental factors are modifiable with sufficient planning, finances, or diligent observation; however, other factors such as large disparities in size, skill, or strength between competing individuals are not always under anyone's control.

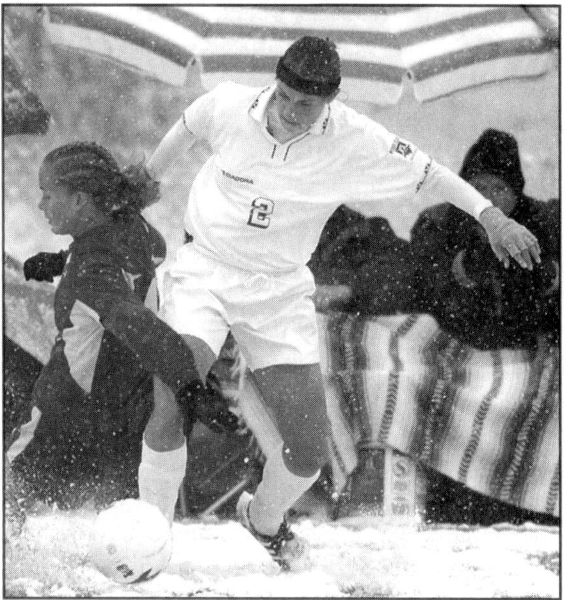

Figure 2-3 | Environmental risk factors. *(Courtesy of Weber State University Athletics)*

Psychological Risk Factors

Later, in Chapter 3, you will learn in greater detail about psychological factors that contribute to injury risk. However, it deserves mention now that athletes' mood states and levels of stress can contribute to injury susceptibility. When individuals are under high levels of stress, they experience increased levels of muscle tension that can interfere with their fluidity of movement and thus alter their movement biomechanics. Over time, the changed mechanics can contribute to overuse injuries. Furthermore, when under high levels of stress, individuals experience a decrease in peripheral vision, a concept commonly known as "tunnel vision." When athletes experience tunnel vision, they are unable to pick up performance cues in the periphery, potentially increasing their risk for injury. Consider a football running back in the open field who fails to pick up a linebacker approaching quickly from the side. If the running back is caught unprepared for the imminent contact and does not have time to brace for impact, he may be at an increased risk for injury. In addition, a lack of coping resources can also be detrimental, as can certain goal orientations, beliefs, and attitudes, as these often affect the amount of stress that individuals experience. See Chapter 3 to learn more about psychological risk factors for injury.

Sociocultural Risk Factors

Several social and cultural factors affect injury risk in sports. Coaches can affect injury risk through both their level of expertise and the style of play they endorse.

Young, inexperienced, or volunteer coaches may lack basic knowledge of injury mechanisms and prevention. It is doubtful that any coach would intentionally subject athletes to situations that might injure them; however, there are many stories of athletes sustaining injury as a result of coaches' actions or inactions. For example, heat-related illness/injuries, and even fatalities, can result when coaches lack understanding of proper hydration protocols or insist on practicing during high-heat and humidity conditions. Inexperienced coaches might fail to correct improper technique, contributing to biomechanical forces that ultimately lead to injury. Furthermore, coaches who encourage or endorse an aggressive style of play may contribute to athletes' injury risk by inadvertently condoning dangerous or illegal actions. For instance, football coaches who reward and praise athletes for making "punishing" hits may unwittingly encourage their athletes to make head-to-head contact or use their helmets as a weapon in tackling in hopes of earning their coaches' praise. Coaches may also use words and phrases that perpetuate the culture of risk in sports. Coaches who tell their athletes to "suck it up" may knowingly or unintentionally send messages that their athletes should not report injuries, a practice that may actually increase risk for long-term harm.

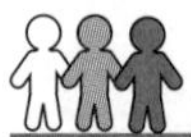

SPECIAL CONSIDERATIONS

The recent revelation of the NFL's New Orleans Saints' bounty system that paid cash rewards for hits that injured opponents called into question the boundaries of tolerable behavior in a sport culture that emphasizes physicality and often intimidation. The unprecedented sanctions meted out to those involved in the bounty program reflected a recognition that the NFL had to take a strong public stand against a part of football culture that threatened player safety. In public statements, NFL Commissioner Roger Goodell emphasized that the league would not tolerate a culture that undermines the health and safety of the players and the integrity of the game. This was further reinforced by his edict requiring every team owner and head coach to certify in writing that no such programs existed in their organizations. Those close to the decisions described this incident as a seminal moment in the culture change for professional football. It is readily apparent that in the current era, fostering, promoting, or condoning behaviors that seek to intentionally injure opposing players will not be tolerated.

Different sports by their very nature have varying levels of injury risk, in essence their own mini-culture of injury. Athletes who participate in contact sports such as football or soccer will be at greater risk for injury than those participating in golf or tennis. The rules of various sports also contribute to the type of injuries to which athletes are most susceptible. Sports that permit greater contact or collisions, like ice hockey or basketball, place athletes at greater risk for **macrotrauma**, whereas sports that involve more repetitive motions, such as swimming or cross-country running, subject athletes to greater risk for **microtrauma**. The types of injuries that athletes are more likely to experience in their sport contribute to the culture.

CLINICAL TIP

Messner, Dunbar, and Hunt (2000) analyzed 23 hours of televised sports programming identified as that most often watched by boys. They found several themes that perpetuate the culture of risk in sport. A few of these themes described that men should give up their body for their team and that they should show guts, and commentators used words to describe the men as warlike. For example, the commentators used a language of weaponry and war such as "kill," "battle," "ammunition," "taking aim," "reloading," and "squeeze the trigger." Awareness of the unique cultures of each sport can assist athletic trainers in understanding and even anticipating the types of behaviors athletes may demonstrate during sport participation.

Officials can also influence injury risk and the culture of sports through the rigor with which they enforce rules to safeguard athletes. Officials' reputations regarding how they call a game enable coaches, athletes, and athletic trainers to make accurate assumptions about how physical a game might be even before it begins. Consistency in rules enforcement, knowledge of game rules, and leniency for physical play by officials all contribute to athletes' injury risk.

Despite the best efforts of the National Athletic Trainers' Association (NATA) to advocate for athletic trainers in all athletic settings, numerous sports events and practices are still not covered by athletic trainers. In these situations where trained medical personnel are not present, athletes who sustain injury are subject to the advice of untrained coaches, parents, or teammates regarding injury care or the wisdom of continuing participation after injury. Unfortunately, research has shown that, in these situations, the desire to win often taints coaches' decisions, and they allow athletes to compete when it may not be safe to do so (Charlesworth & Young, 2004; Murphy & Waddington, 2007; Pike & Maguire, 2003).

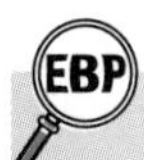

EVIDENCE-BASED PRACTICE

Flint, F. A., & Weiss, M. R. (1992). Returning injured athletes to competition: A role and ethical dilemma. *Canadian Journal of Sport Sciences, 17*(1), 34–40.

Description of the Study

Although an older article, no attempts to replicate the study have been recently conducted. The article describes two studies whose purpose was to investigate the extent to which decisions by coaches and athletic trainers concerning the return of injured athletes to competition were influenced by the player's status and the game situation. Subjects included 126 head coaches and 75 athletic trainers from high school and collegiate basketball programs. Participants were presented with hypothetical game scenarios including winning, losing, or being in a close game when a starter, first substitute, or bench player sustained a mild injury. Participants were then asked to respond yes or no as to whether they would allow a particular athlete in a particular situation to return to competition following injury.

Results of the Study

In both the high school and collegiate samples, coaches' decisions to allow an athlete to return to play were influenced by the game situation and the playing status of the player. In essence, coaches made decisions that increased the likelihood of their team winning the game. The coaches appeared to be more influenced by the player's status and the game situation than by the medical situation. In contrast, athletic trainers did not show a preference for returning players based on player status or game situation. Rather, it appeared that athletic trainers responded primarily to medical factors when making their decisions.

Implications for Athletic Training Practice

The authors concluded that given coaches' limited medical background and the pressures of coaching roles, it is ill-advised for coaches to have decision-making responsibilities where injuries are concerned. It appears that athletic trainers in this study focused on the medical aspects of the situation and were not swayed by external influences when making return-to-play decisions. The authors cautioned, however, that this study involved hypothetical situations and acknowledged that in real-life scenarios, athletic trainers' involvement with the team and the emotional ties developed through this involvement can create difficulties in remaining completely objective in return-to-play decision-making. Athletic trainers must be diligent in ensuring their medical decisions are based on objective medical information.

Sport norms refer to standards, beliefs, or models considered to be normal in sport settings. Table 2-1 provides some examples of sport-specific norms that exist relative to injury risk and injury occurrence. All the slogans highlighted in Figure 2-2 could also be considered sport norms. Athletes are told throughout their sport life about the need to be dedicated, set goals, persevere until those goals are reached,

TABLE 2-1 **Examples of Sport-Specific Norms Relative to Sport Injury**

Sport Situation	Behavioral Norm
Soccer	• Fake an injury to try to draw a card • Kick the ball out of play to allow an injured player to be evaluated
Baseball	• "Brush-back" pitch used as a retaliatory weapon
Ice hockey	• Role of the "enforcer" present on most teams
Football	• Glorification of the "big hit"
Athletic training	• Shield injured athlete from fans and/or media while receiving sideline care

Make sacrifices for "The Game"
Strive for distinction
The Sport Ethic
Accept no obstacles in the pursuit of success
Accept risks and play through pain

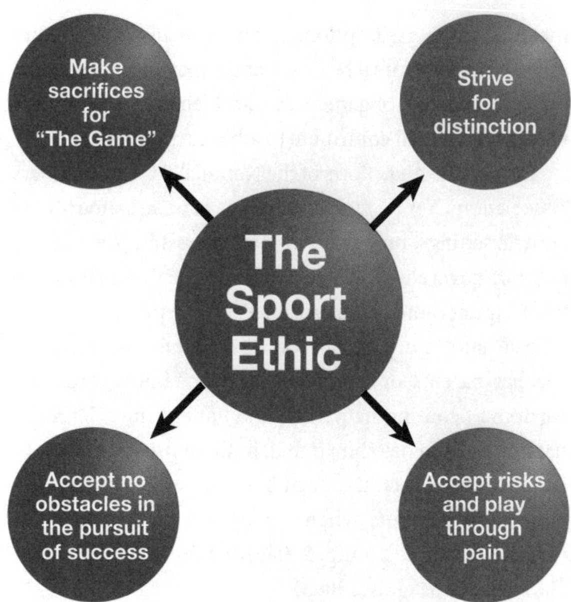

Figure 2-4 | Components of the sport ethic.

accept adversity as a challenge to overcome, and be willing to make sacrifices and put aside other interests to focus on sports. Although these norms contribute to the culture of sport as we know it today, some of these normative beliefs or standards impact injury risk directly or indirectly.

THE SPORT ETHIC

The ***sport ethic*** (Coakley, 2009; Hughes & Coakley, 1991) is society's criteria for what it takes to be identified as an athlete in sports today. The sport ethic suggests that athletes are expected to engage in four types of ***normative behavior*** (Fig. 2-4):

1. *Make sacrifices for "the game."* Athletes are expected to have a devoted love for "the game" and prove it by giving sports a position of top priority in their lives. This is reflected in athletes displaying the "proper attitude" (a term frequently used by coaches), living up to the expectations of their teammates and coaches, showing unwavering commitment, and facing the demands of sports without question. This norm is manifested in athletes consistently doing whatever is necessary to meet the demands of the coach, the team, or the competition. The concept of "paying the price," whatever that price might be, is inherent in this norm.

   Consider the case of Trevor Wikre, a college football player at Mesa State College, who severely dislocated his little finger during his senior season. Rather than endure corrective surgery and the 6-month recovery time recommended, he asked his surgeon to instead cut off his finger so he could play in the game on Saturday. The surgeon reluctantly agreed (there was a possibility of arthritis and other medical complications). The athlete stated about his team and his decision, "This team is too good, and there's too much love....There was no way I was missing out" (Ballard, 2008, p. 72). Although this seems rather extreme, it does demonstrate the lengths to which athletes will go to play the game they love.

2. *Strive for distinction.* Athletes are expected to have an irrepressible desire to be the best and to achieve top honors in their sport. Winning becomes exceptionally important in that it establishes distinction and represents continuous efforts toward improvement. Athletes are constantly pushing limits and doing what it takes to be the best they can be. For example, Michael Phelps commented after his 2008 Olympic gold-medal, world-record time of 1:52.03 in the 200 butterfly that he was still disappointed, "I know I can go faster than that" (Casey, 2008, p. 72). Phelps' coach

said of him: "He's addicted to the excitement. It's like any addiction: You have to have more, you have to have higher" (Casey, 2008, p. 73). Evidently, even the most decorated athlete ever in a single Olympic Games still desires to strive for distinction as evidenced by his return to Olympic competition in the 2012 games.

3. *Accept risk and play with pain.* As discussed earlier, sport participation involves the risk for injury or bodily harm. It also presents the risk for failure. However, this norm suggests that true athletes willingly accept these risks and dismiss any fear of them. Athletes do not give in to pain or the physical and psychological pressures present in sport. It is expected that athletes face challenges with calm, cool composure and accept the risks for failure and injury with courage.

   Brett Favre, former quarterback in the NFL, had almost every part of his body listed on an NFL injury report: hand, neck, toe, hamstring, head, elbow, back, side, chin, thigh, shoulder, forearm, thumb, hip, ankle, and heel. Yet, over 19 consecutive seasons, he never missed a start—that's 297 consecutive games. He even played with a broken thumb on his passing hand in the game after his father died. Undoubtedly, many of those starts required him to play with pain and accept the risks of doing so.

4. *Accept no obstacles in the pursuit of possibilities.* Athletes are reluctant to accept obstacles without trying to beat the odds and overcome them. Athletes often feel obligated to pursue their dreams without reservation and without concern for the cost. Athletes have a profound belief that dreams are always attainable if they never give in to the obstacles that stand in their way. For example, Bethany Hamilton was born into a family of surfers. She entered her first surf competition at the age of 8 and won two events in her division. At the age of 13, Bethany was attacked by a 14-foot tiger shark while surfing off the North Shore of Kauai. The shark attack severed her left arm just below the shoulder. After losing more than 60% of her blood and making it through several surgeries, Bethany returned to the water just 1 month after the attack to continue to pursue her goal of becoming a professional surfer. After teaching herself to surf with one arm, she returned to competitive surfing, winning her first national title in 2005. In 2007, Bethany turned professional and she continues to compete successfully. Bethany's perseverance in the face of dramatic obstacles continues to be an inspiration to many.

THE SPORT ETHIC AND ATHLETES' BEHAVIOR

The degree to which individuals accept the norms of the sport ethic and internalize them as what it takes to be considered a true athlete varies greatly. Acceptance of these norms can be viewed as a continuum of behavior (Fig. 2-5), with most athletes falling in the midrange, or "normal" range, of the continuum. Athletes who reject or dismiss the norms of the sport ethic fall along the left end of the continuum and are labeled as ***underconformers***, whereas those who unconditionally accept these norms fall at the far-right end and are labeled as ***overconformers***.

Society seems to value and reward those who fall in the middle to right end of the behavioral continuum. Athletes who skip sport practices because of other obligations (e.g., music lessons, speech tournaments, club meetings) often have their commitment questioned by coaches and teammates. Similarly, high school athletes who do not participate in their sport year-round (e.g., summer teams, travel teams) often find themselves reprimanded, ignored by coaches, or cut from the team. Unless they possess exceptional sport skill, they may be excluded from elite teams or advanced leagues. In contrast, athletes who accept the sport ethic norms unconditionally or without limits are often hailed as role models by coaches because of their unquestioning commitment to the team and willingness to withstand pain and discomfort to achieve their goals.

When these expectations or norms are applied to the sport injury setting, an interesting continuum of behaviors results (see Fig. 2-5). Athletes are taught from early on that pain is normal in sports, and the normative culture of sports encourages ignoring or minimizing injury in the pursuit of victory. Most athletes fall in the middle, or "normal," range of the sport ethic continuum and have been called "gamers" (Kotarba, 1983). They seem to understand that sport participation comes with some pain and

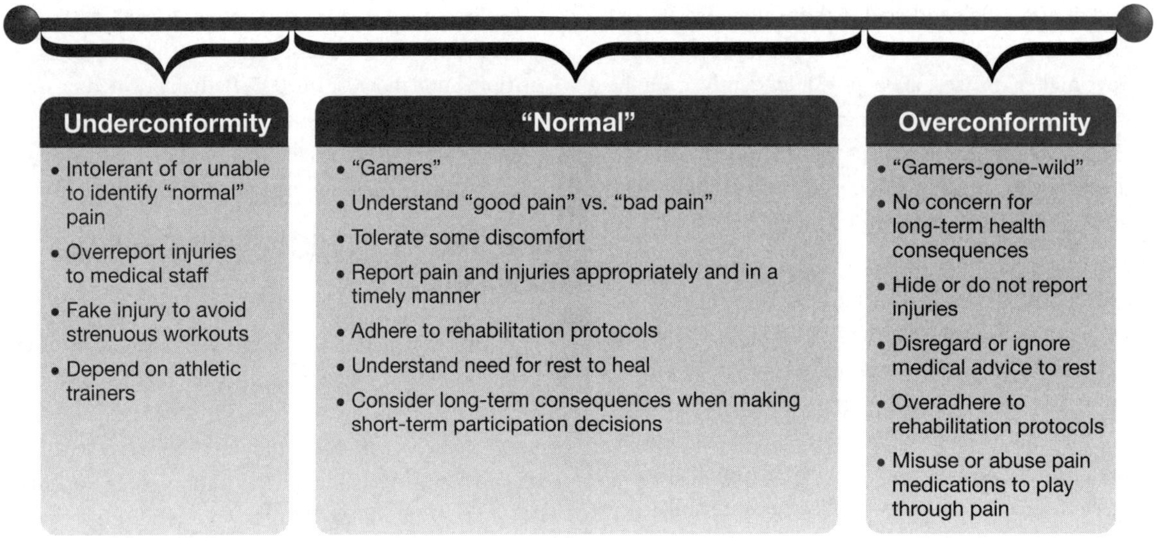

Underconformity	"Normal"	Overconformity
• Intolerant of or unable to identify "normal" pain • Overreport injuries to medical staff • Fake injury to avoid strenuous workouts • Depend on athletic trainers	• "Gamers" • Understand "good pain" vs. "bad pain" • Tolerate some discomfort • Report pain and injuries appropriately and in a timely manner • Adhere to rehabilitation protocols • Understand need for rest to heal • Consider long-term consequences when making short-term participation decisions	• "Gamers-gone-wild" • No concern for long-term health consequences • Hide or do not report injuries • Disregard or ignore medical advice to rest • Overadhere to rehabilitation protocols • Misuse or abuse pain medications to play through pain

Figure 2-5 | Continuum of sport ethic behaviors related to athletic injury.

discomfort they must endure. These athletes demonstrate an ability to distinguish between "good pain" (i.e., pain that is benign to long-term health) and "bad pain" (i.e., pain that signifies injury or potentially damaging health consequences). They are tolerant of some discomfort during sport participation but report pain and injuries to medical personnel in a timely manner and under appropriate circumstances. These athletes comply with the medical decisions of athletic trainers or doctors and are adherent to rehabilitation plans, even if that means sitting out for a while to allow injuries to heal. Athletes in this range of the behavioral continuum openly consider possible long-term health consequences of playing in pain before making daily decisions regarding whether they should participate.

At the left end of the behavioral continuum are athletes who openly reject or dismiss the norms of the sport ethic (i.e., underconformers). These athletes are either intolerant of or unable to identify "normal pain" of physical activity, such as bumps and bruises, fatigue, delayed-onset muscle soreness, or the discomfort of intense physical activity. Instead, these athletes report all cases of discomfort to the medical staff. Underconformity behaviors can be intentional or unintentional. For example, some athletes will intentionally fake an injury to avoid hard or intense workouts, behavior referred to as ***malingering***. Often these athletes are participating in sports for reasons other than their own personal love of the game (e.g., to be with friends, to please their parents, to keep the financial benefits of a scholarship), and being injured allows them to be a part of sports without having to endure the training, pressure, or work.

In contrast, young or novice athletes may unintentionally underconform to the sport ethic because of their inexperience with pain and injury in sport. Without having a comparative framework against which to judge pain, they tend to assume every ache is a signal of something bad and report all pain to medical personnel. An example occurred at a Pop Warner Tiny Mite (age 5–7 years) football game. A player remained down on the field at the end of a play. The athletic trainer could hear him crying from the sideline and jogged onto the field when the official determined the player would not get up on his own. Upon reaching the player, the athletic trainer asked him what was wrong, fully expecting to hear about pain in one of his lower extremities. Instead, he looked at her with his tear-filled doe eyes and said that his finger got squished between two helmets. After assuring the athlete and herself that there was no significant injury to his finger, the athletic trainer asked him if he could get up and walk off the field with her. He innocently responded, "Do you think we need the stretcher like on TV last night?"

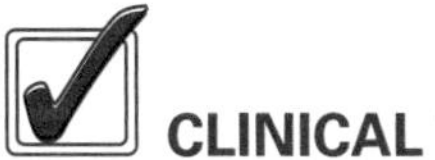

CLINICAL TIP

Athletes often base their perceptions of appropriate behavior in the face of pain and injury on what they have seen modeled by high-profile athletes portrayed in the media. The media includes newspapers, magazines, the Internet, radio, television, video games, and movies. This media content is "re-presented" to us by others including editors, producers, writers, commentators, bloggers, and journalists. When members of the media present stories of athletes pushing through pain and injury, those involved in the media reproduce a culture of risk. Athletes then continue to push through pain and injury because that is expected and even glorified. Athletic trainers should be aware of the media influence and be prepared to educate athletes on why such behavior may not always be appropriate or healthy.

Underconforming athletes can challenge athletic trainers by needlessly, or naively, seeking treatment; being overly dependent on instruction, feedback, and reassurance during rehabilitation; and insisting on modalities or high-tech treatments that are not clinically indicated. Furthermore, the intentionally underconforming athletes who feign injury test the levels of trust and rapport with athletic trainers. In all cases of underconformity, these athletes consume a great deal of the athletic trainers' limited time with health concerns that are nonexistent or benign to short- and long-term health.

CLINICAL TIP

Working with underconforming athletes can be challenging and frustrating for athletic trainers. However, they must refrain from jumping to conclusions that athletes are faking injury or malingering. Faulty assumptions can irreparably damage the trust and rapport athletic trainers have with athletes. Patience and a patient-centered, educational approach to such situations are discussed later in this chapter.

Athletes who behaviorally fall along the far-right end of the continuum can be described as "gamers-gone-wild." These athletes throw out concern for their long-term health in favor of the short-term goal of participation. These athletes can be challenging for athletic trainers for a number of reasons. The overconforming athletes may hide or not report signs and symptoms of athletic injury to the athletic training staff, often risking their future health in the process. If these athletes do report injuries to the athletic trainers, they often disregard or ignore medical advice to rest or limit participation to allow time for healing. To play through their pain and injury, these athletes may misuse or abuse pain medications. These athletes discount or deny potential long-term health consequences of their decisions to play through pain and injury regardless of the likelihood of additional harm.

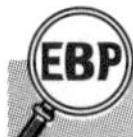

EVIDENCE-BASED PRACTICE

Tricker, R. (2000). Painkilling drugs in collegiate athletics: Knowledge, attitudes, and use of student athletes. *Journal of Drug Education, 30*(3), 313–324.

Description of the Study

The purpose of this study was to examine the knowledge, attitudes, use, and sources of supply for painkilling drugs among collegiate student–athletes. Subjects included 563 student–athletes at two NCAA Division I universities, representing almost all of the male and female athletes from all the sports in which the two universities participated. Participants completed the King Drug in Sport Questionnaire (Dunavant-King, 1991), which includes painkilling drugs as one of its eight subscales. A subset of 165 participants deemed "at-risk" athletes was selected from this group for closer analysis.

Results of the Study

Results from the responses of all participants ($n = 563$) indicated that 58% of the respondents self-reported that they used painkilling drugs regularly throughout their competitive season. In addition, 55% of this group self-reported that they felt they overused painkilling drugs. Strikingly, although 14% stated they obtained painkilling drugs from a physician, 58% reported obtaining drugs from their teammates, and

Continued

60% reported obtaining drugs from their friends. From the smaller cohort (n = 165), 29% stated they would take painkilling drugs to be able to continue to compete through injury instead of resting from sport or after a course of progressive rehabilitation.

Implications for Athletic Training Practice

The author concluded that external influences to win (e.g., from coaches, teammates, friends, family) and internal pressures athletes place on themselves to achieve combine with the readily available access to pain medications from both legitimate and illegitimate sources to create many powerful inducements that may lead to abuse of painkilling drugs among student–athletes. Athletic trainers who work with collegiate athletes should be familiar with the pressures on student–athletes to achieve success and the attitudes of many collegiate student–athletes regarding the use or abuse of painkilling drugs to reach their goals.

Although coaches often favor and praise athletes whose behavior places them farther along the right end of the sport ethic continuum, research has shown that more frequent displays of these overconforming behaviors are associated with more frequent and severe injuries. It seems strange, then, that athletes would willfully subject themselves to increased injury risks by playing through pain and injury; however, many reasons exist why athletes do just that (Box 2-1).

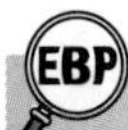

EVIDENCE-BASED PRACTICE

Kenow, L. J., & Wiese-Bjornstal, D. M. (2010, October). *Risk Behavior Conformity in Sport Injury Questionnaire (RBCSI): Preliminary evidence in support of a new measure.* Paper presented at the meeting of the Association for Applied Sport Psychology; Providence, RI.

Description of the Study

The purpose of the study was to assess the relationship between sport ethic conformity and sport injury occurrence among collegiate student–athletes. Subjects included 343 male and female student–athletes from an NCAA Division III institution, representing 11 different sports. Participants completed the Risk Behavior Conformity in Sport Injury Questionnaire (RBCSI), which measures the degree to which athletes conform to the norms of the sport ethic. Higher scores on the RBCSI reflect greater behavioral conformity to the sport ethic. The institution's athletic training staff reported the number and severity of injuries each athlete sustained that year.

Results of the Study

Results of the study indicated that in their past behavior, injured athletes had engaged in greater degrees of behavioral conformity to the norms of the sport ethic than noninjured athletes. In addition, injured athletes indicated they were more likely than noninjured athletes to engage in greater degrees of behavioral conformity to the norms of the sport ethic in their future behavior.

Implications for Athletic Training Practice

This study provides some preliminary evidence that differences exist in sport ethic conformity behaviors among collegiate student-athletes who have been injured versus those who have not. Shipherd (2010) found similar results using a different questionnaire in high school athletes. Taken together, the results suggest that injury prevention strategies should include seeking a reduction in the sport ethic conformity behaviors among those athletes who fall along the far-right end of the behavioral conformity continuum. Injury prevention strategies should include philosophical interventions, such as seeking to alter the "no pain, no gain" mentality in sports, as well as practical interventions such as demonstrating caution in making return-to-play decisions for injured athletes.

BOX 2-1 | Reasons Athletes Risk Playing Through Pain and Injury

Love of the game
Sense of time urgency
Sense of fraternity with teammates who have done the same ("foxhole mentality")
Fear of being labeled weak
Fear of losing their position or playing time
Fear of being overlooked in team selection
Pressure from coaches, teammates, management, or themselves
Insulation from medical opinions outside the sports network

One of the most obvious reasons athletes continue to play through pain and injury is their love of the game. Sport philosopher Yotam Lurie (2006) states, just as in love, the more committed athletes are to their sport, the more they care about it, the more passionate they are to be with it, and the more willing they are to take risks to participate in it. The excitement and exhilaration inherent in sport participation entice athletes to deny or ignore injuries that may separate them from their beloved sport. A collegiate football player, who had endured three knee surgeries, stated, "I love the game so much. I'd do anything and endure any pain just to be a part of it" (N. Rawlins, personal communication, September 14, 2010).

Athletes often voice desires to "play now and heal later." In most sports, opportunities for high-level, organized competition decrease significantly beyond the collegiate years. Thus, athletes often perceive a chronic sense of time urgency in their sport. They hear the clock ticking on their competitive career, and as a result, they frequently view each competition and practice as a chance that cannot be forfeited. Athletic trainers have encountered many discussions with athletes similar to the following:

Athletic Trainer: Your sprained ankle could really benefit from a week of rest.

Athlete: Yeah, but this is the last time we'll play [opponent] *this* year.

Each competition becomes the *last* chance for *this* competition, and athletes never want to miss any of them. Ultimately, injuries that have the potential to further reduce an already limited supply of participation opportunities are seen as inconveniences that should be tolerated, put off to a later time, or ignored completely if at all possible. An example of this mentality can be seen in athletes' attempts to schedule needed surgeries around their competitive schedules. Whenever possible, they decide either to have surgery immediately so they can return in time for important competitions or to postpone surgery until the conclusion of the season so they do not miss out on any competitions.

Athletes' willingness to give their all to stay in the game creates a type of "foxhole mentality." As athletes play through pain and injury, they earn the badge of courage that integrates them into a tightly knit fraternity of athletes who have willingly done the same. An "us versus them" mentality forms that underlies a perceived sense of duty and desire to do what it takes to stay in the trenches with their teammates. Athletes fear that failing to play hurt could result in being labeled weak or a wimp, and thus banish them from the fraternity of those who have played through pain. Subtly, this fear coerces athletes to play through pain and injury to retain their reputation and their identity.

Members of the media often contribute to this fear when they question athletes' decisions to sit out due to injury in front of a larger audience. For example, a great deal of controversy arose when Chicago Bears quarterback Jay Cutler pulled out of the second half of the 2011 NFC title game against the Green Bay Packers because of a medial collateral ligament sprain in his knee. Media outlets and even some players openly questioned his toughness and commitment to the team despite having little information regarding his health status. Impulsive fans are often quick to jump on the bandwagon of condemnation in such instances, creating even greater challenges for the injured player.

Athletes also may willingly play through pain and injury out of fear of losing their position to someone else if they take time off to allow injuries to heal. It has been stated that Brett Favre's previously mentioned streak of consecutive starts as quarterback resulted as much from his desire to never give someone else a chance at the starting quarterback role as anything else. Favre's brother has been quoted as saying, "Part of the thing he [Favre] has always thrived on, part of that streak, is that if you go down, you give somebody else an opportunity…If you don't go down, you don't give somebody that chance" (Rosenberg, 2010, p. 47). Consider the case of Brett Elliott, a talented football player who had earned the starting quarterback position at the University of Utah in 2003. When a fractured wrist forced him to the sideline, Alex Smith (now the starting quarterback for the Kansas City Chiefs) stepped in to replace Elliott and never gave the job back. To get back onto the playing field, Elliott transferred to Linfield College, an NCAA Division III school, and led them to a national championship in 2004. After working so hard to earn their role or position on a team, athletes are reluctant to take time off to heal from injuries out of fear that they may never be able to regain their position once their health has been restored. As one female collegiate volleyball player stated, "Rest isn't an option for me. My spot will get taken, and I'll be resting on the bench" (Sander, 2011, p. 4).

Athletes also fear being overlooked if they take time off for injuries to heal. Selection to elite-level teams, earning scholarships, or promotion up the depth chart is dependent on performing in practices and competitions. During preseason tryouts, new athletes can be especially hesitant to report injuries or sit out of practices because they perceive the need to be seen by and show what they can do to their new coaches. Logical reasoning that it is difficult to make a good physical impression while playing hurt seldom carries much weight with athletes.

SPECIAL CONSIDERATIONS

Within an athlete population, "rest" is often considered a nasty four-letter word. This negative connotation often derives from the assumption that rest automatically means absolute rest, or doing nothing. Actually, athletic trainers more often recommend the concept of relative rest, where injured athletes are requested to reduce or modify, but not eliminate, activity. Injured athletes may be more receptive and adherent to relative rest to facilitate the healing process.

Athletes can feel pressured by coaches, teammates, or management to continue to participate through injury. In the current high-pressure atmosphere of competitive sport, job security for many people is dependent on producing wins. Coaches and management may coerce (intentionally or not) athletes to play through pain to assure that the team continues to win, and thus they continue to earn a paycheck. At the professional level, athletes' marketability is often affected by their ability to remain healthy and productive. Thus, concerns for job security among coaches, as well as injured athletes, further pressure athletes to minimize injury, pain, and physical disability.

Sport sociologist Howard Nixon (1994, 1996) stated that athletes, as they advance to higher sport participation levels, become increasingly isolated from individuals outside of sport. This isolation enhances the socialization process of normalizing pain and injury as a part of sports. Failure to hear dissenting opinions to the sport norms of accepting risks and playing through pain strengthens athletes' resolve to play through pain and injury. This socialization process is becoming more prevalent in youth sports today.

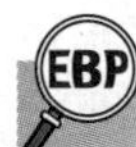

EVIDENCE-BASED PRACTICE

Malcom, N. L. (2006). "Shaking it off" and "toughing it out": Socialization to pain and injury in girls' softball. *Journal of Contemporary Ethnography, 35*(5), 495–525.

Description of the Study

The purpose of the study was to examine how young girls were socialized into the normative behavior associated with the sport ethic as they participated in recreational softball. In this ethnographic study, the author observed preadolescent and adolescent girls for three seasons as they participated in a recreational slow-pitch softball league. Her observations served as the data points for conclusions on how young girls were socialized into normative behavior for dealing with pain and injury.

Results of the Study

Malcom discovered that first-time players and younger girls were often reluctant to place themselves in the way of the ball for fear of getting hurt and often used minor injuries as attention-getting devices. She concluded that these girls did not enter the league socialized to the norms of the sport ethic. However, over the course of the study, coaches knowingly or inadvertently used several strategies to socialize these girls into the sport culture:

- *Reframe pain as a positive thing.* The sting of the bat or a ball caught in the palm elicited comments such as "Doesn't it feel good?"
- *Model downplaying and not complaining about minor injuries.*
- *Directly instruct the girls to "shake off" minor injuries.*
- *Ignore the girls' complaints about minor injuries.*
- *Tease or joke about minor injury complaints.*

Implications for Athletic Training Practice

Malcom concluded that through these processes, most girls learned to adopt the "traditional ballplayer approach" to injuries and pain. Similar instances of socialization can be seen in all youth sport activities. Athletic trainers need to understand and be aware of the socialization process young athletes experience as they move through sports. This process understates the importance of having trained medical personnel or coaches knowledgeable about youth sports injuries present at practices so that athletes' injury behaviors are addressed in an age-appropriate manner.

Approximately 27 million children and adolescents (age 6–17 years) participate annually in team sports in the United States, and several million more are involved in individual sports (DiFiori, 2010). The sport culture in the United States today, which emphasizes excess and early specialization, fosters ever-increasing requirements and desire for success. The professionalized approach to sport, commonly seen in elite-level environments, is drifting down into youth sport organizations as well. As a result, increasingly more youngsters are involved in year-round sports activity, which has the potential to increase injury risk in youth sport participants. Whether fueled by parental dreams of collegiate scholarships or visions of Olympic glory or professional contracts, many youths begin to specialize in a single sport at a young age. To acquire greater competition frequency, enhanced levels of training, more sophisticated coaching, or greater exposure to college coaches, youths often choose to compete with travel or club teams either as a complement to or a replacement for their participation in their school-based teams. As a result, young athletes are subjected to increased duration and intensity of training sessions, early specialization and year-round training, and increased technical difficulty of skills taught and repetitively executed. Given this environment, it is no surprise that overuse injuries occur with great regularity. Young athletes may be particularly vulnerable to injury in these situations because of factors such as immature skeletal development, underdeveloped coordination and skill, and muscular imbalances produced by nondiverse training strategies, such as extensive running, throwing, kicking, or swimming.

Unfortunately, little is known about the long-term health consequences associated with many of the injuries seen in youth sports (e.g., physeal injuries, anterior cruciate ligament reconstruction), and what is known is not very promising for these athletes' long-term health. For example, long-term follow-up of young athletes with meniscus surgery indicates that more than 50% of the patients will have knee osteoarthritis and associated pain and functional impairment (Maffulli, Longo, Gougoulias, Loppini, & Denaro, 2010). Athletic trainers should be concerned over these trends and the lack of knowledge regarding long-term repercussions. Further research investigating the short- and long-term health consequences of early specialization in youth sports is definitely needed to provide evidence-based guidance as to healthy participation strategies for youths.

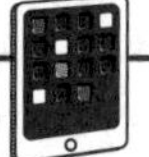

VIRTUAL FIELD TRIP

As seen in the preceding description of youth sport injury, the sport culture can lead to an increased risk for sport injury for young athletes, particularly overuse-type injuries. Visit Davis*Plus* (http://davisplus.fadavis.com) to view the NATA Position Statement: Prevention of Pediatric Overuse Injuries (Valovich McLeod et al., 2011).

Issues of gender in the sport culture are also important to consider. Athletic trainers will discover that gender impacts their interactions with athletes on a daily basis. Gender is a central component of our society. Consider the gendered perceptions of the appropriateness of male athletes wearing pink (other than during breast cancer awareness month), or community reactions to girls participating on the boy's wrestling or football teams. Gender impacts everything we do. It also impacts athletes' experiences with pain and injury. Early research had indicated that male athletes may be more likely to experience pressure from their coaches and fans to play while hurt, and that male coaches were more likely to say that playing hurt deserved respect and were impressed with athletes who did so. However, more recent studies (Charlesworth & Young, 2004, 2006; Sabo, 2004) have found striking similarities among both male and female athletes relative to their willingness to place their bodies at risk for injury, to play through pain, or to attempt to return to sport before being fully recovered. Consistent with early studies of male athletes, female athletes also faced a range of overt and covert pressures to play through pain and injury.

Male and female athletes do retain some differences in their pain and injury experiences, however. Many times, male athletes play through pain and injury because of the social messages that come along with being a male individual in our society. Male athletes push through pain because they do not want to be seen as a "sissy"; instead, they play through pain to demonstrate their manhood and masculinity. The culture of physically aggressive masculine sports (i.e., football, ice hockey) even glorifies pain and injury to the point of separating male from female athletes. Although women's ice hockey is now an NCAA-sanctioned sport, rules restrict body checking in the women's game out of concern for health and safety. On the other hand, female athletes may be concerned with perceived inconsistencies of being "athletic" and being a woman in that some consider that injuries and their resultant scars have a negative impact on being attractive or sexy. Female athletes also differ from male athletes in that they are more likely to discuss their injuries openly with others versus male athletes who tend to deal with them privately. Furthermore, even though Title IX has gone a long way to improve sport equality, the availability and quality of medical treatment and rehabilitation facilities for women sometimes still lags behind what is available to male athletes (Charlesworth & Young, 2004, 2006; Hogshead-Makar & Zimbalist, 2007).

For athletic trainers, it is important to understand and accept that there is no single explanation of pain and injury experiences for all men and women. It is also important for athletic trainers to avoid generalizing or stereotyping what they expect to see regarding pain and injury responses across genders.

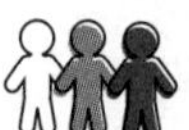

SPECIAL CONSIDERATIONS

Although male and female athletes are becoming increasingly similar in their willingness to play through pain and injury or return to sport before being fully recovered, the media coverage and the public's reaction to male versus female athletes playing though pain and injuries are rather different. When Curt Schilling pitched a game in the 2004 World Series in his "bloody sock," this act was celebrated throughout the nation and the media. In contrast, after Kerri Strug vaulted in the 1996 Olympic Games on a severely injured ankle, this act was both celebrated and critiqued. Newspapers, television, and magazines all questioned her decision, and many suggested that she should have declined her vault and accepted her injury. These are not isolated examples; indeed, there are numerous other examples to suggest the media coverage is different for male and female athletes when they are injured. Athletic trainers should refrain from allowing the media's representation of athletes' actions based on gender to influence treatment or return-to-play decisions.

ATHLETIC TRAINERS' ROLE IN THE SPORT CULTURE

In this sport culture, athletic trainers face a daunting task. The NATA Code of Ethics and Board of Certification (BOC) Standards of Professional Practice (2006) emphasize that athletic trainers must keep the athletes' health and well-being as the foremost priority. However, the win-at-all-costs mentality makes it difficult to preserve the primacy of the patient. Too frequently, the long-term health and well-being of athletes are compromised for the short-term thrill of victory. Complicating this process will be athletes who want to play, coaches and management who want to win and therefore need their star athletes to quickly return from injury, members of the media who glorify incidents where athletes endure pain and injury, and athletic trainers' own strong bonds with the athletes and teams with whom they work. At these times, athletic trainers will encounter difficult ethical challenges.

The daily contact athletic trainers have with athletes, coaches, and teams results in strong bonds and identification with the team and their goals. As will be discussed in Chapter 9, these bonds assist in producing trust and rapport with athletes. Although this is important, it is even more important that athletic trainers avoid getting caught up in the hysteria of fandom, or being a fan of the team, while making return-to-play decisions. Athletic trainers must maintain a reserved objectivity during professional decision-making to protect the best interests of the athletes, even if that means making return-to-play decisions that compromise the likelihood of the team's success.

It is the athletic trainers' responsibility to be a voice of reason in the culture of risk created by sports norms. Their training and expertise in the physical, psychological, and sociocultural aspects of injury and the injury rehabilitation process should encourage them to make objective assessments regarding the risks athletes face for sustaining injury and how many of those risks are reasonable. Sport sociologist Parissa Safai (2003) stated that sports medicine personnel are responsible for creating a "culture of precaution"—or sensible risk taking. Understanding the physical, environmental, psychological, and social risk factors inherent in sport participation allows athletic trainers to objectively determine and then negotiate a safe level of risk for athletes' participation. Athletic trainers may determine that there are times when playing through injury is acceptable and times when it is not. An 800-meter runner might be cleared by an athletic trainer to participate with a sprained elbow, whereas a basketball player with the same injury might not. The degree of risk inherent in each injury situation is based on several factors (Box 2-2). Athletic trainers must objectively analyze these factors and use them as the foundation for their decisions regarding playing "safely" in sport. Outside influences, such as pressures from coaches, teammates, fans, members of the media, and athletes themselves, must not cloud the ultimate priority of assisting athletes to compete as safely as possible. Athletic trainers must keep the long-term health and safety of the athletes prioritized over the short-term glory of winning.

Athletic trainers will be challenged in this process. In addition to the outside influences mentioned earlier, athletic trainers may experience their own personal pressures to encourage athletes to play through pain and injury. For example, when athletic trainers find themselves understaffed to provide the type of care desired and needed, triage becomes a necessity. Minor injuries or injuries to nonstarters may be minimized to provide care for more severe injuries or injured starters. Unfortunately, these decisions and actions, although sometimes unavoidable, send messages that some injuries are not worthy of the athletic trainer's time and attention, or that those athletes most critical to team success are more deserving of proper care. In both cases, the neglected athletes may resort to playing through pain and injury because care is not available to them, thereby promoting the win-at-all-costs mentality and the culture of risk in sport.

Athletic trainers may also be personally motivated to quickly return injured athletes to play to please coaches or management, or both, thus making their own job more

BOX 2-2 | Factors That Influence Reasonable Risk in Playing Through Sport Injury

Sport played (e.g., football, track, swimming, lacrosse)

Body part injured (e.g., injured finger for a pitcher vs. a soccer player)

Developmental level of the athlete (e.g., youth sport participant, professional athlete)

Time in the season (e.g., preseason, off-season, end of season)

secure. Athletic trainers concerned about establishing a reputation for getting athletes back in the game or keeping athletes on the playing field may also engage in decision-making that enhances the culture of risk taking in sport. In all of the earlier situations, athletic trainers will face many ethical dilemmas regarding when they should allow athletes to play with pain and injury.

CLINICAL TIP

Athletic trainers need to be conscious of how their reactions to athletes and various situations may contribute to a culture of risk in sport. Consider your reactions to the following scenarios:

- How do you react when athletes "overreport" pain?
- How do you react when you think an athlete is malingering?
- How do you react when an athlete continuously presents with an injury right before conditioning time in practice?
- How do you handle multiple injured athletes when you are understaffed? Does this contribute to an athlete playing through pain?
- How do you react when coaches pressure you to return their star athletes to play for a big game even when you think they are not yet ready?
- How does your desire to establish "a good reputation" as an athletic trainer impact your decisions regarding athletes participating through pain and injury?
- How might concerns for your job security impact critical decisions about whether an athlete can continue to participate with injury?

Athletic trainers must be certain that their decision-making in the earlier scenarios does not actually contribute to a culture of risk.

ASSESSMENT OF CONFORMITY BEHAVIORS IN SPORT

Assessment of athletes' degree of conformity to the norms of the sport ethic is still in its infancy. Little research has been done to this point on conformity behaviors and sport injury risk and occurrence. Several assessment tools under development include:

Rehabilitation Over-Adherence Questionnaire (ROAQ; Podlog et al., 2013). This questionnaire is designed to assess injured athletes' tendency toward overadherence behaviors and beliefs. Participants are instructed to respond to 10 items on a 5-point Likert scale. Each item is prefaced by the stem "To what extent do you…" Preliminary work on this 10-item questionnaire suggests two overadherence subscales. The first subscale includes items assessing athletes' tendency to attempt an expedited return (e.g., "try to catch up with other athletes who are further ahead in their rehabilitation" and "perform more rehabilitation exercises than your athletic trainer recommends"). The second subscale includes items assessing athletes' tendency to ignore practitioner recommendations (e.g., "ignore your athletic trainer's advice to avoid pushing through unwanted pain" and "hide pain about your injury from doctors or other rehabilitation experts"). Higher scores on the ROAQ indicate greater tendencies to overadhere to rehabilitation. The ROAQ is a valid and reliable instrument for use in research and applied settings.

Risk Behavior Conformity in Sport Injury (Kenow & Wiese-Bjornstal, 2010). This questionnaire measures athletes' attitudes and behaviors relative to the sport ethic norms. This 17-item questionnaire assesses athletes' past and self-predicted future attitudes and behaviors (e.g., "Continued participation against the recommendation of medical professionals" and "Used prescription drugs to play through pain of injury"). For the past behaviors scale, participants respond to items on a 5-point Likert scale (1 = never, 5 = always) based on the trunk, "In your past sport experience, how often have you…" Participants' self-reported future behaviors are assessed by having them respond to the same items using the trunk, "If you did this before, how likely is it you would do it again in the future…" Responses are again on a 5-point Likert scale (1 = not at all likely, 5 = very likely). Total possible scores range from 27 to 135 for each scale, with higher scores indicative of greater behavioral conformity to the norms of the sport ethic.

Notably, both of these questionnaires are still being refined and need further validation and testing; however, they offer promise for future research in the link between sport ethic conformity and injury.

Another option for subjectively assessing athletes' degree of conformity behavior would be to ask them to place themselves along a continuum similar to Figure 2-6. Although not scientifically based, this subjective assessment will enable athletic trainers to visualize where athletes think they stand regarding their willingness to tolerate pain and injury to participate in sports. An interesting basis for conversation would be for athletic trainers to independently mark where they would position the athlete on the continuum. Discrepancies in the marks should be discussed with the athlete.

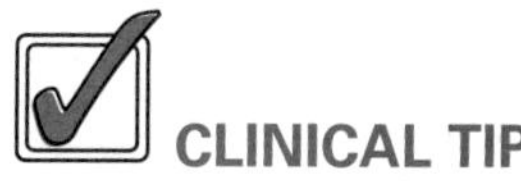

CLINICAL TIP

Athletic trainers who have never personally participated in competitive sports may feel challenged to empathize with injured athletes' motives to play through pain and injury. In these situations, athletic trainers should strive to educate themselves on the culture of sport to gain an appreciation for the injured athletes' perspectives regarding playing through pain and injury. Athletic trainers' ability to demonstrate empathy to athletes' beliefs and values is essential in developing rapport and positive therapeutic relationships.

CLINICAL TIP

The personal beliefs and experiences athletic trainers had as former athletes or performers may influence their professional decision-making. If, as athletes, they tended to play through pain and injury, they may find it difficult to understand and express empathy toward their patients, who may not share similar views about playing through pain and injury. Athletic trainers should make a concerted effort to understand their own beliefs and behaviors relative to the sport ethic so they can avoid letting personal biases impact their work with injured athletes.

PSYCHOSOCIAL STRATEGIES

This section focuses on psychosocial strategies for working with athletes in the sport culture. As mentioned earlier, athletes will disperse along a continuum of behaviors relative to the norms of the sport ethic. Of greatest concern for athletic trainers will be athletes who fall near either end of the continuum (i.e., the underconformers and the overconformers). The different strategies athletic trainers will need for working with these two groups are reviewed in the following subsections.

Never **Sometimes** **Most of the time** **Always**

On the continuum above, place a mark that indicates how often you engage in one or more of the following behaviors when injured:

- Hidden or not reported an injury to coaches or medical staff
- Continued sport participation against the wishes of medical providers
- Used prescription medications to play through pain
- Performed more than the prescribed amount of rehabilitation activities
- Disregarded long-term health consequences so you could play now

Figure 2-6 | Self-assessment of sport ethic conformity.

Strategies for Overconformity

As mentioned earlier, greater degrees of conformity to the sport ethic are associated with more injuries and more severe injuries. Education and communication will be the athletic trainer's primary weapons in combating overconformity behavior; however, goal setting with an appreciation of the time urgency athletes often feel to get back to their sport is also essential. A more global intervention technique involves trying to impact the media's representation of playing through pain and injury (Box 2-3).

Education

Education is perhaps the most valuable intervention athletic trainers can use when dealing with overconformity behaviors. It is important to educate not only athletes but also their support network (e.g., coaches, family members, friends) regarding risks and dangers associated with overconformity to the sport ethic. The education process should focus on five key issues: (1) the meaning of pain, (2) the potential long-term consequences of playing through injury, (3) the degree of risk present in playing with pain and injury, (4) an awareness of athletes' beliefs and attitudes regarding pain and injury, and (5) a unified approach to the situation among the support network and the athletic trainer.

In athletes who tend to overconform to the sport ethic, pain is normalized as a part of sport that should be denied, tolerated, or ignored. It is essential that these athletes and their support network are educated that all pain is not necessarily good pain. Athletic trainers will want to help athletes effectively identify the pain that serves the protective function of discouraging them from participation that could exacerbate injuries or be hazardous to their long-term health or well-being. To do this, athletes could be encouraged to assess their experienced pain along a pain continuum with concrete markers (Fig. 2-7). Athletic trainers can then educate athletes that participating when their pain rises above a certain level (e.g., a 2 or 3 on the pain continuum) could be dangerous to their long-term health and should be reported to the athletic trainers.

The education process must include teaching athletes the long-term consequences of playing through pain and injury. This will be a challenging task for athletes who frequently think only in the present and often consider themselves to be indestructible. Peer modeling can be very effective in getting the message across. Athletes who have suffered irreparable harm from trying to hide injuries or playing through them may be most convincing in communicating with their peers the necessity to consider the long-term consequences of short-term decisions. Athletic trainers can also point to retired professional athletes who now struggle with long-term consequences from injuries that they attempted to ignore or play through.

BOX 2-3 | Intervention Strategies for Working With Overconforming Athletes

Education

- Meaning of pain
- Potential long-term consequences of playing through injury
- Degree of risk present in playing through pain and injury
- Athletes' beliefs and attitudes regarding playing through pain
- Support network role

Communication

Goal setting with appreciation for athletes' perceived sense of time urgency

Decreasing media glorification of playing through injury

CLINICAL TIP

When using role models, athletes are more apt to give credibility to a peer model they find similar to themselves in some way. Videotaping interviews with injured athletes or choosing a retired professional athlete from the athlete's sport to serve as peer models may be particularly powerful in this process. For example, one former NFL player describes his current life as like being locked in a torture chamber because of the injuries sustained during his playing career: "I guess I'm proud about being a champion, giving everything I had. Even if it ruined me" (Leahy, 2008, p. W08).

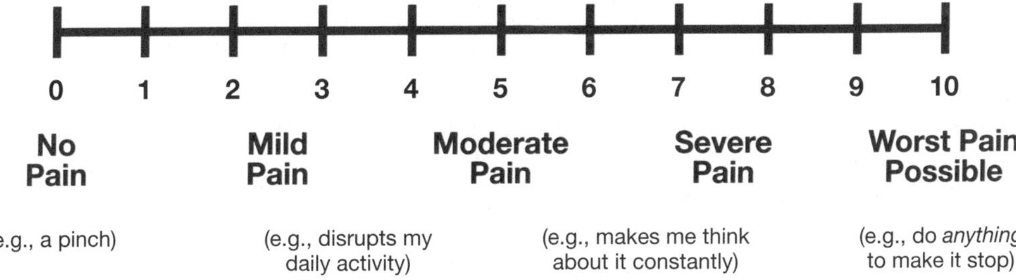

Figure 2-7 | Pain continuum.

An effective technique to assist athletes in recognizing the risks of playing through pain and injury is to assist them in placing their current situation on a risk-assessment grid (Fig. 2-8). The risk-assessment grid locates the likelihood of future harm if the athlete plays through his or her pain or injury along the x-axis, ranging from low to high, and the severity of such harm along the y-axis, ranging from low to high. Points that fall closer to the upper right quadrant indicate greater likelihood for long-term consequences or serious repercussions resulting from trying to play through pain. This process may help athletes visually see the risk inherent in their decisions to play through pain and injury. Athletic trainers can then discuss choices that may minimize long-term risks or consequences. It should be noted, however, that in these discussions, overconforming athletes often hear only a dichotomous "play or no play" message and may choose to play even if the consequences appear to be dire.

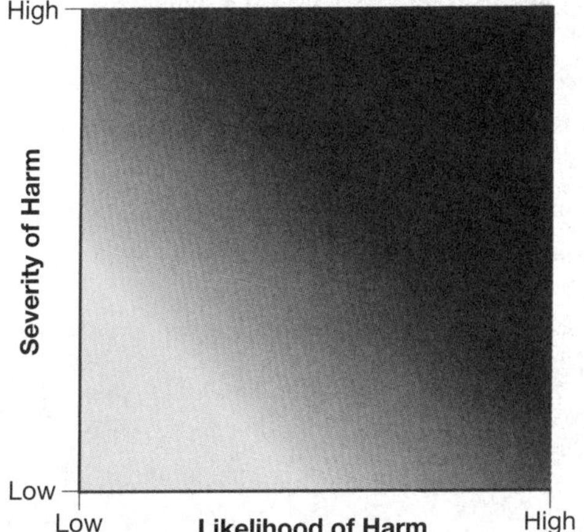

Figure 2-8 | Risk-assessment grid. *(Adapted from Anderson, L. [2007]. Doctoring risk: Responding to risk-taking in athletes. Sport, Ethics, and Philosophy, 1[2], 119–134)*

Athletes' beliefs, attitudes, and behaviors regarding conformity to the sport ethic, and in particular their willingness to play through pain and injury, can be assessed by having athletes complete Figure 2-6. Their resulting self-assessment can serve as a basis for discussions about why they feel the need to play through pain and injury, and how those choices can possibly compromise their long-term health.

Coaches, family members, and other individuals in the athletes' support network may have a strong influence on athletes' decisions regarding whether to play with pain and injury. Therefore, these individuals must also be educated on the long-term consequences that accompany short-term decisions regarding whether to participate. The impact the words and actions of these individuals have on athletes should also be highlighted. What might seem to be an innocent comment regarding the team needing a win or the desire to see the athlete play could be interpreted by injured athletes as pressure to play. For example, a parent who states, "I really miss being able to see you play," or a coach who states, "We really need a win tonight," may unknowingly encourage the injured athlete to attempt a premature return from injury just to please them. Hopefully, coaches, family members, and significant others have the athletes' best interests in mind and will serve as effective advocates to help them see the big picture regarding decisions to play with pain and injury.

Communication

In addition to education, it is essential that athletic trainers communicate effectively with coaches and athletes regarding athletes' participation status following injury. As mentioned earlier in this chapter, overconforming athletes tend to disregard medical advice to rest following injury or attempt to overadhere to rehabilitation protocols. Therefore, rationale for limits placed on athletes should be clearly communicated so everyone understands the "why" behind the restrictions and will hopefully adhere to the recommendations given by athletic trainers. As will be discussed in Chapter 5, two-way communication is essential in this process because it provides an opportunity for coaches and athletes to rephrase what they have heard the athletic trainers say regarding limits and ask questions for clarification of athletes' status. It is critical to include injured athletes in these discussions so that there is no appearance of a conspiratorial alliance between coaches and athletic trainers to needlessly minimize athletes' playing opportunities. Athletes should again be encouraged to paraphrase what they have heard the athletic trainers and coaches say regarding their playing status and limits. Athletes can also ask questions of both athletic trainers and coaches to clarify any concerns they may have regarding their status or situation.

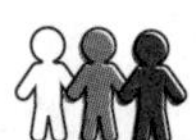

SPECIAL CONSIDERATIONS

Athletic trainers who work with youth and adolescent athletes must include the athletes' parents or legal guardians in all communication and education efforts regarding the injury and the rehabilitation choices because the parents/guardians are the legal decision-makers. In these situations, the education and communication processes discussed earlier in this chapter become at least three-way conversations rather than the two-way communication typically seen between athletic trainers and legally independent athletes. As more individuals join these conversations, the potential for conflicting opinions increases. Athletic trainers should seek to build consensus among all informed parties whenever possible, but in cases where differing opinions exist, athletic trainers must remain a strong advocate for the welfare of the injured athlete above all other concerns.

Goal Setting With an Appreciation for Time Urgency

Goal setting to establish safe and concrete benchmarks for returning to play or activity following injury can effectively combat overconforming behaviors so long as athletes are enlisted as collaborative partners in the process. Chapter 10 will discuss effective goal setting more explicitly. Overconforming athletes are anxious to return to play quickly following injury; however, athletic trainers will need to assist them in planning the safest schedule for that return. For example, athletic trainers can discuss the importance of a gradual functional progression with an athlete who is anxious to return to play following a hamstring strain. Educating the athlete on the need to be able to perform pain-free jogging and then running before attempting an explosive full sprint may be critical in stopping the athlete from doing too much too soon.

Many athletes have a mind-set gained from their physical training that "more is better." To get stronger and faster, they train harder and more frequently. Unfortunately, when it comes to injury and injury rehabilitation, more is not always better. Injured tissue does not respond to the overload principle the same way healthy tissue does. In fact, in rehabilitation, doing more than what is prescribed can actually slow the healing process. Athletes need to be educated that prescriptions for rehabilitation exercises are not minimum guidelines; rather, they are a bull's-eye that needs to be accurately hit every time. Athletes need to be educated that there is an optimal tissue-healing process for each injury that cannot be accelerated; however, athletes can get in the way of this process by making poor choices, such as trying to do too much too soon. Instead, athletic trainers can assist injured athletes in setting appropriate goals that direct the use of their excess energy to working out the *uninjured* parts of their body so they stay prepared to return to sport as soon as the injured part will allow.

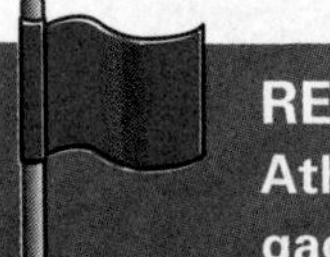

RED FLAG

Athletes who persistently engage in more rehabilitation exercise than prescribed and consequently end up compromising the healing process may benefit from referral to a mental health professional.

When appropriate, athletic trainers can assist injured athletes with negotiating surgical schedules to minimize missed competition time. For example, an athlete with a small meniscus tear in her knee may choose to undergo surgery as quickly as possible during a playing season to rehabilitate and return to play in time for upcoming playoff competitions. On the other hand, she may choose to finish the season and postpone surgery until she has downtime for surgical recovery. It is important that athletic trainers discuss the pros and cons, as well as the long-term risks and consequences, of such decisions with injured athletes. However, allowing athletes some guided autonomy in making these choices can help promote better adherence to rehabilitation goals and recovery timelines.

Decreasing Media Glorification of Playing Through Injury

As mentioned earlier in this chapter, the media's representation of athletes playing through pain and injury can have a dramatic effect on athletes' perceptions of what is expected behavior. Although this is a huge hurdle to overcome, athletic trainers can attempt to make some progress by working with local media outlets on how they portray athletes' postinjury behavior. Athletic trainers can encourage these outlets to promote stories where athletes make wise choices about giving injuries adequate time to heal and use discretion about trying to play through pain and injury rather than glorify and glamorize athletes' warrior-like efforts to persist in the face of injury.

For example, during the 2009 season, the Portland Trail Blazers NBA team experienced a rash of injuries to key players. The local newspaper, *The Oregonian*, published a feature article in the sports section highlighting the lessons learned by the team and head athletic trainer, Jay Jensen, about exercising caution and patience when rehabilitating from injury. The article discussed how previous decisions to quickly return their players resulted in exacerbation of injury, and had convinced the team and athletic trainer to exercise greater caution and patience in their later return-to-participation decisions. The article applauded the more conservative process that resulted in the healthy return of several key players without injury flare-up. The article had great impact on the attitudes of Portland-area athletes and fans regarding the wisdom of trying to play through pain and injury (Quick, 2009).

Strategies for Underconformity

Athletes who underconform to the norms of the sport ethic will be challenging to work with because of the time demands such behaviors place on athletic trainers. In these situations, it is important for athletic trainers to do three things: (1) educate athletes, (2) assess and identify sources of secondary gain, and (3) look for indications that athletes' motives for participation are not their own (Box 2-4).

Education

Athletes who unintentionally underconform to the norms of the sport ethic by reporting all instances of pain and discomfort need education to understand the differences between "good pain" and "bad pain." Contrary to overconforming athletes, these athletes often make the assumption that all pain is bad or indicative of injury. Many times, these athletes lack a frame of reference by which to judge the pain they are experiencing. As discussed in the overconformity strategies section, using a pain continuum (see Fig. 2-7) with concrete markers of what might indicate reportable pain (e.g., 3 or 4) can assist athletes in determining which pains should be reported to the medical staff.

It is important for athletic trainers to remain patient, particularly with young or inexperienced athletes, as they report their pain. Each event should be approached as an opportunity to educate athletes on the differences between

BOX 2-4 | Intervention Strategies for Working With Underconforming Athletes

Education

- Define "good" pain versus "bad" pain
- Assess and identify sources of secondary gain
- Assess athletes' motives for participation

Assess secondary gain

pain that indicates tissue damage or injury versus pain that accompanies intense physical activity. A patient-centered, educational approach will establish strong rapport with athletes and build a sense of trust. Athletes will know that their athletic trainers will listen to their concerns without passing judgment, and they will gradually learn which pains necessitate medical attention. It is important to remember that losing patience with underconforming athletes or assuming that a pain complaint is unsubstantiated without fully evaluating the condition can irreparably destroy athletes' trust and confidence in athletic trainers, and may be medically negligent.

Assessing Secondary Gain

Situations where athletes intentionally underconform to the sport ethic, such as malingering or faking injury to avoid hard or strenuous workouts, create equal challenges. In these instances, it is important to look for the ***secondary gain*** athletes may be experiencing from being injured. Athletes may be expressing pain as a means to get attention from the athletic training staff, coaches, or significant others (e.g., family members, teammates, friends) that they don't receive when playing, or they may be using their injury to escape from a perceived stressful situation.

Consider the case of Jill. She was a star player throughout her high school career. Her coach doted on her because she was always the standout player. Her family and community knew her as the star athlete. Now, at college, Jill finds herself in the middle to bottom of the pack in athletic ability. Where she was once the apple of her coach's eye, she is now hardly even noticed. After a mild ankle sprain, Jill's coach is now checking in with her daily and asking how she is doing. Her teammates ask how she is doing and when she will be able to return to play. They share how sorry they feel for her and sympathize with how difficult it must be for her to sit out from a sport she loves. Jill's parents, whom she misses a great deal, are now calling on a daily basis to check in on how she is doing. Instantly, Jill is receiving social attention as an injured athlete that she was missing as a healthy athlete. It is easy to see that, if the reward she feels from this increased attention is greater than the reward she perceives from playing, she may choose to remain injured.

Situations such as these are challenging situations for athletic trainers. In some cases, athletes may benefit from referral to a mental health professional or a certified sport psychology consultant (AASP-CC) to sort out some of these secondary gain issues. However, athletic trainers who feel comfortable in gathering additional information can try the following as a first step before resorting to referral:

- Treat these instances of underconformity as an exercise in building trust.
- Find a place to speak with the athlete in confidence.
- Acknowledge confusion with the discrepancy between the athlete's symptoms and behaviors and the physical findings (e.g., "I want to talk with you about your injury. I'm perplexed by the lack of progress we've achieved with our rehabilitation plan.").
- Present concerns honestly; ask the athlete how he or she feels about the situation and if he or she has any additional information that might help to better understand the lack of progress (e.g., "I'm wondering if you can help me understand how you're feeling about our lack of progress. What do you think we can do differently in the way we're doing rehabilitation?" As a follow-up question, you could ask, "What would you like to see happen with your healing and rehabilitation?").

This will hopefully open the door to productive conversations. Even if the athlete has little to offer, the athletic trainer now has created an opportunity to seek agreement on how rehabilitation will proceed. If the athlete expresses a strong desire to return to play as soon as possible, athletic trainers can discuss with the athlete how to collaborate to help him or her assume greater self-control in the rehabilitation process so the athletic trainers can also assist other athletes. Athletic trainers may choose to set up contracts that specify what rehabilitation behaviors must be seen in the athlete to participate in competitions. These contracts may be especially helpful when dealing with athletes suspected of malingering to avoid strenuous workouts but who then apparently heal quickly before competition.

However, if the athlete seems hesitant or reluctant to return to play, some factors should first be ruled out before assuming that secondary gain is the driving cause. Fear, uncertainty, or lack of intrinsic motivation can also cause reluctance to return to play. Athletic trainers should look for these indications and be ready to intervene:

- *A lack of sufficient knowledge about the rehabilitation plan or the injury itself:* If athletic trainers notice this, they can educate the athlete on what has happened, what needs to heal, and the link between prescribed daily exercises and the long-term goal of returning to play.
- *A lack of confidence in the ability to rehabilitate or return to preinjury form:* If athletic trainers notice this, they can use the intervention techniques outlined in Chapter 11, such as functional progressions, goal setting, affirmation statements, or performance imagery, to restore the athlete's confidence.
- *A fear of reinjury:* If athletic trainers notice this, they can use the intervention strategies outlined in Chapter 11, including normalizing the fear response, educating athletes on the adaptive value of their fear, reframing the arousal that fear produces as something potentially beneficial to performance, identifying safe limits for athletes' return to play, and reviewing the functional progressions that will enable them to return safely.
- *Participation in sport for other than intrinsic reasons:* To assess athletes' motivation for participation, athletic trainers can ask them why they are participating in sport (e.g., "I'm struck by your willingness to continue participating in sport considering the amount of pain and injury you keep experiencing. What drives you to keep doing it?"). Athletic trainers can look for explanations that indicate extrinsic motives for participating (e.g., parental or other external pressure, desire for social connections, wanting to impress others, fear of failing). If athletic trainers identify external reasons for participating that are concerning, it may be wise to refer athletes to a mental health professional or an AASP-CC who can help them sort out their motives and decide whether they truly want to continue participating.

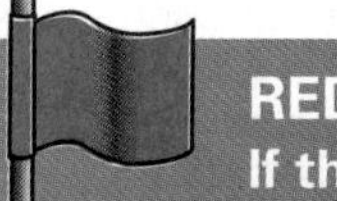

RED FLAG

If the described initial steps to clarify athletes' underconformity behavior do not result in beneficial information, referral to a mental health professional is warranted and highly recommended.

ATHLETE INSIDER CONCLUSION

After crossing the finish line to clinch the bronze medal, Petra collapsed in pain and had to be carried off the course. Later, at a Vancouver hospital, doctors diagnosed Petra with five broken ribs and a collapsed lung. That night, Petra was at the medal ceremony. She arrived in a wheelchair with a tube in her chest to relieve the air pressure built up around her collapsed lung; she left proudly with an Olympic bronze medal hanging around her neck.

Petra's story offers a concrete depiction of many of the sociocultural aspects of injury and injury response. With her story in mind, reflect on the following questions:

1. What sociocultural factors (social norms/pressures) can you identify that may have contributed to Petra's decision to persist despite her injury and pain?
2. As an athletic trainer, do you think it was wise to allow Petra to continue to compete despite her pain experiences? Why or why not?
3. What pressures do you think Petra's coaches and medical support team faced in deciding whether to allow her to compete?

Effective Psychosocial Strategies for the Athletic Trainer to Use With Petra

Based on the psychosocial strategies discussed previously in this chapter, the following interventions would be appropriate when working with Petra:

1. Using the risk-assessment grid (Fig. 2-8), help Petra calculate the expected risk of continuing to race through the "ominous clicking sound."

2. Ask Petra to rate her pain using the pain continuum (Fig. 2-7).
3. Educate Petra and her support team about the potential health consequences of racing through the "ominous clicking sound."
4. Encourage Petra's support team to be certain they are considering Petra's health over the glory of an Olympic medal before allowing her to continue racing.

Considering the culture, media exposure, initial medical diagnosis, and pressure associated with the Olympic Games, as well as the reality that this really was Petra's last chance to compete for an Olympic medal, it is doubtful that Petra could have been swayed from making the participation choices she did. However, for other athletes who are considering playing through pain and injury in less dramatic situations, the earlier described techniques may be very helpful.

CONCLUSION

This chapter has described the sociocultural aspects of injury and injury rehabilitation. Athletic trainers should familiarize themselves with how the sport culture contributes to injury risk and athlete behaviors following injury. Understanding the behavioral norms of the sport ethic should enable athletic trainers to identify, understand, and work more effectively with athletes who conform to these norms in varying degrees. This chapter also cautions athletic trainers against jumping to conclusions regarding malingering athletes, as erroneous assumptions could be deleterious to the relationships that must be maintained. Athletic trainers are encouraged to use the psychosocial strategies outlined within the chapter to intervene with athletes who may be engaging in behaviors that could compromise their long-term health or interfere with optimal healing from injury. This chapter also highlights the importance of athletic trainers gaining an awareness of their own personal biases toward normative behaviors reflected in the sport socioculture.

REFERENCES

Anderson, L. (2007). Doctoring risk: Responding to risk-taking in athletes. *Sport, Ethics, and Philosophy. 1*(2), 119–134.

Ballard, C. (2008). Digital revolution. *Sports Illustrated. 109*(15), 72.

Board of Certification (BOC). (2006). *BOC Standards of Professional Practice.* Retrieved November 16, 2011, from www.bocatc.org/images/stories/multiple_references/standardsprofessionalpractice.pdf.

Casey, S. (2008). We are all witnesses. *Sports Illustrated, 109*(7), 69–73.

Charlesworth, H., & Young, K. (2004). Why English female university athletes play with pain: Motivations and rationalizations. In K. Young (Ed.), *Sporting Bodies, Damaged Selves: Sociological Studies of Sports-Related Injury* (pp. 163–180). London: Elsevier.

Charlesworth, H., & Young, K. (2006). Injured female athletes: Experiential accounts from England and Canada. In S. Loland, B. Skirstad, & I. Waddington (Eds.), *Pain and Injury in Sport: Social and Ethical Analysis* (pp. 89–106). New York: Routledge.

Coakley, J. (2009). *Sports in society: Issues and controversies* (10th ed.). New York: McGraw Hill.

DiFiori, J. P. (2010). Overuse injury of the physis: A "growing" problem. *Clinical Journal of Sport Medicine, 20*(5), 336–337.

Dunavant-King, N. (1991). The development of an instrument to determine the knowledge, behavior and attitude of college athletes about sport-performance drugs and sport-coping drugs. Unpublished Doctoral Dissertation, University of Kansas, Lawrence, Kansas.

Epstein, D. (2011). The truth about pain: It's in your head. *Sports Illustrated, 115*(5), 58–66.

Flint, F. A., & Weiss, M. R. (1992). Returning injured athletes to competition: A role and ethical dilemma. *Canadian Journal of Sport Sciences, 17*(1), 34–40.

Hogshead-Makar, N., & Zimbalist, A. (2007). *Equal play: Title IX and social change.* Philadelphia: Temple University Press.

Hughes, R., & Coakley, J. (1991). Positive deviance among athletes: The implications of overconformity to the sport ethic. *Sociology of Sport Journal, 8*, 307–325.

Kenow, L. J., & Wiese-Bjornstal, D. M. (2010, October). *Risk Behavior Conformity in Sport Injury Questionnaire (RBCSI): Preliminary evidence in support of a new measure.* Paper presented at the meeting of the Association for Applied Sport Psychology; Providence, RI.

Kotarba, J. A. (1983). *Chronic pain: Its social dimensions.* Newbury Park, CA: Sage.

Leahy, M. (2008, February 4). The pain game. *Washington Post,* W03. Retrieved December 9, 2011, from www.washingtonpost.com/wp-dyn/content/story/2008/01/31/ST2008013101655.html?sid=ST2008013101655.

Lurie, Y. (2006). The ontology of sports injuries and professional medical ethics. In S. Loland, B. Skirstad, & I. Waddington (Eds.), *Pain and Injury in Sport: Social and Ethical Analysis* (pp. 200–210). London: Routledge.

Maffulli, J., Longo, U. G., Gougoulias, N., Loppini, M., & Denaro, V. (2010). Long-term health outcomes of youth sports injuries. *British Journal of Sports Medicine, 44*(1), 21–25.

Malcom, N. L. (2006). "Shaking it off" and "toughing it out": Socialization to pain and injury in girls' softball. *Journal of Contemporary Ethnography, 35*(5), 495–525.

Messner, M. A., Dunbar, M., & Hunt, D. (2000). The televised manhood formula. *Journal of Sport & Social Issues, 24*(4), 380–394.

Murphy, P. & Waddington, I. (2007). Are elite athletes exploited? *Sport in Society, 10*(2), 239-255.

National Athletic Trainers' Association (NATA). (2005). *NATA Code of Ethics.* Retrieved November 16, 2011, from www.nata.org/insets/about_NATA/index.htm.

Nixon, H. L. (1994). Social pressure, social support and help seeking for pain and injuries in college sports networks. *Journal of Sport & Social Issues, 18*, 340–355.

Nixon, H. L. (1996). Explaining pain and injury attitudes and experiences in sport in terms of gender, race, and sports status factors. *Journal of Sport & Social Issues, 20*(1), 33–44.

Pike, E. C. J. & Maguire, J. A. (2003). Injury in women's sport: Classifying key elements of "risk encounters." *Sociology of Sport Journal, 20*, 232–251.

Podlog, L., Gao, Z., Kenow, L., Kleinert, J., Granquist, M., Newton, M., & Hannon, J. (2013). Injury rehabilitation overadherence: Preliminary scale validation and relationships with athletic identity and self-presentation concerns. *Journal of Athletic Training, 48*(3), 372–381.

Quick, J. (2009, February 1). Walking 'a fine line' on comeback from injury. *The Oregonian*, D3.

Rosenberg, M. (2010). A long, painful farewell. *Sports Illustrated, 113*(22), 44–48.

Sabo, D. (2004). The politics of sport injury: Hierarchy, power, and the pain principle. In K. Young (Ed.), *Sporting Bodies, Damaged Selves: Sociological Studies of Sport-Related Injury* (pp. 59–79). Oxford, U.K.: Elsevier.

Safai, P. (2003). Healing the body in the "Culture of Risk": Examining the negotiation of treatment between sport medicine clinicians and injured athletes in Canadian intercollegiate sport. *Sociology of Sport Journal, 20*, 127–146.

Sander, L. (2011). An epidemic of injuries plagues college athletes. *The Chronicle of Higher Education*. Retrieved November 16, 2011, from http://chronicle.com/article/An%20-Epidemic-of-Injuries/129313.

Shipherd, A. M. (2010). *Overconformity to the sport ethic among adolescent athletes and injury*. Unpublished master's thesis, Florida State University, Tallahassee, FL.

Tricker, R. (2000). Painkilling drugs in collegiate athletics: Knowledge, attitudes, and use of student athletes. *Journal of Drug Education, 30*(3), 313–324.

Valovich McLeod, T. C., Decoster, L. C., Loud, K. J., Micheli, L. J., Parker, J. T., Sandrey, M. A., & White, C. (2011). National Athletic Trainers' Association position statement: Prevention of pediatric overuse injuries. *Journal of Athletic Training, 46*(2), 206–220.

BOARD OF CERTIFICATION STRATEGIES AND COMPETENCIES

This chapter has addressed many of the sociocultural issues that surround athletes' participation in organized sports. In particular, for the Athletic Training Education Competencies (Fifth Edition), this chapter has reviewed how sociocultural factors play a significant role in athletes' and athletic trainers' decisions regarding return to play following injury (PS-3), as well as how these factors influence athletes' experiences with pain and injury (PS-9). It has further touched on sociocultural issues that influence the type and quality of health care received by injured athletes (PS-10) and the sociocultural influences that challenge athletic trainers in providing such care. Finally, the chapter offers suggestions for psychosocial intervention strategies to minimize the deleterious effects of the sport culture and normative sport behavior (PS-8). Athletic training students should feel well prepared to respond to questions on the BOC examination relative to these competencies.

Board of Certification Style Questions

1. Overconformity to the sport ethic is evident in which of the following athlete behaviors? (Choose all that apply.)
   a. Hiding or not reporting injuries to athletic trainers
   b. Faking injury to avoid strenuous workouts
   c. Doing more than the prescribed rehabilitation exercises
   d. Misusing or abusing pain medications

2. The dominant sport culture in high-intensity sport today includes which of the following normative behaviors? (Choose all that apply.)
   a. Limit obstacles that interfere with injury rehabilitation.
   b. Accept risks and play with pain.
   c. Strive for extinction.
   d. Make sacrifices for the game.

3. The athletic trainer notices that an athlete seems willing to return to sport participation following injury even though her pain is sufficient to suggest that doing so would exacerbate her injury. What should the athletic trainer provide in this situation to prevent further injury?
   a. Referral to a mental health-care professional
   b. Education and goal setting
   c. Taping and bracing
   d. Assessment of secondary gain

4. Underconformity behaviors can result from which of the following factors? (Choose all that apply.)
   a. Lack of sufficient knowledge about the injury itself
   b. Desire to avoid stressful situations
   c. Lack of experience with injury
   d. Assumption that all pain is good

5. Athletes may risk additional injury and play through pain because of which of the following factors? (Choose all that apply.)
   a. Fear
   b. Pressure from external sources
   c. Insulation from medical opinions outside the sports network
   d. Secondary gain

END-OF-CHAPTER EXERCISES

1. Consider an athlete you are currently working with in one of the sports you cover who you think could be categorized as an overconformer to the sport ethic. Develop a list of behaviors and/or beliefs that make you identify this athlete in this way. After you have compiled this list, discuss strategies you might use to help alter those behaviors/beliefs.
2. Outline the behaviors and/or attitudes that lead you to suspect that an athlete with whom you are working is malingering. With a classmate, role-play a discussion you would have with such an athlete to identify whether your suspicions are correct. Continue your discussion to include how you would work with the athlete to make any needed changes to his or her behaviors.
3. Identify locker room or team slogans used by athletic teams at your institution that may be problematic if applied to the injury rehabilitation setting. Describe how you can work with teams and coaches to understand the impact such statements might have on injured athletes.
4. Assess the physical, environmental, psychological, and sociocultural injury risk factors present for a particular sport team or individual athlete at your institution. Identify which of these injury risk factors are modifiable and develop recommendations on how such factors could be modified to reduce injury risk.
5. As described in this chapter, each sport has varying levels of injury risk and its own culture of injury risk. Choose a sport to consider. Describe the culture of that sport and how this culture impacts injuries. Which types of injuries are more likely to occur in this sport? Which types of injuries are athletes more or less likely to report in this sport? How do others (e.g., coaches, parents, media) involved in the sport impact athletes' decisions to report an injury?
6. Reflect on your own experiences as an athlete (if applicable). Did you play through injuries during your athletic experiences? If so, why or why not? How did the culture of your sport and others around you (teammates, coaches, parents, etc.) impact your decision to continue to play through pain and injury? How do your personal experiences when deciding whether to play through pain and injury help you to understand the experiences of athletes with whom you work as an athletic trainer?
7. Interview an athlete at your institution who has played through multiple injuries during his or her athletic career. Ask that person to discuss the reasons for choosing to play through pain and injury, and compare those reasons with the ones described in the literature. Also, ask the athlete to discuss whether he or she would make similar choices regarding playing through pain and injury in the future. Why or why not? Consider taping these interviews for future use in a modeling library.

8. Consider each of the following scenarios and use the risk-assessment grid (Fig. 2-8) to evaluate the level of risk present if athletes were to participate with their injuries. First, identify the factors that determine the level of risk and whether that risk is reasonable. Next, discuss the recommendation you would offer athletes regarding the wisdom of their participation. Describe which factors influenced your decision.
   a. An athlete, who has a contract with a professional football team, broke his radius a week ago. A physician not associated with the team told him to stop playing for 6 weeks to allow the fracture to heal. However, the player asks the team doctor to pad the cast and prescribe painkillers so he can play this coming Saturday. The team is in the playoffs and is facing possible elimination without a win, and this player is clearly integral to the success of the team.
   b. A masters' level athlete facing retirement from racing in the coming year has hip arthritis. He has completed 11 marathons and really wants to complete his 12th so he can have an even dozen. He knows that the trauma of the competition is almost certain to cause more damage to his joint surfaces; however, he wants to complete "one more race."
   c. A collegiate softball player was beaned in the face during batting practice on Monday. She suffered a fractured mandible that was wired shut. Her physician has advised that she take a little time off but said that she could participate so long as she doesn't get hit in the face again. She is willing to wear whatever protective device you recommend. She just really wants to play in the game on Saturday.
   d. A high school senior cross-country runner has a gastrointestinal illness that has caused vomiting and diarrhea for the past 48 hours that has left him struggling to remain hydrated. He is scheduled to run in the regional finals tomorrow. If he can place in the top six for the race, he will be able to compete in the state meet next weekend—a goal he has had since he was in fifth grade.

9. Select a media (newspaper, magazine, radio, television, or Internet) presentation of a sport injury. Based on the presentation, answer the following questions: (a) What kind of light (i.e., favorable or not) does the media portrayal cast on the situation and/or the injured athlete's actions? (b) How does this media portrayal of the injury and the injured athlete support or discourage a "culture of risk" in sport? (c) As an athletic trainer or athletic training student committed to the health and well-being of injured athletes, what is your impression of the media's portrayal of this injury experience? and (d) What impact will this media portrayal have on readers' or observers' views regarding acceptable and expected behaviors when athletes are injured in sport?

Chapter 3

Psychosocial Antecedents to Injury

Megan D. Granquist and Jennifer Jordan Hamson-Utley

CHAPTER OUTLINE

KEY TERMS

Acute Of short onset or duration.

Adrenocorticotropic hormone A hormone secreted by the anterior pituitary gland in response to stress.

Antecedent A preceding event or condition, or a preexisting factor.

Athletic identity The degree to which a person identifies the self as an athlete.

Chronic Of long onset or duration.

Cognitive appraisal Interpretation of a situation.

Cognitive relaxation A relaxation method that includes verbal and visual cues, which lead individuals to a relaxing time and place.

KEY TERMS *continued*

Cortisol A naturally occurring stress hormone in the human body that is associated with the fight-or-flight response.

Mood Emotional state (e.g., happy, sad).

Motivational Strategies that influence an individual's desire or drive.

Pain-spasm cycle Pain that causes vasoconstriction and muscle spasm, which, in turn, causes more pain, which, in turn, exacerbates the cycle; sometimes referred to as the *pain-spasm-pain cycle*.

Positive affirmation A positive declaration of truth; used in rehabilitation and healing to improve mind-set and to motivate.

Primary appraisal Initial assessment of a situation to evaluate it as a threat or challenge.

Progressive muscle relaxation (PMR) A technique for learning to monitor and control muscle tension.

Rehabilitation nonadherence The athlete working either too little (i.e., underadherence) or too much (i.e., overadherence) based on recommendations of the athletic trainer.

Rumination Cyclic nature of the thought process, where thoughts that one ignores resurface more often; stable trait, linked to depression.

Secondary appraisal Secondary assessment of a situation, including assessment of available coping resources.

Self-talk Internal and/or external statements to the self, multidimensional in nature, that have interpretive elements associated with their content; it is dynamic and serves at least two functions (instructional and motivational).

Social support Includes the feeling or sense of being supported by others, the act of supporting others, and social integration.

Somatic relaxation A relaxation method that leads the participant to a relaxed state through focus on the breath and breathing patterns.

Stress Response of the body to any demand made upon it; physiological (i.e., body, muscle tension) or psychological (i.e., overwhelming feelings that are good or bad).

Stressor Stress producer; may be positive (eustress) or negative (distress).

Thought stopping A psychological strategy that allows the athlete to gain control over the thought process, changing negative thoughts to more productive positive thoughts.

Trait anxiety A stable personality construct of worry (includes high and low).

CHAPTER OBJECTIVES

After reading this chapter, you will be able to:

1. Describe the physiological, behavioral, and emotional impact of psychological stress.
2. Describe the role that stress plays in the risk for injury.
3. Describe how to identify and measure athlete stress.
4. Summarize the impact that the athletic trainer can have in regard to an athlete's management of stress and injury prevention.
5. Identify psychosocial strategies to reduce injury risk.
6. Implement psychosocial strategies to reduce injury risk.

ATHLETE INSIDER

It is the first home game of the season, and Susan, a catcher for the university softball team, is making her return following successful anterior cruciate ligament (ACL) rehabilitation of her right knee. It was a frustrating end to last season for her when she felt her knee give way as she followed through with her batting swing. Susan was adherent to her rehabilitation program and now feels very strong physically. In recent weeks, however, she has been arguing with her boyfriend and feels distracted because of the emotional toll the arguing has been taking on her, as well as feeling tired because of lack of sleep. Susan has limited social support but feels she can talk to her team's athletic trainer. Before the game, she expresses to the athletic trainer that she feels quite stressed and nervous about her return to the sport. It is now Susan's turn to bat. She swings, follows through, steps to run toward first base, and *pop*, she feels a familiar pain in her previously healthy left knee.

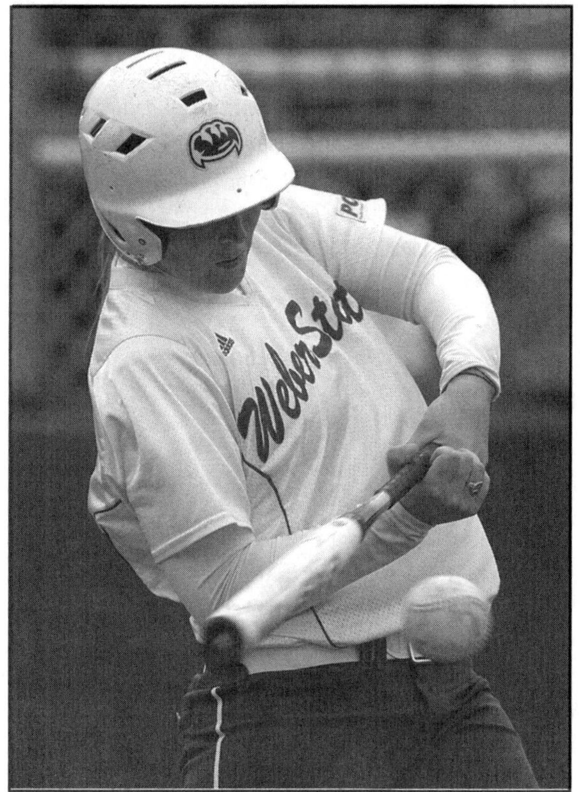

Figure 3-1 | Athlete Insider *(Courtesy of Weber State University Athletics)*

INTRODUCTION

This chapter encourages a holistic view of injury prevention by highlighting potential contributors to injury beyond physical factors (such as physiological and biomechanical) and environmental factors (such as playing surface and protective gear) by investigating psychosocial factors (psychological and social). This chapter will encourage athletic training students and athletic trainers to critically examine sources of stress and monitor stress for the athletes with whom they work, and to take an integrated approach to the reduction of injury risk. Readers will learn how to apply various psychosocial strategies to reduce stress and injury risk, such as promoting positive thinking, and how to enhance coping resources, such as facilitating social support networks. This chapter focuses on settings in which the athletic trainer can have the most impact on reducing injury risk by interacting with the athlete before an injury occurs.

It is important to acknowledge that not all stress is associated with negative repercussions (i.e., distress); stress may have positive implications (i.e., eustress). Stress is what drives us to take action, to be motivated toward a task, to avoid procrastinating. It is important to emphasize that stress is not necessarily a property of the situation, but rather how a person views (i.e., cognitively appraises) the situation (i.e., perceives that the demands of the situation outweigh one's resources). However, in the context of this chapter, distress is typically referred to simply as stress and has a negative implication.

STRESS RESPONSES: THE MULTIDIMENSIONAL EFFECTS OF STRESS

Hans Selye described the body's ***stress*** response as the "fight-or-flight response": "Whatever the problem, it can be met only through one of two basic reaction forms: . . . through fight, or . . . by running away" (Selye, 1975, p. 1). He went on to describe how, no matter the ***stressor***, the body reacts physiologically. Interestingly, he provides the example of "the athlete who desperately wants to win the race. . . ." (pp. 12–13).

More recent research has demonstrated that psychological stress influences us in multiple ways: (1) physiologically (such as increased heart rate, respiration, blood pressure, and inflammation; immunosuppression; decreased healing; impaired sleep), (2) cognitively (such as increased worries, intrusive thoughts or images, attention and focus difficulties), (3) emotionally (such as frustration, depression, anxiety), and (4) behaviorally (such as poor choices, sleeping difficulties, self-medication, ***rehabilitation nonadherence***; Box 3-1). These responses are all interrelated and have different effects on each individual based on that person's held coping resources (Fig. 3-2). For example, individuals with physiologically impaired sleep may have trouble with cognitive focus, which may lead them to experience emotional frustration, which may, in turn, cause them to make poor decisions leading to poor behavioral choices. Alternatively, people with elevated stress may make poor choices or decisions, leading to increased worries, which impairs their sleep, which causes emotional or attentional difficulties.

The effects of accumulated stressors can take a physiological toll on an athlete in many ways. Specifically related to performance, impaired sleep, decreased ability to heal, and depression of the immune system are of great concern for the healthy athlete. Physiologically, when an individual experiences stress, a reaction starts in the cerebral cortex of the brain, and the hypothalamus releases the ***adrenocorticotropic hormone***. Evidence shows that, following stress, there is a subsequent release of ***cortisol*** as a result of adrenocorticotropic hormone stimulating the adrenal cortex. An increase in cortisol

BOX 3-1 | Effects of Stress

Physiological: increased heart rate, increased respiration, increased blood pressure, increased inflammation, immunosuppression, decreased healing, impaired sleep

Cognitive: increased worries, intrusive thoughts or images, attention and focus difficulties

Emotional: frustration, depression, anxiety

Behavioral: poor choices, sleeping difficulties, self-medication, poor rehabilitation adherence

Figure 3-2 | Multidimensional effects of stress.

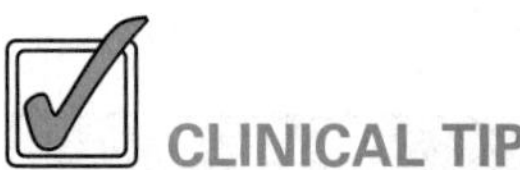

CLINICAL TIP

When working with elite athletes, athletic trainers should be aware of their strong ***athletic identity***, self-motivation, and need to maintain a high fitness level. These elements are likely to affect how the athlete perceives and responds to preinjury stressors. Research supports the iceberg profile (Morgan, 1980), which neatly displays the differences in ***mood*** states between elite and nonelite athletes.

CLINICAL TIP

Athletic trainers should be aware of how stress may influence their professional practice. Burnout in athletic training is a widespread problem among both clinicians and educators. Research by Kania, Meyer, and Ebersole (2009) measured burnout in athletic trainers and found that personal characteristics (emotional exhaustion, depersonalization, and personal accomplishment) significantly predicted burnout as compared with environmental characteristics. Research by Walter et al (2009) found gender differences in burnout, including female athletic trainers experiencing significantly more emotional exhaustion as compared with male athletic trainers. Athletic trainers experience on-the-job stressors every day. It is important that athletic trainers pay attention to their own physical and mental health needs, so they are able to deliver effective therapies to the populations they serve. This involves noticing sources of stress, and learning and using coping skills to handle the stressors; these practices can be shared with the athlete during daily care routines.

has been linked to adverse health effects including chronic stress, depression, and a suppressed immune system. Conversely, the benefit of a decrease in cortisol demonstrates increases in positive mood and decreases in perceived stress levels and anxiety levels. As a result of lower levels of stress, individuals may experience a decrease in pain and reinjury anxiety, as well as an increase in healing. Research shows that female athletes are more susceptible to stress throughout the duration of practice and competition than their male counterparts. Women may report higher levels of stress as a result of physiological differences involving the hypothalamic-pituitary-adrenal axis surrounding the menstrual cycle. The hypothalamic-pituitary-adrenal axis response may affect the manner in which women's autonomic nervous system responds to stress. Due to female athletes reporting higher levels of stress, athletic trainers need to be sensitive to the specific needs of female athletes. How athletes perceive their stress will undoubtedly have an effect on how the body will respond physiologically; the response will influence the athlete's ability to fight off sickness and injury, and will affect overall health.

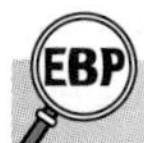

EVIDENCE-BASED PRACTICE

Dawson, M., Hamson-Utley, J. J., Hansen, R., & Olpin, M. (in press). Examining the effectiveness of psychological strategies on physiologic markers: evidence-based suggestions for holistic care of the athlete. *Journal of Athletic Training.*

Description of the Study

The aim of this study was to quantify the effects of psychological strategies (two types of relaxation) on both physiological (saliva cortisol) and subjective assessments of stress. The randomized, double-blind study (with a control group) included 97 college-aged participants who met the criteria for no prior use of imagery or relaxation strategies. Participants were randomly assigned to the somatic treatment condition (37.1%, $n = 36$), the cognitive treatment condition (35.1%, $n = 34$), or the control condition (27.8%, $n = 27$). Participants consisted of male (33%, $n = 32$) and female individuals (67%, $n = 65$). Outcome measures included saliva cortisol level, blood pressure, and heart rate, all of which were measured before and after the intervention. Salivary cortisol was analyzed using an enzyme immunoassay kit. Two samples for both pretests and post-tests were analyzed; an average was used in statistical analysis. Additional variables measured included subjective reports of stress using the Stress-O-Meter (SOM) and the Perceived Stress Scale (PSS); the SOM is an ***acute*** measure of stress and was used both pretest and post-test, whereas the PSS is a ***chronic*** measure of stress and was used as a pretest only.

Results of the Study

There was a significant difference in reduction of cortisol between the treatment groups ($F_{2,97} = 15.62$, $P < .000$). Post hoc Tukey's test revealed that together the cognitive (–.424) and somatic (–.561) groups were significantly different from the control group, but not significantly different from each other. Participant reports of stress were significantly different before and after the intervention ($F_{2,97} = .693$, $P < .000$); however, the subjective report was uncorrelated with physiological stress (cortisol). Female participants (5.15 ± 1.796) reported higher scores on both the SOM (pretest) and the PSS (18.31 ± 5.833) as compared with male participants (15.272 ± 5.390).

Implications for Athletic Training Practice

Relaxation interventions have an effect on cortisol levels in college-aged students. Cortisol levels were unrelated to subjective reports of

Continued

stress; however, female participants reported higher levels of stress. Athletic trainers should consider gender differences when handling stress in rehabilitating athletes. In addition, athletic trainers should look to use stress-reduction strategies with athletes as prevention and care tools.

The ***cognitive appraisal*** of a stressful event will directly impact how that stressor affects the athlete's attentional focus, emotional stability, and general health. To put it very simplistically, when something stressful happens to an individual, he or she can respond to solve the stressor or not respond and ignore the stressor. When someone ignores the responsibility of handling a stressor, worry often results. Worry causes ***rumination*** of negative thoughts and likely increases negative self-talk, resulting in a negative mood state. If the athlete attempts to participate in a sport during a time of worry, the risk for injury increases because of attentional focus being burdened by worry and negative thoughts associated with the stressor.

A cognitive appraisal model of psychological response to sport injury best explains how athletes' personality factors, as well as their prior experiences with stress, interventions, and coping resources, affect how they will respond to a new source of stress. The model presents personality factors (e.g., optimism, pessimism) and situational factors (e.g., sport type, time in season, coach influences, playing status) that influence how athletes see the stressor (i.e., as something they can overcome or as something that they will not be able to defeat). When athletes have ample coping resources at their disposal (such as those provided by the athletic trainer and other support avenues), they will likely have a greater sense of control over the stressor and view the stressor as a challenge. On the contrary, if an athlete is lacking in social support and coping skills, the stressor is likely to be viewed as a threat and take an increased physiological toll, thus increasing the risk for injury. The way the athlete cognitively appraises stress influences both the emotional and behavioral responses to the stressful event.

Mental stressors also have an emotional effect on athletes that can change the way they function and place them at high risk for athletic injury. Emotions have been described as the by-products of cognitive appraisal, when athletes have assessed the situation and made a decision about how this stress will impact them individually. Research suggests that accepting, internalizing, and taking personal responsibility for or ownership of the stressor results in a more positive, driven approach to managing the stress and improving an athlete's overall outlook.

CLINICAL TIP

Research by Tracey (2003) suggests that both thoughts and cognitive appraisal strongly influenced an athlete's emotional response to the stress associated with athletic injury. She found that the cognitive appraisal was more important than the stressor itself (injury), and that early acceptance of the stress assists in effective management and improvement of state of mind of the athlete. Athletic trainers should be mindful of each athlete's individual characteristics and how these might influence that person's cognitive appraisal of stressful events. They should target those athletes who face extreme stress and who lack coping skills to improve social support systems and increase coping skills, thus facilitating stress management and reducing injury risk.

Stress has an effect on how an athlete responds behaviorally to daily and novel events. For instance, when an individual is "stressed out," he or she may act angry or make rapid decisions leading to incorrect judgments or negative outcomes. Stress can cause behaviors that are out of the ordinary, including defensive actions, dysfunctional actions, and expressive actions. Defensive actions include those that attempt to counteract the stressor. Examples of this include practicing a breathing technique on the spot to calm down or yelling at a teammate to release the stress. Dysfunctional actions are those that cause impaired or abnormal functioning. An example of this type of behavior is a "mental block" in the athlete that leads to an unsuccessful performance; athletes commonly report that they "forgot what to do" in a high-pressure situation. Finally, expressive actions are those that physically display stress.

Examples of this are swinging arms, shaking fists, and moving around. Such overt behaviors are seen as highly effective in reducing stress, but they can take a dangerous turn on the athletic field.

Behavioral displays related to stress have an impact on the athletic field; stress has been linked to aggressive play, which is likely to increase injury risk. Behaviorally, male individuals are held to different standards by society when it comes to handling stress. Female individuals are allowed to cry and express emotions associated with weakness and lack of strength to endure stress, whereas males are required to endure stressors without a trace of emotional evidence. This gender difference may result in the greater incidence of male athletes displaying aggressive behaviors on the athletic field as compared with female athletes, also leading to increased injury risk. Behaviorally, establishing an array of counterbehaviors, or coping skills, is the best way to manage stress. Both male and female athletes can benefit from time-management skills, taking "me" time, and identifying other ways to limit stress (e.g., planning ahead for exams, traveling, and financial obligations). These coping skills are discussed in more detail later in the Psychosocial Strategies section.

STRESS–INJURY RELATIONSHIP

Research has indicated that individuals with higher levels of psychological stress may have as much as two to five times greater risk for injury than those with lower levels of stress. Because injury prevention is a primary responsibility of athletic trainers, the reduction of injury risk warrants serious consideration. To understand how best to reduce injury risk, it is beneficial to have an understanding of the psychosocial factors thought to be related to risk. What is the relationship between psychosocial factors and injury? Which factors have researchers examined, and what are their conclusions? Although physical and environmental predictors of injury have been widely researched, there is limited research on psychosocial aspects related to injury risk. This section discusses the theoretical basis for the relationship between stress and injury.

A stress–injury model, developed by researchers Mark Andersen and Jean Williams (1988), has been the classic example demonstrating how stress influences athletic injury risk. The premise of this model is that psychosocial ***antecedents*** influence how an individual interprets and responds to stress; in turn, this stress response influences injury risk (Fig. 3-3). Three major categories of antecedents influence the interpretation of the stressors and, therefore, the response to stress. These are personality, history of stressors, and coping resources.

Personality includes constructs such as hardiness, optimism, and pessimism. Psychologists generally consider personality to be a stable trait; thus, intervention research does not generally focus on personality as a modifiable factor. Personality traits, however, should not

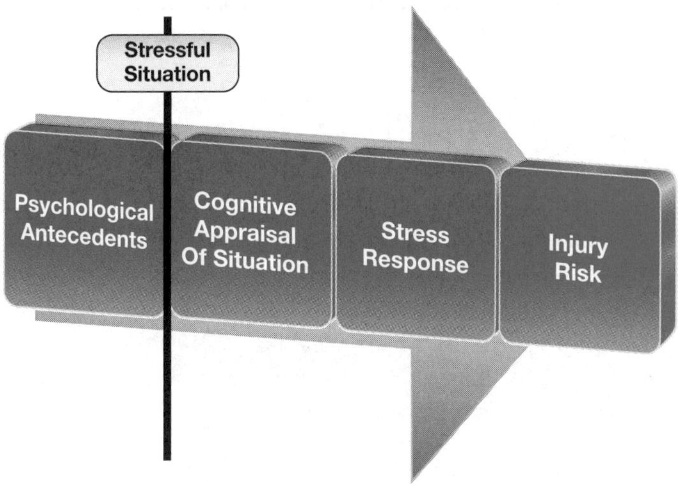

Figure 3-3 | Antecedents and responses to stressors.

be confused with mood states such as happiness or anger, because moods regularly fluctuate. Mood states are based on both an individual's personality and his or her environment.

An individual's response to stress is influenced by stressors previously experienced to that point. A person's history of stressors includes overall life stress (major events such as moving, financial issues, etc.), daily hassles (such as being stuck in traffic, being late for practice, etc.), and previous injuries. Although the quantitative amount of life stress (i.e., number of stressors) that an individual experiences influences current stress response, the qualitative measure of the stressor (i.e., positive or negative) is perhaps more important because negative stressors have a greater influence on stress response. For example, moving is a stressful event for many people. In that case, the event occurrence is the quantitative measure, and the interpretation of the move (i.e., positive experience, negative experience) is the qualitative measure. For an athlete, being benched after 2 years of holding a starting spot is the quantitative aspect, and the negative interpretation of being benched (i.e., being angry and demotivated) is the qualitative aspect. The Life Events Survey for Collegiate Athletes (Petrie, 1992) is used to measure stress in student–athletes; it is discussed further later in the Measuring and Monitoring Stress in Athletes section.

SPECIAL CONSIDERATIONS

The athletic trainer must pay close attention to freshmen collegiate athletes, those who are heavily recruited out of high school, and those who are far away from home because these factors might predispose an athlete to experience higher levels of stress. It is common for an outstanding high school athlete to become a "small fish in a big pond" in college athletics. Managing this change in playing status and the lack of attention regarding outstanding sports abilities from others might be a stressor for an athlete whose social support network is thousands of miles away.

Coping resources are tools that individuals have at their disposal to handle stressful situations. Examples of coping resources include social support and stress-management techniques. Coping resources, also commonly referred to as coping skills, can buffer the influence of an individual's personality and history of stress on his or her stress response. Coping skills, together with the other antecedents of personality and history of stressors, influence an individual's cognitive appraisal of the situation.

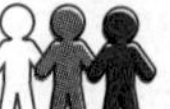

SPECIAL CONSIDERATIONS

It is common for high school and freshman-level university athletes to lack a developed, practiced set of coping skills for use in the face of stress. Thus, it becomes the job of the athletic trainer to provide education on the usefulness of such skills with athletes attempting to balance the demands of sports, school, and life.

When individuals encounter a stressful situation, they cognitively appraise whether they perceive it as a threat or a challenge (also referred to as ***primary appraisal***). As discussed, the direct influences on cognitive appraisal are the psychosocial antecedents of personality, stress, and coping resources. If individuals appraise the situation as a threat, they next evaluate whether they have adequate resources to deal with the situation (also referred to as ***secondary appraisal***). If they appraise the situation as threatening and determine they are not capable of handling it, then they have an increased stress response leading to an increased risk for injury. For example, an individual may have high life stress but have a hardy personality and ample coping resources, thus minimizing the stress response and reducing the risk for injury. In contrast, an individual may have high ***trait anxiety***, may experience much life stress and many daily hassles, and have inadequate coping resources; such a person may have a greater stress response and be at an increased risk for injury.

It is important to keep in mind that the athletic trainer is in a prime position to equip athletes with the coping skills they need to manage their stress better. Athletic trainers, more than other allied health-care professionals, are in daily contact with athletes. This consistent presence allows them to participate as a coping resource, by providing social support, and allows a better opportunity to notice athlete stress and to teach athletes effective skills to manage that stress. Developing a relationship with the athletes they care for is instrumental in opening lines of communication between the athletic trainer and the athlete, which exposes the stress the athlete experiences, calling for intervention to take place. Again, it is the role of the athletic trainer to provide such support, including education on coping skills, with the goal of decreasing overall risk for injury. Chapter 5 provides a detailed discussion regarding communication skills for the athletic trainer, and Chapter 9 examines social support.

Antecedents influence an athlete's cognitive appraisal of a stressful situation. How the athlete cognitively appraises the stressor influences the stress response, which, in turn, influences injury risk. Psychosocial strategies to reduce stress aimed at cognitive appraisal and stress response, as Williams and Andersen (1998) have proposed, may also be aimed at antecedents. Athletic trainers should recognize these psychosocial strategies as part of their scope of practice.

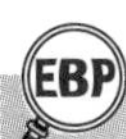

EVIDENCE-BASED PRACTICE

Maddison, R., & Prapavessis, H. (2005). A psychological approach to the prediction and prevention of athletic injury. *Journal of Sport & Exercise Psychology, 27,* 289–310.

Description of the Study

Based on the stress–injury model by Williams and Andersen (1998), this article covers two related prospective studies. In study one, male rugby players (n = 470, age range 16–34 years, M = 20.69 years) completed the Life Events Survey for Collegiate Athletes, Sport Anxiety Scale, modified Ways of Coping Scale, and Social Support Questionnaire, and reported the number of injuries they had sustained the previous season. In study two, players from the first study who were identified as possessing psychological characteristics for high injury risk (n = 48) were randomly assigned to either a cognitive behavioral stress-management intervention group or a control group. The intervention consisted of six 90- to 120-minute weekly sessions and provided training in somatic and cognitive relaxation, cognitive mental strategies (e.g., imagery), and additional strategies (e.g., goal setting). Participants in study two completed the Sport Anxiety Scale and the Athletic Coping Skills Inventory. In both studies, they tracked the number of injuries and time missed. Injury was recorded if an athlete had to modify at least one game or practice, or receive treatment before or after practice. Although published in 2005, researchers still commonly cite this study today.

Results of the Study

Study one found that negative life events (r = .11, P < .05) and problems coping (r = .12, P < .05) were related to injury time missed. Further analyses revealed that social support, coping type, and previous injury interacted and maximized the relationship between life stress and injury. Study two found that those who participated in the stress-management intervention reported less time lost because of injury compared with those in the control group. Upon completion of the intervention, participants also had an increase in coping resources and a decrease in worry.

Implications for Athletic Training Practice

To reduce injury and time loss because of injury, athletic trainers should help athletes incorporate stress-management strategies into their daily routines and assist athletes in identifying coping resources. Athletic trainers can also provide social support for their athletes.

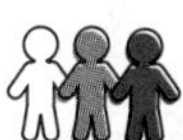

SPECIAL CONSIDERATIONS

Female athletes experience higher levels of stress compared with their male counterparts. Athletic trainers need to be mindful of

Continued

perceived stressors when working with female athletes or athletic teams. It might be more difficult to assess stress in male athletes; thus, a daily or weekly measure of experienced stress might be useful to assist in the prevention of injury.

VIRTUAL FIELD TRIP

Many universities have resources where athletes can receive services for stress management.

Visit http://davisplus.fadavis.com for examples of such resources.

HOW CAN ATHLETIC TRAINERS INTERVENE TO REDUCE INJURY RISK?

Athletic trainers are perfectly situated to monitor athlete stress early on and to intervene with psychosocial strategies aimed at reducing injury risk. In an ideal scenario, they can identify athlete stress in its earliest stage and introduce psychosocial strategies to decrease injury risk. One early-identification method is preseason screenings.

During the preseason, when athletes are participating in physicals and getting medical clearance to participate in their sport, they could also complete stress and coping inventories (Box 3-2). These inventories can serve as a baseline for stress status and coping ability, and be used to monitor changes. They can also be used to identify athletes who may benefit from education on and training in psychosocial strategies. It is important to point out that the use of these inventories for mental health purposes (such as identifying depression or clinical anxiety) is outside of the scope of athletic training practice, and the intent of these inventories is not to diagnose mental illness but to gather information. If qualified mental health professionals (i.e., licensed psychologists) are part of the sports medicine team, they may play a role in identifying mental health issues. This will be discussed further in Chapter 6.

BOX 3-2 | Stress and Coping Inventories

Life Events Survey for Collegiate Athletes
Perceived Stress Scale
Sport Anxiety Scale
Stress-O-Meter
Brief COPE

The psychosocial strategy intervention model (Fig. 3-4) serves as a visual representation of where athletic trainers can intervene with psychosocial strategies related to stress. As the schematic shows, stress contributes to a variety of physical outcomes, such as increased tightness, spasm, and guarding of the muscles. These conditions, in turn, contribute to additional outcomes such as decreased range of motion and increased pain. Athletic trainers may recognize the interplay between the spasm and pain as the well-known ***pain-spasm cycle***. These physical pain-spasm factors are known to be related to injury. This schematic will be expanded in Chapter 8 to describe its use in the rehabilitation process. In addition, pain will be discussed in detail in Chapter 7.

CLINICAL TIP

Many counseling centers within the college or university offer free stress-management workshops for students. Athletic trainers can inquire about and advertise these workshops to their athletes. Athletic trainers may also work with their institution's counseling center to conduct stress-management workshops specifically for their student–athletes. They may also schedule these workshops for entire teams or offer them as part of an NCAA CHAMPS/Life Skills Program.

MEASURING AND MONITORING STRESS IN ATHLETES

With injury prevention in mind, it is important for athletic trainers to be aware of how much stress athletes are experiencing. Sometimes this can be as easy as paying attention to the athlete. Oftentimes the athletic trainer is

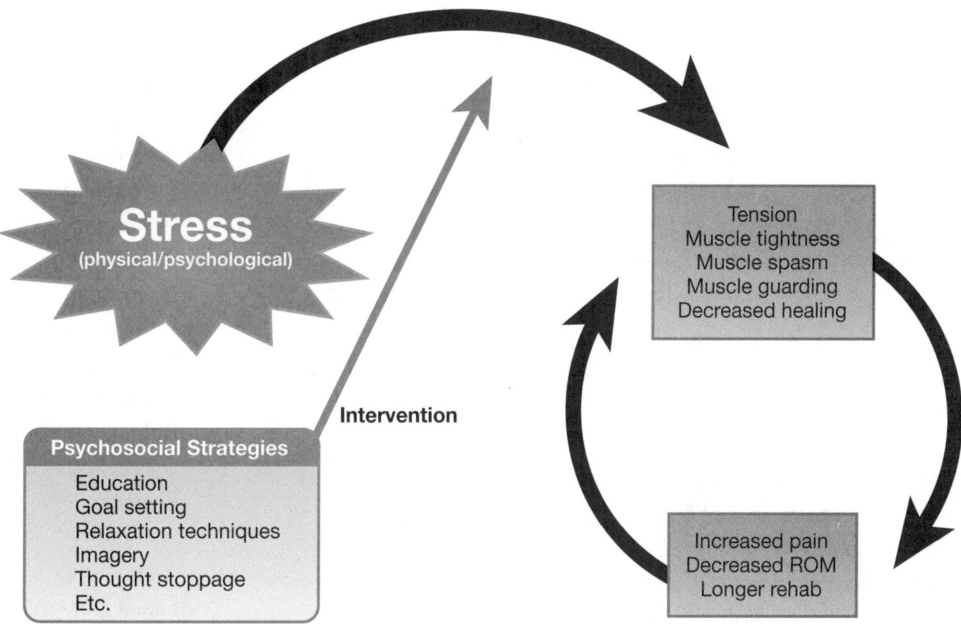

Figure 3-4 | Psychosocial strategy intervention model.

busy doing many things like taping, bandaging, preparing medical kits for practice, providing treatments, and overseeing prepractice stretching. Being aware of the athlete's stress level can place the athletic trainer in a position to act as a preventative measure by providing ways to reduce stress. There are also other ways to become aware of an athlete's stress in a busy athletic training room; these include using stress inventories or surveys to assess the athlete's acute and chronic levels of stress. Following are four stress inventories that the athletic trainer may wish to use in the athletic training room.

Life Events Survey for Collegiate Athletes (Petrie, 1992): The Life Events Survey for Collegiate Athletes is one measure to use in rating the overall life stress of student–athletes. This measure contains both a quantitative measure (i.e., which events happened within the last year) and a qualitative measure (i.e., positive to negative).

Perceived Stress Scale (Cohen, Kamarck, & Mermelstein, 1983): The Perceived Stress Scale is a global measure of perceived stress commonly used to evaluate an individual's chronic stress level, including his or her thoughts and feelings over the past month. Participants answer 10 questions on a scale from 0 to 4 (0 = never, 4 = very often). The Perceived Stress Scale has a possible total of 40 points. A score of 0 to 13 indicates a low stress level, 14 to 26 is a moderate stress level, and 27 to 40 is a high stress level. The Perceived Stress Scale is a valid and reliable inventory, and is widely used to measure chronic stress levels.

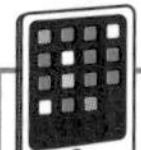

VIRTUAL FIELD TRIP

The Perceived Stress Scale (PSS) is a global measure of perceived stress commonly used to evaluate an individual's chronic stress level. Visit http://davisplus.fadavis.com for a link to this valuable resource and activities associated with it.

Stress-O-Meter (Olpin & Hessen, 2010): The Stress-O-Meter is a personal evaluation of acute or daily levels of stress. The survey is a Likert scale that ranges from 1 to 10 (1 = extremely relaxed and peaceful, 10 = very high levels of stress). This measure has been widely used and has good validity and reliability.

Stress Symptom Checklist (modified from Romas & Sharma, 1995): The Stress Symptom Checklist is an additional tool for measuring and monitoring stress in athletes (Table 3-1). Athletic trainers can use it as a screening tool with otherwise healthy or injured athletes to identify sources of stress. (Refer to the Psychosocial Strategies section later in this chapter for more information on the Stress Symptom Checklist and how athletic trainers can use it to determine effective psychosocial strategies for athletes experiencing stress.)

CLINICAL TIP

To manage the awareness of stress in a busy athletic training room, place the Stress-O-Meter at the sign-in desk so athletes must report their current level of stress daily. Periodically throughout the day, examine the sign-in sheet and look for those athletes who reported high levels of stress (from 7 to 10) and talk to them about providing a stress-management strategy. Having an iPod with relaxation audio scripts that is easily accessible, while remaining secure, is an initial offering athletic trainers can provide for their athletes.

PSYCHOSOCIAL STRATEGIES

Knowing that stress, together with personality and coping resources, influences how an individual appraises a situation, athletic trainers can incorporate psychosocial strategies into their practice as tools to reduce athletic injury risk. Just as athletic trainers tailor physical injury-prevention programs to individual athletes, they should also create psychosocial strategies for individual athletes who may be at increased risk for injury. Athletic trainers can play a vital role in teaching athletes how to manage stress; some athletes may already have the coping skills but are unaware of how best to apply those skills in the face of a new stressor. As already mentioned, because personality is generally considered a stable trait, psychosocial strategies typically focus instead on reducing athlete stress and enhancing athletes' coping resources. Athletic trainers can teach athletes stress-management techniques and ways to strengthen their coping skills.

TABLE 3-1 Stress Symptom Checklist

When you are feeling stressed, what do you usually experience? *Check all that apply.*			
Increased heart rate	☐	Difficulty controlling troubling thoughts	☐
Sweaty but cold hands	☐	Reoccurring worrying thoughts	☐
Increased sweating	☐	Difficulty concentrating	☐
Diarrhea	☐	Difficulty making decisions	☐
Difficulty staying still	☐	Envision negative scenarios	☐
Abdominal aches	☐	Feel a lack of control	☐
Fidgeting	☐	Envision disturbing events	☐
Difficulty moving	☐	Think of escaping the situation	☐
Upset/nervous stomach (i.e., "butterflies")	☐	Uncertain of how the situation will end	☐
Fatigue	☐	Headache	☐
Physical reaction score:	**/10**	***Psychological reaction score:***	**/10**
Total reaction score:	**/20**		

Adapted from Romas, J. A., & Sharma, M. (1995). *Practical Stress Management: A Comprehensive Workbook for Managing Change and Promoting Health* (pp. 37–38). Needham Heights, MA: Simon & Schuster.

Athletic trainers should take the opportunity to educate their athletes on the effects of stress. Athletes seem to be more receptive to stress management when athletic trainers discuss the physical aspects associated with psychological stress. Connecting the dots for athletes regarding how these physical aspects might affect their training and athletic performance may better convince them to attempt to manage their stress. This can be done through individual conversations between the athletic trainer and the athlete (such as while the athletic trainer is stretching the athlete before practice) or through team meetings (such as the preseason meeting when other preventative measures such as hydration are discussed). Often athletes will deny they are "stressed." However, when the athletic trainer normalizes stress and portrays it to athletes as something that everyone deals with, they may be more willing to admit they feel stress and more open to hearing about and/or trying stress-management techniques (e.g., deep breathing, relaxation).

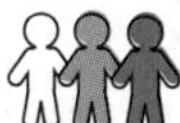

SPECIAL CONSIDERATIONS

Considering the unique traits and experiences of the high school athlete, the athletic trainer should pay specific attention to the environment of the athletic training room and the availability of services. Often, the high school athletic training area is very crowded, with no room to move or to get services. It also may be loud and have an overlying busy feeling, which might turn some athletes away when they really need help. Another consideration is that there is often only one athletic trainer helping both genders with all sports and covering team games while other team practices are occurring. This limits the ability of the athletic trainer to pay attention to the individual needs of high school athletes and to provide what they perceive as quality care.

CLINICAL TIP

Preparing a "stress-management tool kit" for the athlete or the team would be an excellent way to attempt to minimize stress and the injuries that result from it. The contents of this tool kit might look like this:

1. Stress symptom checklist (which increases awareness about levels and sources of stress)
2. Relaxation podcasts (with and without visual cues)
3. Positive self-talk podcast to identify stressors and negative self-talk
4. Simple breathing exercises podcast
5. Sleep-induction podcasts

With this tool kit, athletes can learn to identify their stressors and practice the skills that will help them manage their stress. Having a tool kit already packaged will increase the likelihood that the athletic trainer will use the kit with athletes as a prevention measure, thus reducing injury risk.

An important part of the athletic trainer's job is helping athletes prevent injury. They do this in many ways including educating athletes on proper nutrition and hydration, monitoring warm-up and training techniques, providing preventative taping/bracing, and monitoring environmental field and equipment conditions (Fig. 3-5). Athletic trainers can further reduce/prevent injury by addressing the psychological antecedents that contribute to athletic injury, such as stress and coping resources. Athletic trainers can serve as coping resources for athletes. They may provide social support in the form of listening and information. Depending on the amount of time athletic trainers have and the type of relationship they have with athletes, they may also help with basic life and coping skills related to avoiding substance use/abuse, which some athletes may rely on to deal with stress.

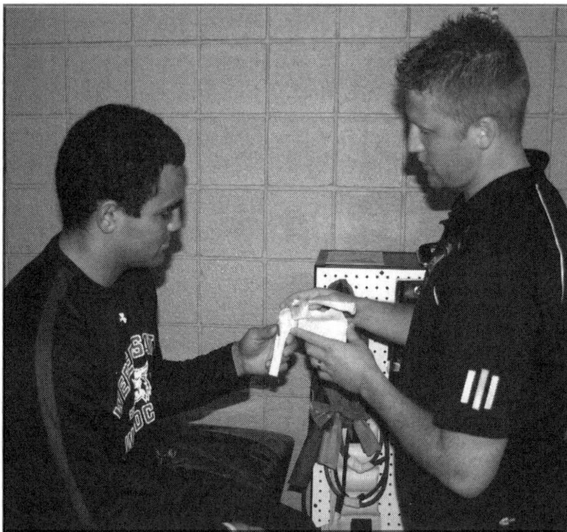

Figure 3-5 | Providing education as an injury-prevention tool.

As part of their role related to injury prevention, athletic trainers should implement psychosocial strategies aimed at reducing stress and increasing coping resources. Common stress-management techniques athletic trainers can implement include relaxation, positive self-talk, and thought stoppage. They can also easily implement coping resources such as social support and positive affirmations.

As mentioned previously, there are several tools that athletic trainers can use to measure and monitor stress in their athletes. For example, athletes can complete the Stress Symptom Checklist and share with their athletic trainer how their stress manifests: cognitively, somatically, or both. Athletic trainers then can target stress-management relaxation techniques to address cognitive, somatic, or combination symptoms.

Coping Resources

Various networks can provide athletes with ***social support*** including family, friends, significant others, coaches, teammates, the college or university counseling center, and the athletic trainer (including athletic training students). Athletic trainers can provide social support by communicating with athletes about daily events, school, or any injuries they might have. Chapter 9 is focused specifically on social support. Research suggests that athletes expect athletic trainers to provide social support and to provide a positive environment within which to rehabilitate after injury (Fig. 3-6). ***Motivational*** techniques such as goal setting, personal best podcasts (i.e., video highlight compilations set to the athlete's favorite music), positive affirmations, and positive self-talk can serve as useful skills for stress reduction.

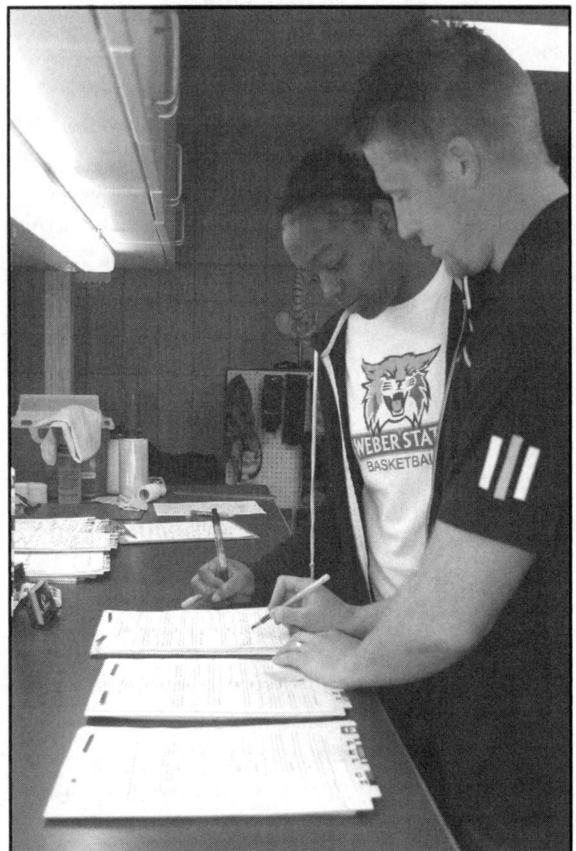

Figure 3-6 | Being supported by the athletic trainer.

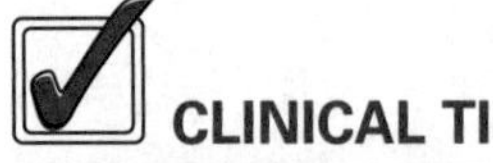

CLINICAL TIP

Research by Hayley Russell and Jill Tracey (2011) suggests that athletes expect their athletic trainer to educate them about their injury and to provide an atmosphere in which they: (1) feel comfortable enough to ask questions, (2) spend quality time, and (3) feel positively supported by the athletic trainer.

Positive affirmations can also be effective for the unmotivated athlete. Because it is common for the athletic trainer to be present on the sideline at practice, he or she is in prime position to hear negative self-talk as a result of poor technique or after a missed shot by the athlete. It is likely that these persistent negative comments damage the athlete's confidence in his or her ability to perform. Thus, it may be helpful for the athletic trainer to assist athletes by providing guidance on incorporating affirmation statements into their prepractice routine. This might be a set of 6 to 10 statements that are positive and motivational in nature; the athlete listens to these before practice (or rehabilitation) as a way to focus on the tasks at hand. This improved focus is a key element of injury prevention.

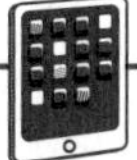

VIRTUAL FIELD TRIP

To study examples of positive self-talk strategies and positive affirmation routines involving motivational goal setting, go to http://davisplus.fadavis.com and complete the critical listening exercises.

Stress-Management Techniques

Common stress-management techniques include relaxation (cognitive and somatic), positive self-talk (thought-stopping techniques), and positive affirmations. A ***cognitive relaxation*** strategy is a guided approach that may include listening to an imagery script that leads the participant through a rain forest or alongside a calm lake, observing nature. It also might take the athlete up a staircase of colors or a moving escalator that brings him or her to a relaxing place. In contrast, ***somatic relaxation*** focuses on physiological techniques such as breathing that lead the participant to a state of relaxation. Common breathing exercises include counting and focused inhalations or exhalations. For example, counting backward from 30 with deep inhalations anchored by each number or holding the breath for a count of 5 before exhaling are useful in promoting a state of relaxation. Focused inhalations or exhalations are those that promote relaxation through focusing on bringing in calm warm air on the inhale and releasing stress through an exhale.

Progressive muscle relaxation (PMR) is another somatic relaxation technique. PMR is a useful technique for decreasing or eliminating tension in the skeletal muscles of the body. Developed by American physician Edmund Jacobson in the early 1920s, it was originally used to treat anxiety, which has been related to high levels of muscle tension. Anxiety is often a response to a stressor due to a primary appraisal of insufficient coping skills. Progressive relaxation of the muscles is a systematic contracting and relaxing technique that can be a useful coping skill for athletes who experience stress or injury. The athletic trainer can act to prevent injury by reducing muscle tension that often accompanies stress by teaching the athlete how to use PMR. An example of PMR is in Box 3-3.

BOX 3-3 | Progressive Muscle Relaxation Strategy

by Andi Pigeon, Athletic Training student, Weber State University

Being an athlete requires a lot from a person. Oftentimes athletes overlook the mechanics and the uniqueness of their physical makeup. In other words, they are unaware of their body and what it is doing. Learning how to actively relax the muscles of the body is a perfect way for the athlete to explore and become more aware of his or her body's tension. The technique is easy to learn; an athlete can do it just about anywhere, and its effects are almost immediate if performed properly. PMR is truly the mind–body connection at work.

As you begin learning more about muscle relaxation, keep in mind four things that are necessary for the relaxation to occur. First, you must be able to find a comfortable place and position to relax. Do try to dim the lights and put on relaxing music if it is available to you. Second, make sure you become aware of your body; otherwise, it will be hard to relax the muscles. It is important to be able to focus on the things that are happening on the inside of your body rather than on the outside in the environment surrounding you. Third, be able to consciously regulate the depth and rhythm of your breathing. By focusing on breathing deeply, you'll be able to become more relaxed and more aware of your internal state. Lastly, it is important to be able to actively contract and relax your muscles along with your breathing. Counting is often

Continued

BOX 3-3 | Progressive Muscle Relaxation Strategy—cont'd

a helpful aid. Also, be sure to work each muscle group one at a time, not all at once.

Now, let's begin by doing an actual muscle-relaxation exercise.

First, close your eyes and get into a comfortable position either lying down or in a chair.

Begin by breathing in slowly through your nose, pulling air down into your stomach, and feeling your stomach rise slowly. Hold the air you have taken in and now very slowly exhale that breath through your nose, allowing for your lungs to empty and then your stomach to slowly collapse as you empty out all of the air. Good. Let's try that one more time. This time, breathe in slowly through your nose, imagining the air reaching deep down into your stomach, filling your stomach with air. Hold that breath and now slowly exhale through your nose, allowing your lungs to empty and then your abdomen to sink slowly back down. Let all the tension melt away as you exhale more deeply with each breath. Continue to breathe slowly and gently throughout the rest of the exercise. Now, let's begin muscle relaxation by closing your right hand into a fist. Squeeze tightly, feeling the tension in the muscles of your hand and lower arm. Hold as you breathe in ... and relax as you breathe out. Let all the tension go.

Now, tighten your left hand into a fist; squeeze tightly. Feel the muscles of your hand and lower arm as they are very tense. Breathe in, holding the tension ... then relax as you slowly breathe out.

Concentrate now on your shoulders. Slowly raise them up toward your ears, holding your arms tight against your sides. Tense the muscles of your upper arms and your shoulders. Hold that tension. Breathe in ... and then relax as you breathe out, letting all the tension go.

Notice the difference in how your muscles feel. Notice what it feels like for your muscles to be tense and what it feels like to be relaxed.

Let's proceed now to the muscles of your back. Arch your back slightly and pull your shoulder blades together, tightening the muscles of your back. Hold this tension. Breathe in, continuing to hold the tension ... and exhale as you let all the tension go. Let the muscles of your back relax. Allow these muscles to be loose and comfortable.

Concentrate on the muscles of your chest and stomach. Bend forward slightly and cross your arms in front of you, tightening your chest and stomach muscles. Hold the tension. Breathe in ... and breathe out. Relaxing. Letting go. Feel the muscles relaxing. Notice the feeling of tension and then relaxation.

Tighten now the muscles of your buttocks, feeling your body raise up slightly as you do so. Hold the tension. Feel the tension in the muscles. Breathe in ... hold ... and relax. Breathe out. Let the muscles become relaxed and loose. Let all the tension go. Focus your attention on the muscles of your thighs. Tighten these muscles on the front, sides, and back of your upper legs. Hold ... breathe in ... and now breathe out. Let the tension leave your body as you exhale. Now tense the muscles on the front of your lower legs by raising your feet and toes upward. Breathe in, holding the tension. Now breathe out. Relax.

This time point your toes down and feel the tension in the back of your lower legs and feet. Hold this position tightly. Feel the tension. Breathe in ... and exhale. Allow your muscles to relax. Feel the relaxation.

BOX 3-3 | Progressive Muscle Relaxation Strategy—cont'd

Notice the muscles throughout your body.

You can use this method to relax any areas of your body that remain tense. Scan your body now for any areas of tension and focus on relaxing each area as you breathe.

If there are any remaining areas that are still tense, tighten the muscles in this area. Hold the tension tighter, tighter ... breathe in ... and relax. Feel the area relaxing as you breathe out.

Let your body relax even further... deepening the state of relaxation. With each breath, you can become even more relaxed. Deeper and deeper... very peaceful ... comfortable ... relaxed ... free from tension ... No cares ... No worries ... Just relaxation.

Enjoy this feeling of relaxation you are experiencing.

Take note of this feeling of relaxation. Memorize the feeling, so in the future you can picture this relaxed state and feel calmer simply by remembering how relaxed you were. Take a moment now to observe the relaxation you are experiencing and memorize it.

Now it is time to reawaken your body.

Turn your attention to your body ... feel the energy flowing through your body as your muscles reawaken but remain free of tension. Gently move your muscles as you feel a state of wakefulness returning.

Take a few moments to continue slowly reawakening your mind and body. Feel your mind returning to its usual level of alertness.

When you are ready, open your eyes and return to your day, feeling calm and energetic.

Muscle-relaxation exercises can be done anywhere at any time. Notice the feeling that you had after this script. Repeating it in the future or building a muscle-relaxation script of your own could help you to relieve tension in the future. It is important as an athlete to know that tension is not always beneficial and can sometimes be detrimental. Having a way to wind down and relax your muscles is ideal to help be effective on and off the field.

Positive ***self-talk*** increases relaxation by promoting a positive thought process and combating negative stress-producing thoughts. It is common for athletes to dwell on the negative effects of stressors in their lives (e.g., a failed exam, relationship difficulties) and of sports situations (i.e., not training well, losing their spot on the team). They can use the ***thought-stopping*** technique to gain control over negative thoughts and change them into positive, stress-reducing cognitions. When athletes are preoccupied with negative thoughts, they become distracted, unfocused, and prone to injury.

CLINICAL TIP

When the athletic trainer hears the athlete saying, "I can't do this" or "I just can't get it done today," he or she should introduce the thought-stopping and positive self-talk techniques to the athlete as ways to change negative thoughts to positive, more productive, even motivational thoughts and phrases. These are effective methods of dealing with the negative thoughts that can distract athletes and make them more prone to injury.

CLINICAL TIP

Athletic training students have an advantage because the athletes are their peers. As a result, they may be familiar with the stressors the athletes face due to academics and busy schedules, and they understand the personal life and financial stressors that are common in the college-aged population. In addition, athletes may be more apt to share personal stressors with their athletic training student peers than with seasoned athletic trainers.

ATHLETE INSIDER CONCLUSION

Susan has several psychosocial factors that influence her risk for injury. Her history of stress, including life stress (arguments with her boyfriend) and previous injury history (ACL injury of the right knee), as well as a lack of adequate coping resources (limited social support) all influence her cognitive appraisal of her current stressful situation (returning to competition). These psychosocial factors created an increased stress response, which influenced her risk for injury and possibly contributed to the ACL injury of her left knee.

Effective Psychosocial Strategies for the Athletic Trainer to Use With Susan

The following psychosocial strategies, aimed at factors related to the stress response, can be used with Susan:

1. Pregame or prerehabilitation mental routine with positive self-talk (2–5 minutes in length, using the athlete's language and cue words; Box 3-4)
2. Somatic relaxation at night to achieve restful sleep (15–45 minutes of guided relaxation by focusing on breathing); several different types of somatic relaxation can help achieve the relaxation response: diaphragmatic breathing, rhythmic breathing, ratio count breathing, and PMR (Box 3-5)
3. Personal best podcast to improve overall self-confidence (5–10 minutes of the athlete's best performances to focus them on their abilities and returning to play)
4. PMR to improve physical and mental stress (10–15 minutes in a quiet, relaxed atmosphere; Box 3-3)

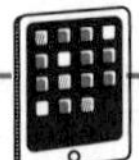

VIRTUAL FIELD TRIP

Find a sample of psychosocial strategies (e.g., relaxation scripts, personal best scripts, etc.) at http://davisplus.fadavis.com.

BOX 3-4 | Positive Self-Talk Strategy

Sit or lie down comfortably.

Relax your shoulder muscles in particular. Relax your whole body and empty your mind.

Close your eyes.

Take 10 deep, slow breaths. Breathe from the pit of your stomach and feel your lungs filling.

Focus on your breathing. Feel it getting deeper and slower. Feel yourself relaxing and any muscle tension drifting away.

Relax your shoulders and neck again. Feel the muscle tightness reducing, leaving you relaxed.

Visualize yourself being happy, succeeding, winning, being loved, laughing, feeling good.

Relax your forehead, feeling the creases from the day's worries melting away.

Relax your mouth, allowing it to drop slightly open, to a restful position.

Relax your eyes, feeling the weight of your eyelids pressing down, heavy.

Allow a gentle smile to appear on your face as you feel a calmness enter your mind.

Now, focus on your rehabilitation plan for the day and say these words to yourself:

I will be successful today.

I will complete all exercises, at full effort.

I have the determination to return to the (field).

I will work hard today to reach my goals.

I choose to be here, and I choose to endure anything that comes my way.

I will become stronger today.

I am in control of my destiny and my success.

CONCLUSION

This chapter has described psychosocial contributors to injury risk. Athletic training students and athletic trainers are encouraged to integrate psychosocial strategies into their clinical practice and should recognize that, as part of injury prevention, they should address the psychosocial aspects of injuries. The management of stress should involve aspects of the physiological, cognitive, emotional, and behavioral components of the stress experience.

BOX 3-5 | Somatic Relaxation Strategy

1. *Diaphragmatic breathing* helps to regulate breathing and facilitates oxygen delivery and waste removal from systemic musculature. Have the athlete rest his or her hand on the lower abdomen and pay attention to the rising and falling of the area.
2. *Rhythmic breathing* requires the athlete to breathe in and out to a specific count. Have the athlete sit or lie down in a comfortable position and begin to breathe. Then, move his or her attention to the in-count and out-count of the breath. Have the athlete breathe in for four counts and out for four counts, establishing a rhythm in his or her breathing.
3. *Concentration breathing* is great for athletes who have difficulty focusing on the relaxation process because of unwanted or intrusive thoughts. Have the athlete focus on the rhythm of his or her breathing; following the pattern of the breath helps to keep the athlete on track.
4. *5-to-1 ratio count breathing* uses imagery of numbers as athletes anchor the thought process to the relaxation response. Have the athlete imagine a number 5 and inhale for a count of 5, followed by an exhale to a count of 5. Continue counting down to the number 1, with an inhale of 1 and an exhale of 1. A general affirmation statement should follow the 5-to-1 count breathing: "I feel more relaxed; I feel ready to play my game."
5. *1-to-2 ratio count breathing* involves inhaling for 1/2 of the exhale count. Have the athlete inhale for 2 counts and exhale for 4 counts. With practice, the athlete can build to 4-to-8 or 6-to-12 counts.
6. *PMR* is a type of somatic relaxation (Box 3-3). It involves systematic, purposeful tension release from the muscles with a resulting relaxation response.

Athletic trainers are encouraged to examine the athlete's personal and situational factors to provide or encourage the use of coping skills that will likely alter the cognitive appraisal and minimize the negative impact of the stress experience. This chapter also highlighted various psychosocial strategies for use with athletes experiencing stressful events with the aim of preventing injury. Relaxation, positive self-talk, positive affirmation statements, and PMR are a few tools suggested for use to gain control over and reduce stress. It is also important to be mindful of individual differences, such as gender, in noticing and handling stress.

REFERENCES

Andersen, M. B., & Williams, J. M. (1988). A model of stress and athletic injury: Prediction and prevention. *Journal of Sport & Exercise Psychology, 10*(3), 294–306.

Cohen, S., Kamarck, T., & Mermelstein, R. (1983). A global measure of perceived stress. *Journal of Health and Social Behavior, 24*(4), 385–396.

Dawson, M., Hamson-Utley, J. J., Hansen, R., & Olpin, M. (in press). Examining the effectiveness of psychological strategies on physiologic markers: evidence-based suggestions for holistic care of the athlete. *Journal of Athletic Training.*

Kania, M. L., Meyer, B. B., & Ebersole, K. T. (2009). Personal and environmental characteristics predicting burnout among certified athletic trainers at National Collegiate Athletic Association institutions. *Journal of Athletic Training, 44*(1), 58–66.

Maddison, R., & Prapavessis, H. (2005). A psychological approach to the prediction and prevention of athletic injury. *Journal of Sport & Exercise Psychology, 27,* 289–310.

Morgan, W. P. (1980). Test of champions: The iceberg profile. *Psychology Today,* 92–99.

Olpin, M., & Hesson, M. (2010). *Self-assessment: Stress management for life: A research-based, experimental approach* (2nd ed., pp. 17–19). Belmont, CA: Wadsworth, Cengage Learning.

Petrie, T. (1992). Psychosocial antecedents of athletic injury: The effects of life stress and social support on female collegiate gymnasts. *Behavioral Medicine, 18*(3), 127–38.

Romas, J. A., & Sharma, M. (1995). *Practical Stress Management: A Comprehensive Workbook for Managing Change and Promoting Health* (pp. 37–38). Needham Heights, MA: Simon & Schuster.

Russell, H. & Tracey, J. (2011). What do injured athletes want from their healthcare professionals? *International Journal of Athletic Therapy & Training, 16*(5), 18–21.

Selye, H. (1975). *Stress without distress.* New York: Penguin Books.

Tracey, J. (2003). The emotional response to the injury and rehabilitation process. *Journal of Applied Sport Psychology, 15*(4), 279–293.

Walter, J. M., Van Lunen, B. L., Walker, S. E., Ismaeli, Z. C., & Oñate, J. A. (2009). An assessment of burnout in undergraduate athletic training education program directors. *Journal of Athletic Training, 44*(2), 190–196.

Williams, J. M., & Andersen, M. B. (1998). Psychosocial antecedents of sport injury: Review and critique of the stress and injury model. *Journal of Applied Sport Psychology, 10*(1), 5–25.

BOARD OF CERTIFICATION STRATEGIES AND COMPETENCIES

As the sixth edition of the Board of Certification's Role Delineation Study outlines, athletic trainers are involved in the prevention and care of athletic injury (Domain 1). Athletic trainers must educate athletes regarding potential risks of participation and guide them to participate in a safe manner. In addition, it is the duty of the athletic trainer to be aware of potential stressors faced by athletes and to offer assistance and strategies to counteract the stressors, thus helping to prevent injury. Athletic training students may provide assistance in buffering stress without the athletic training students knowing it. They do this through supportive communication, active listening, and injury or health education. Because stress is a common antecedent of injury, effective athletic trainers must be equipped with the tools to assist athletes in dealing with stress to avoid or reduce injury occurrence. Beyond the communication skills mentioned earlier for use in the clinical setting, knowledge of strategies to assist the athlete with stress reduction is also a useful tool for the athletic trainer. Relaxation, positive self-talk, and goal-setting strategies can all play a role in the prevention of injury by reducing physical and mental stress, increasing the ability to focus, and improving the mind state of the athlete (i.e., positive thoughts). Specific to the Fifth Edition Athletic Training Education Competencies, this chapter has introduced psychosocial antecedents of athletic injury risk (PS-1) and discussed the function of education to enhance the psychological well-being of the athlete (PS-6).

Board of Certification Style Questions

1. The athletic trainer notices that an athlete seems stressed out and distracted during practice and is not acting like herself. What should the athletic trainer provide in this situation to aid in the prevention of injury? (Choose all that apply.)
   a. Referral to mental health-care professional
   b. Communication and social support
   c. Sport-specific drills
   d. Taping and bracing

2. The athlete is experiencing stress and anxiety when considering readiness to return to play following rehabilitation of the ACL. What psychological strategies could the athletic trainer use to minimize the risk for reinjury? (Choose all that apply.)
   a. Performance imagery
   b. Somatic relaxation
   c. Positive self-talk
   d. Goal setting

3. Gender differences in needs and expectations related to the care provided by the athletic trainer exist. Examples of these differences are:
   a. Male athletes' needs focus on injury and stress-management education, whereas female athletes' needs focus on the caring and compassion shown by the athletic trainer.
   b. Male athletes' needs focus on the caring and compassion shown by the athletic trainer, whereas female athletes' needs focus on injury education.
   c. Both genders have the same needs when it comes to athletic training services.
   d. Male athletes seek social support, whereas female athletes seek information from the athletic trainer.

4. A social work referral is prudent for the following stressors experienced by an athlete (choose all that apply):
   a. Financial concerns
   b. Shelter concerns
   c. The ability to buy food and eat nutritionally as required by the sport
   d. Relationship issues with the coaches

5. Identify effective stress-management strategies for an athlete who has lost his place on the starting lineup (choose all that apply):
   a. Performance imagery
   b. Thought stopping
   c. Goal setting
   d. Systematic desensitization

END-OF-CHAPTER EXERCISES

1. Choose a variety of preinjury factors and discuss how they influence the risk for sport injury. In your response, be sure to include discussion of:
   a. the antecedents of injury.
   b. cognitive appraisal.
   c. useful interventions.

2. Consider an athlete you are working with right now in the athlete training room. Brainstorm potential antecedents that may have placed that athlete at risk for injury.

3. Outline the factors that affect cognitive appraisal for an achievement-oriented freshman athlete, far from home and new to the university setting, with a first-time ACL injury that occurs during the first week of the sport season. Also consider the role of the team's athletic trainer and highlight how he or she might assist the athlete.

4. Analyze the effects of gender on antecedents. Explain how male and female athletes may have a different set of psychological antecedents. Which ones are sometimes shared across genders?

5. Consider a typical freshman student–athlete who is from out of state and is experiencing a moderate-to-severe injury for the first time. Complete the diagram in Figure 3-7 (page 78).

6. Create a stress-management tool kit for an athletic team. Consider common sources of stress presented in this chapter and from your work with these athletes, and how best to manage these stressors. Include the Stress Symptom Checklist (or another way of increasing awareness about sources of stress). Include at least three different exercises and options for each exercise (i.e., two relaxation podcasts). Finally, introduce your tool kit to your athletic team or individual athlete and practice implementing psychosocial strategies with the athlete(s).

7. Outline how situational factors such as playing status, time in season, type of sport, level of competition, and scholarship status can affect how athletes perceive various stressors. Use a chart form to list the common stressors of college athletes and then blend in each of the situational factors listed earlier in your responses.

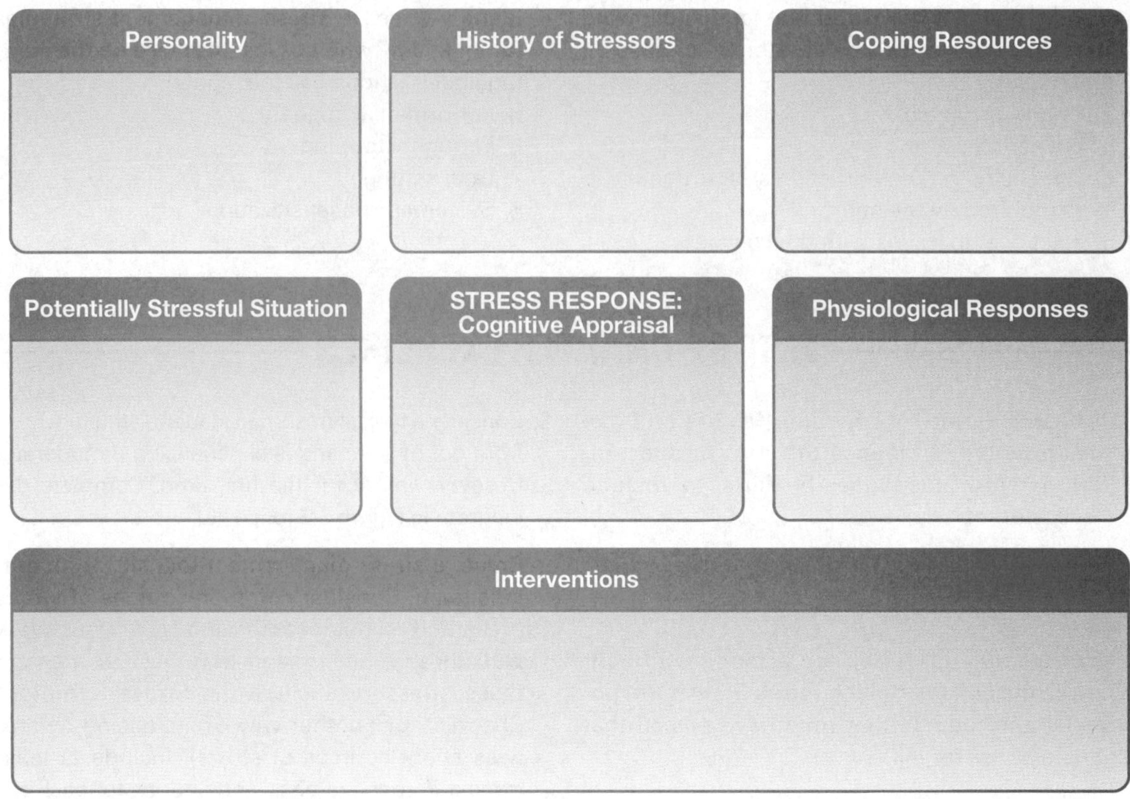

Figure 3-7 | Antecedents to athletic injury.

Chapter 4

Emotional Responses to Injury

Jennifer Stiller-Ostrowski with Jill Tracey

CHAPTER OUTLINE

KEY TERMS

Active listening Communication technique that requires the listener to feed back what is heard by restating or paraphrasing; to confirm what was heard and to confirm the understanding of both parties.

Athletic identity The degree to which a person identifies the self as an athlete.

Cognitive appraisal Interpretation of a situation.

Cognitive rest Stopping activities that require concentration and attention; may include a temporary leave from academic/work responsibilities, reduced school day/workload, and/or additional time allowed to complete tasks or tests.

KEY TERMS *continued*

Cognitive restructuring A cognitive behavioral strategy used to identify and replace irrational or maladaptive thoughts that often occur in anxiety-provoking situations.

Concussion A complex pathophysiological process that affects the brain, induced by traumatic biomechanical forces.

Countering A technique used to challenge the veracity of irrational and/or maladaptive thoughts by using logical counterstatements.

Dissociative imagery A relaxation strategy to distract the athlete from focusing on injury-related pain.

Emotion-focused coping Strategies aimed at reducing the negative emotional response associated with stress; may be the only realistic option when the source of stress is outside of the person's control.

Healing imagery Focusing attention on a target visual stimulus to produce a specific physiological change that can promote healing.

Instrumental coping Strategies that target the causes of stress in practical ways that address the stress-producing problem or situation, consequently directly reducing the stress; examples include finding out about the injury, attempting to alleviate sources of stress and discomfort, and listening to the advice of health professionals.

Malingering Intentionally pretending to have or exaggerating physical or psychological symptoms, especially to avoid work or a return to participation.

Postconcussion syndrome (PCS) A complex disorder in which a variable combination of postconcussion symptoms (such as headache and dizziness) last for weeks and sometimes months after the concussive event.

Post-traumatic growth (PTG) A positive psychological change experienced as a result of highly challenging life events and circumstances.

Primary appraisal Initial assessment of a situation to evaluate it as a threat or challenge.

Secondary appraisal Secondary assessment of a situation, including assessment of available coping resources.

Secondary gain Favorable consequences, such as increased attention from significant others and escape from stressful situations, or medication use, that occur in conjunction with the generally undesirable injury.

Self-efficacy Confidence in one's ability to perform a particular task in a specific situation.

Self-talk Internal and/or external statements to the self, multidimensional in nature, that have interpretive elements associated with their content; it is dynamic and serves at least two functions (instructional and motivational).

Social support Includes the feeling or sense of being supported by others, the act of supporting others, and social integration.

Thought stopping A psychological strategy that allows the athlete to gain control over the thought process, changing negative thoughts to more productive positive thoughts.

Trait anxiety A stable personality construct of worry (includes high and low).

CHAPTER OBJECTIVES

After reading this chapter, you will be able to:

1. Integrate applicable theoretical models of emotional response to injury and forced inactivity.
2. Identify what may affect athletes' postinjury emotions and subsequent behaviors, including personal situations and injury characteristics.

3. Describe the cognitive and emotional impacts of catastrophic and career-ending injuries.
4. Summarize the unique emotional impact of concussive injuries.
5. Describe the influence of athletic identity on appraisal and emotional/behavioral response to injury.
6. Implement strategies designed to aid athletes in managing emotions and facilitating positive responses to injury, including emotion-focused and instrumental coping strategies.
7. Describe the concept of post-traumatic growth and understand the potential for developing it within the rehabilitation environment.
8. Identify athletes who may be intentionally or unintentionally prolonging the injury process.
9. Implement strategies to help athletes maintain athletic identity throughout the injury and rehabilitation process.
10. Identify scenarios in which maladaptive emotional response necessitates psychosocial referral.

ATHLETE INSIDER

Maryn is a senior on the girls' varsity basketball team at the local high school. She had an incredible junior year and was contacted by elite Division I collegiate women's basketball programs. Maryn knows that a scholarship is probably her only opportunity to receive a college education—an education that she would be the first in her family to earn. She worked hard all throughout the off-season, playing in pickup games with local college players who were home for summer break. The season opener is today. With the stands packed with college recruiters, Maryn gets the ball from the opening tip. As she easily weaves her way through the opposing team, she makes a cut and feels a sharp pain as her knee buckles underneath her. A magnetic resonance imaging scan 3 days later reveals a grade 3 anterior cruciate ligament (ACL) sprain, damage to her lateral meniscus, and a large osteochondral defect on her femur. Following her diagnosis, college recruiters stop pursuing her. Although not clinically depressed, Maryn experiences significant negative emotions postinjury. She stops attending practices and begins to isolate herself from her teammates.

INTRODUCTION

Anecdotally, emotional disturbance is common following injury, yet the extent to which these disturbances affect the injured athlete vary greatly. The common nature of emotional disturbance might lead to underattention by the allied health professional who is treating the athlete. Using a theoretical approach, this chapter identifies the common emotional responses of athletes following injury. This chapter helps the athletic trainer differentiate typical responses from responses that require psychosocial strategies or referral. Injury type (i.e., acute vs. chronic), severity (i.e., mild, moderate, or severe), and frequency (e.g., first time vs. 10th time) are addressed. In addition, this chapter presents research findings regarding which responses might interfere with rehabilitation and require the use of psychosocial strategies or referral for psychosocial intervention. The chapter guides the athletic trainer to recognize emotional disturbance following sports injury, including ***concussion***, and provide management strategies to facilitate athletes' rehabilitation and their return to sport participation.

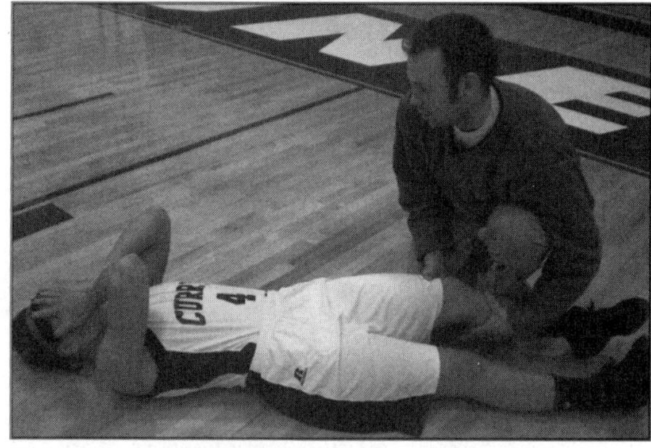

Figure 4-1 | Athlete Insider *(Courtesy of Christy Eason)*

PSYCHOLOGICAL COMPLEXITY OF INJURY

During their training, athletic trainers learn to accept the fact that injury is a natural part of athletic participation. Although injury is commonplace, athletic trainers must consider the impact each injury has on the individual athlete. Although this may be the fifth ACL tear that the athletic trainer has seen this year, it is likely the first for the individual involved. For this reason, the athletic trainer needs to be conscious of typical emotional responses following injury to help the athlete cope with what is happening (both physically *and* emotionally) and to move forward in the most positive manner possible. Although many injured athletes cope well with injury, a significant subset experiences serious cognitive and emotional disruption. The negative psychological impact of sport injuries has been well documented in the literature and includes high school, college, and elite sport athletes (for a review of psychological impact of injuries, see Brewer, 1994; Evans, Mitchell, & Jones, 2006; or Gallagher & Gardner, 2007).

An athlete may view injury in many different ways, and athletic trainers must remember that there is no "right" or "wrong" way to react. Athletes may view the injury as either a positive or a negative experience, as a disappointment, or as an opportunity to show courage, or they may attempt to avoid acknowledging the degree to which they have been injured. Athletic trainers know that negative stress occurring in athletes' lives at the time leading up to the injury is a significant predictor of the degree of emotional distress. Common psychological problems associated with injury include fear and anxiety, identity issues, confusion, isolation, and perhaps even depression.

As a general rule of thumb, athletes' emotions often form a U-shaped pattern, with periods of the greatest emotional disturbance occurring immediately after injury and just before return to play (when anxiety may be high and confidence in the involved body part and in overall ability to perform may be low). As athletes make progress throughout the course of rehabilitation, emotions generally become more positive. In other words, athletes' moods tend to parallel their perception of recovery. It is essential for athletic trainers to understand typical emotional reactions following injury so they can help to facilitate emotional recovery and identify when an athlete may benefit from referral to other professionals who have expertise with emotional issues following injury. Such issues may include failure to adapt, post-concussion issues, extreme malingering, and career-ending or catastrophic injury.

CLINICAL TIP

For athletes undergoing ACL reconstruction surgery, studies have found significant differences in negative mood state and coping with pain at 2 weeks and 2 months postsurgery. Greater mood disturbance should also be expected in competitive athletes (vs. recreational; Morrey, Stuart, Smith, & Wiese-Bjornstal, 1999). Athletic trainers should be aware of these differing mood states during various phases of rehabilitation and in various patient populations, and they should be prepared to assist athletes in identifying and implementing appropriate coping resources. Athletic trainers can be active in demonstrating empathy by talking with athletes about how they are feeling in an attempt to focus them on coping proactively. Athletic trainers can continue to help athletes set realistic rehabilitation goals, encourage the practice of healing imagery, and seek out social support from various resources.

THEORETICAL MODELS OF EMOTIONAL RESPONSE TO INJURY

Athletic trainers and other allied health-care providers have recognized that the mental aspect of sports injuries existed, but they may not have considered this when the priority is to return athletes to the field as quickly as possible. They believed that there were grieflike phases, or stages, that athletes progress through following injury; however, there is little education about what is "typical" for athletes during these stages or about ways to help athletes get through the injury-and-recovery process mentally strong. An understanding of the typical cognitive and emotional profile following injury can be helpful in identifying athletes who may benefit from the use of psychosocial strategies.

Theories explaining emotional responses following injury have evolved greatly over time. Early researchers believed that postinjury stages followed a similar pattern as those postulated by Kübler-Ross (1970) in her grief response model. This model focuses on a perceived loss (e.g., death, job, marital separation) and asserts that grief is an active process that changes over time through a sequential series of steps or stages. The theory asserts that individuals progress from denial to anger to bargaining to depression, finally reaching a stage where they accept the diagnosis and its repercussions. This loss-of-health model was derived from patient populations (e.g., terminally ill cancer patients) who are significantly different from injured athletes, and researchers have found little support for the existence of the bargaining or depression stages with injured athletes.

From this early model, Brown and Stoudemire (1983) developed their own three-stage model of the typical grief process. They theorized that athletes enter a shocklike stage immediately after injury, followed closely by a stage of intense preoccupation with the injury and its effects. Once athletes are able to accept the injury, they enter a reorganization state. Although researchers applied this model successfully in the past, it is not generalizable to all injured athletes. It is through the work of Brown and Stoudemire that we get our first glimpse into potential variations of these strict stagelike models; however, these concepts were not applied within an injured athlete context for another decade.

In 1990, Hardy and Crace modified the original grief response model, resulting in four stages with extremes that better reflected the typical magnitude of emotional response to athletic injury. This theory suggests that athletes progress from initial denial ("It's OK; I'll run it off.") to anger ("I wasn't supposed to be in that play in the first place!") to sadness ("I'm not going to be able to play for weeks.") to acceptance and reorganization ("I can't change the fact that I got hurt; now what can I do to help myself?"). However, research with an athletic population has been unable to identify such stagelike emotional patterns. Stagelike models have received criticism because they do not consider individual differences that may affect how an individual reacts to injury (e.g., severity of injury, individual's perception of injury as threatening/nonthreatening), nor do they address potential cognitive disruptions in response to stress (addressed in Chapter 3). We now recognize that emotional response to injury does not necessarily follow a sequential stagelike progression.

An alternative to the stage models was further evolved by Heil (1993) in his description of the affective cycle of emotional response. The sequential nature was replaced by a cyclical process for which injured individuals could maneuver back and forth. The components include distress, denial, and determined coping. The distress element acknowledges the disruptive aspect of an injury and how it can place an emotional imbalance such as anxiety, depressed mood, or helplessness. Denial involves a sense of lacking acceptance of the severity of the injury and the subsequent rehabilitation involved. Denial is complex because it can be both adaptive, serving as a protective mechanism to limit overwhelming emotions, or maladaptive if emotions are ignored and not processed. Determined coping implies a perspective whereby athletes not only accept the severity and prognosis of their injury, but proactively incorporate coping strategies (i.e., seeking social support, applying instrumental coping) to process through recovery. At the onset of injury it is understandable to experience the distress and denial elements and as rehabilitation progresses, generally athletes adopt determined coping. The unique feature of the affective cycle is the potential to repeat or cycle back and forth with all three elements.

Brewer's cognitive appraisal model (1994) is a significant deviation from the previous stagelike models that attempted to predict the sequences of emotional responses to athletic injury. As presented in Chapter 3, both personality and situational factors can be antecedents to injury. These factors can also influence an athlete's perception of the meaning of injury. Brewer's model focuses attention on the role and power of ***cognitive appraisal*** and how the individual's perception of the injury affects subsequent emotions and actions. The model also allows for the influence of situational factors (e.g., time of season, starter/nonstarter) and injury characteristics (e.g., severity). Essentially, the appraisal determines the emotional reaction, which then influences the subsequent behavioral response. There are unidirectional arrows between each component (injury → appraisal → emotional response → behavioral response). The foundation of the model is that, although athletes cannot change the fact that injury has occurred, they can change their appraisal of what the injury means to them. As you consider this model, it is important to understand that an arrow indicates that intervention is possible (see Psychosocial Strategies section for more details about this).

Working within an athletic population, Udry, Gould, Bridges, and Beck (1997) developed a model that attempts to sort emotions into three general categories of responses to injury. In the first category—injury-relevant information processing—the focus is on the pain and extent of the injury. The athlete questions how the injury happened and recognizes the negative consequences and inconveniences of being injured. The second category—emotional upheaval and reactive behavior—essentially encompasses the majority of emotions previously broken into separate stages. Athletes may feel agitated, emotionally depleted, isolated, and disconnected; they may experience shock, disbelief, denial, or self-pity. In the final category—positive outlook and coping—the athlete accepts the injury and begins to deal with its consequences. The athlete tends to be optimistic and is relieved to sense progress toward the injury healing. While this model does allow for individual differences, it is still somewhat stagelike.

Although researchers have observed in injured athletes behaviors consistent with the various phases hypothesized in stage models, they have not documented a common sequence of discrete emotional reactions to athletic injury. Athletic trainers should not expect specific "categories" or "progressions" of emotional distress in response to athletic injury. It appears that emotional reactions to injury vary more across individuals than stage models would suggest, and there is no substantial evidence to support the assumption that there is a universal stagelike pattern of response to negative life events.

Cognitive appraisal models have evolved from earlier models and take into account individual differences (e.g., personality), situational and environmental factors (e.g., preseason vs. playoffs), the individual's perception of the injury as either threatening or nonthreatening, the individual's history of stress and coping resources, and the interaction between the two. In cognitive appraisal models, it is the individual's appraisal of the injury that determines his or her emotional response; the emotion is essentially a reaction to the perceived meaning of the injury. There are two basic forms of cognitive appraisal: primary and secondary. ***Primary appraisal*** is an assessment of what is at stake, whereas ***secondary appraisal*** is an assessment of the coping options an individual has available to him or her.

The integrated model of response to sport injury (Wiese-Bjornstal, Smith, Shaffer, & Morrey, 1998) expands on Brewer's model by emphasizing that both preinjury and postinjury factors influence reactions. Rather than stagelike, this model emphasizes that cognitive, emotional, and behavioral responses to injury can and will change over time in a dynamic way, illustrating the athlete's evolving and complex responses to injury. The model encompasses preinjury stress factors and the impact of the athlete's perception of the injury as a stressor, implying that the resultant emotional response depends on the athlete's cognitive appraisal. Finally, the interaction between appraisal and emotional response dictates the behavioral response to injury (see Wiese-Bjornstal et al., 1998).

The progression of emotional response models led to the development of the biopsychosocial model by Brewer, Andersen, and Van Raalte (2002) to offer a broad perspective of sport injury rehabilitation processes. Because we now have a more comprehensive understanding of an athlete's reaction to sustaining an injury, it also helps to be cognizant of the implications the injury can have on overall well-being. The model explores the numerous factors that include characteristics of the injury itself (e.g., type, severity, history), as well as the various biological, psychological, and social correlates. Understanding the influence of these variables on emotional response and subsequent recovery is important for athletic trainers. The model has seven components: injury characteristics, sociodemographic variables, biological variables, psychological variables, social/contextual variables, intermediate biopsychological responses, and rehabilitation outcomes. Viewing emotional response from this multifaceted perspective allows athletic trainers to see the injury process more holistically, as one that involves physical, psychological, and social components. The model does help to integrate existing models and to highlight the connection of biological factors that had not been included to this extent previously. More discussion of this model and its relationship to rehabilitation adherence is in Chapter 8.

As cognitive appraisal models postulate, knowing that an event has occurred is not as important in determining the emotional response as knowing how the individual has interpreted or cognitively appraised the event. Athletes may attribute injury to any number of factors (e.g., themselves, their equipment, bad luck, the inherent risk of the sport), and appraisal involves consideration of the severity of the injury itself, as well as the impact of the injury on their athletic goals. Events may be viewed as threatening or nonthreatening, and how athletes appraise the stressors is thought to have implications for the intensity (moderate vs. intense) and range (relief vs. distress) of emotions they experience and their subsequent behaviors. Obviously, injury severity and rehabilitation length are two factors that would influence reactions, and they are also why researchers dismiss stagelike models. Short-term injuries do not follow the same "stages" as long-term injuries.

With these issues in mind, Hedgpeth and Gieck (2004) developed the progressive reactions of injured athletes based on severity of injury and length of rehabilitation model. This model attempts to predict typical emotional reactions based on the anticipated length of rehabilitation following injury. Injuries that require short rehabilitation (less than 4 weeks), those that require long rehabilitation (more than 4 weeks), chronic injuries, and career-ending injuries each have a different set of typical responses to injury, to rehabilitation, and to return to activity. For example, athletes will likely experience shock and perhaps relief following injury that requires a short rehabilitation (less than 4 weeks), will approach rehabilitation with optimism and likely impatience, and will be eager and anticipate their return to sport. Athletes who experience chronic injury are generally angry and frustrated with the injury, may be apprehensive of the rehabilitation process, and may be alternately confident or skeptical as they approach return to activity. Following a career-ending injury, athletes will likely react with grief or isolation and may experience a loss of ***athletic identity*** during the rehabilitation process, but they should ultimately come through the experience with closure and a sense of renewal.

FACTORS THAT INFLUENCE EMOTIONAL RESPONSE AND SUBSEQUENT BEHAVIORS

These earlier models of response to injury and rehabilitation, particularly cognitive appraisal models, have provided a strong understanding of the significance of how individuals interpret or appraise the injury situation. The factors that influence appraisal of the injury and its effect on emotion include many of the same personal and situational variables that served as antecedents to injury, as well as several additional factors. Personal factors relate to the stable characteristics within the individual, whereas situational factors vary extensively over time, yet both can strongly influence appraisal. Personal factors include aspects of the injury (e.g., history, severity), individual differences (e.g., self-perceptions, history of stressors, coping skills), demographics (e.g., gender, age), and physical factors (e.g., physical health status, disordered eating). Situational factors include sport factors (e.g., type, level), social factors (e.g., team influence, family dynamics), and environmental factors (e.g., rehabilitation environment, accessibility to rehabilitation).

Although models have effectively outlined typical emotional responses depending on the severity of injury and length of rehabilitation, many other factors influence an athlete's emotions and subsequent behaviors following injury. Expectations for recovery and perceptions of injury consequences begin to form soon after injury. Athletes are sponges looking to "soak up" any information that will inform them of possible recovery outcomes. Open, two-way communication between athletes and athletic trainers is vital to the rehabilitation process. The injured athlete is emotionally vulnerable during the recovery process, and the verbal and nonverbal behavior of the athletic trainer can greatly impact subsequent emotional response. Numerous researchers have discussed the role of communication and how combining empathy with honest assessment of the injury is a delicate and often challenging task. The manner and tone in which athletic trainers talk with injured athletes can greatly influence their emotional responses. There is arguably a big difference between saying, "The swelling looks like it is down today, and your range of motion is better," as opposed to "There is still a lot of swelling, and you are lacking 30 degrees of motion." Although essentially communicating the same objective information, an athlete will likely perceive the two statements very differently; one has an optimistic "spin," whereas the other is stating facts that he or she will likely perceive negatively. Athletes are particularly sensitive not only to *what* is said but also to *how* it is said, so athletic trainers need to be aware of both their words and their tone of voice when delivering messages. Research shows that adherence to rehabilitation improves when injured athletes feel they have a positive relationship or alliance with the health-care provider (learn more about effective communication strategies in Chapter 5).

It is during this period shortly following injury that irrational thoughts may begin to surface. These thoughts have a negative effect on the athlete's emotional reaction and behavioral response. Both internal and external factors may influence these reactions, including personality attributes and characteristics (e.g., strong athletic identity), sport context (e.g., starter, senior year), injury history (e.g., 1st time vs. 10th time), and other pressures (e.g., scholarships). Injury context is also an important factor in determining how athletes will respond to injury. Researchers have demonstrated that athletes will react more negatively if they believe their injury was the result of illegal or aggressive behavior than if they attribute it to incidental contact. In addition, athletes who perceive that they caused their own injury may experience greater negative mood states because they believe they were unable to exert personal control over the situation. For injured athletes, grieving results from the loss of some aspect of the self. Although usually not permanent, the loss of participation and all that comes with it may be a traumatic event. Furthermore, psychosocial reactions and emotional responses may be determined to some extent by the way athletes perceive that others *expect* them to respond. Resultant emotional reactions can have a significant impact on athlete receptiveness and adaptation to treatment and rehabilitation intervention, and can either help or hinder these processes.

At a time when the physical injury is causing stress, pain, and potentially a disruption in daily activities, the athlete may also experience a social loss because of a perceived or real disenfranchisement from teammates and coaches. We understand how an injured athlete can feel this way during this phase, because it can be a stressful and emotionally challenging period. To manage during this time, athletes may use emotion-focused or instrumental coping techniques. ***Emotion-focused coping*** involves using self-regulation to manage what is causing stress, and it can be either proactive (i.e., relaxation, meditation) or potentially detrimental (i.e., withdrawal, self-blame). The intention of emotion-focused coping strategies is to soothe the individual and to increase his or her overall quality of life. ***Instrumental coping*** or problem-focused coping involves finding out specific information about the injury and actively incorporating strategies to alleviate the sources of stress or discomfort, such as listening and complying with advice from health-care providers, goal setting, and positive self-talk. Instrumental coping strategies focus on actively finding and implementing solutions to a stressful problem. Perceived controllability is a factor that determines the individual's choice of coping strategy (in other words, if an individual feels they are "better" at one coping strategy than another, they will likely adopt that particular strategy).

CLINICAL TIP

Many situations lend themselves to both emotion-focused and instrumental coping strategies. For example, an athlete who is having difficulty coping with forced time away from her sport may benefit from spending some time reconnecting with friends she does not usually have time for during her sports season (emotion focused), whereas also finding ways to maintain her cardiovascular fitness levels as she allows her injury to heal (instrumental). Athletic trainers can encourage athletes to identify and use many different coping methods at various points during the recovery-and-rehabilitation process.

Athletic Identity

Athletic identity is the degree to which an individual identifies with the athlete role. Individuals with a strong athletic identity are those whose self-worth is tied closely to their identity as an athlete. This predominant perception seems to have a severely negative effect on psychological recovery from injury. When athletic ability is taken away, even temporarily, individuals with strong athletic identity may be unable to adjust to being injured. As a result, athletic trainers should pay special attention to helping them to maintain their identity, as perceived incompetence in this highly valued domain can profoundly affect their feelings of self-worth. Researchers have demonstrated a correlation between individuals with high athletic identity and psychosocial distress following injury and sport career termination (see following Evidence-Based Practice feature).

Consider the case of Maryn in the Athlete Insider section at the beginning of this chapter. Maryn's high athletic identity likely influenced her perception of the meaning of her injury and her subsequent emotional response. The fact that her sense of self-worth was so closely tied to her "identity" as a basketball star caused her to experience significant negative mood states following injury. Athletes with a strong and exclusive athletic identity will interpret injury in terms of its implications for athletic functioning and will therefore likely experience emotional difficulties when injury impairs their ability to perform in their sport. Any athletic injury, particularly a career-threatening injury, disrupts their predominant identity. When athletes lack other sources of self-worth and self-identity, it is likely there is increased risk for emotional disturbance and poor adjustment because they may have a more difficult experience in coping with forced time away from their sport. The Athletic Identity Measurement Scale (AIMS; Brewer, Van Raalte, & Linder, 1993) is a reliable and valid measure of athletic identity, assessing the strength and exclusivity of identification with the athletic role.

RED FLAG

Athletes with a strong, exclusive athletic identity may be at increased risk for negative mood disturbance and depression following injury. The AIMS (Brewer, Van Raalte, & Linder, 1993) is a seven-item Likert scale that can be used to evaluate athletic identity in injured athletes. Individuals rate the extent to which they agree with seven statements regarding identification with the athletic role. This measure encompasses both strength and exclusivity of athletic identity, and researchers found it to be a valid representation of the social, cognitive, and affective aspects of athletic identity. The athletic trainer could have athletes complete this survey to help gain an understanding of their athletic identity and to take steps to ensure that they maintain this important identity throughout the injury-recovery process.

Athletic identity is fairly stable across time; however, it does tend to decrease following severe injuries that threaten sport participation. Researchers have hypothesized that this may be a self-protective mechanism (see Evidence-Based Practice feature on page 93). However, athletes with a strong athletic identity can also learn how to transfer their athletic strategies to the rehabilitation setting, primarily by using some of the same strategies that made them successful in their sport to make them successful during rehabilitation. Although athletic trainers should encourage athletes to stay involved in their sport as much as possible, to adjust to time away from physical activity, they should also be persuaded to focus on other areas of their sport or event. Athletes can be encouraged then to use this physical break as a chance to work on their mental game (see later Psychosocial Strategies section).

Finally, athletes should take advantage of new opportunities that have been presented to them. For example, if a lacrosse player tore his ACL, he could use this time away from the sport to focus on upper-body weight lifting (see more examples of facilitating positive consequences from injury later in this chapter). It is also a period that allows many athletes to focus more on their academic work because they have extra free time available, because they may not be attending practices and competitions.

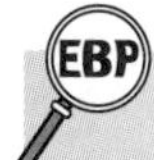

EVIDENCE-BASED PRACTICE

Brewer, B.W., Cornelius, A.E., Stephan, Y., et al. (2010). Self-protective changes in athletic identity following anterior cruciate ligament reconstruction. *Psychology of Sport and Exercise, 11*(1), 1–5.

Continued

Description of the Study

One hundred and eight individuals (47% competitive athletes, 49% recreational athletes, 4% nonathletes) undergoing ACL reconstruction surgery were given the AIMS before surgery and at 6, 12, and 24 months postsurgery. Subjective perception of rehabilitation progress was measured by asking patients to rate their percentage rehabilitated (0%–100%).

Results of the Study

Fifty-eight complete data sets were analyzed. Changes in AIMS scores were examined using a repeated-measures analysis of covariance (controlling for age and gender). AIMS scores decreased significantly over time. Post hoc pairwise comparisons demonstrated the most significant decrease in AIMS scores between 6 and 12 months after surgery; there were no significant decreases from before surgery to 6 months after surgery or from 12 to 24 months after surgery. Hierarchical regression was used to examine the relationship between perceived recovery progress and athletic identity between 6 and 12 months after surgery. Results indicated that the percentage rehabilitated accounted for a significant proportion of the variance in AIMS scores; specifically, individuals who perceived a smaller percentage rehabilitated demonstrated greater decreases in athletic identity.

Implications for Athletic Training Practice

The results of this study imply that athletic identity may decrease over the course of a lengthy rehabilitation process. In this study, the greatest decreases were during the 6- to 12-month period, which is when patients who have undergone ACL surgery typically return to sport. The correlation between poor perceived rehabilitation progress and lowered AIMS scores seems to indicate that the decreased athletic identification serves a self-protective role. Athletic trainers should be aware that high athletic identity can predict poor rehabilitation adherence, and they should implement strategies to help athletes maintain and transfer this identity into the rehabilitation setting. It is important to recognize that this will be a difficult time for athletes and work to help develop realistic expectations of their performance levels as they begin to return to sport.

Secondary Gain and Malingering

Secondary gain refers to a complex phenomenon in which an athlete who is motivated by return to participation may actually prolong the recovery process because of the subconscious benefits of remaining injured. The injured athlete receives personal attention from the athletic trainer (and significant others) and may view the athletic training room as a source of safety and security. Although these "benefits" are often viewed as positive attempts to make an injured athlete's daily life easier, they may actually have a negative impact by encouraging athletes to *remain* injured. Secondary gain is typically explained by one of two causes: need for attention or fear of returning to sport. For example, athletes who are not receiving enough attention from significant others in their personal lives may gain psychological benefits from attention received while injured. Alternatively, the athlete may have a subconscious fear of returning to competition that masks itself as continued physical impairment. Indications of secondary gain include pain that is disproportionate with objective clinical signs (e.g., lack of swelling), resistance to undergoing further evaluation to isolate the sources of newly described pain or symptoms (e.g., claims that they "couldn't get a ride" to their magnetic resonance imaging appointment), and decreased adherence to the rehabilitation program. The athlete receives increased attention following the development of new symptoms, whereas avoidance of diagnostic testing and lack of adherence to rehabilitation will prolong recovery and delay return to participation. Although the athlete may subconsciously perceive these "benefits" of being injured as positive consequences, these secondary gains actually result in delayed physical and psychological recovery. The athletic trainer must take steps to prevent and address secondary gain with injured athletes. This may include finding ways to nurture athletic identity while injured.

Malingering is a term that has appeared in medical literature for nearly half a century, yet researchers do not completely understand this complex phenomenon. Malingering is a conscious attempt to *act* injured because of perceived external incentives for being or remaining injured; the athlete has previously learned that there is a reward for this behavior. The malingering athlete attempts to intentionally deceive the athletic trainer (and physicians, coaches, teammates) about the injury by consciously manufacturing symptoms. The primary motive is to avoid practice or competition, whether because of fear of returning to activity, need for attention, or both. Malingering is different from secondary gain in that secondary gain is an *unconscious* attempt to prolong recovery, whereas malingering involves *conscious* deceit on the part of the athlete. Within the athletic context, suspicions of malingering are most often reported in athletes who have symptoms associated with low back pain or following head injury, because both of these diagnoses rely heavily on subjective information and have courses of recovery that are difficult to predict. However, the potential for malingering exists following any medical pathology (and, in fact, even in the absence of true medical pathology).

The malingering athlete presents a special challenge for the athletic trainer. Because there is no definitive "test" for malingering, it is impossible to know for certain whether the athlete is malingering or exhibiting legitimate physical symptoms that are not textbook characteristics of the injury. This can be frustrating not only for the athletic trainer and the sports medicine team, but also for coaches and teammates. Although determining malingering behavior can be difficult, observing behavioral patterns may indicate obvious red flags (Table 4-1). For example, because malingering is a conscious effort to gain some external incentive, injuries tend to occur only at times that are convenient for the athlete. The malingering athlete will also feel no guilt for "letting the team down" by being injured and has no real motivation to return to participation. These athletes seem emotionally detached from the

TABLE 4-1 **Common Behavioral Observations and Examples of Malingering Behavior**

Cause	Behavioral Observation	Example
Need for attention not received elsewhere	Complaints of new symptoms occur only when attention from athletic trainer staff decreases.	An athlete continues to report symptoms because he enjoys the attention he gets from coaches, teammates, and fans for "playing through the pain."
Escape from athletic/sport pressures	Athlete seems stressed, overwhelmed by athletic participation.	An athlete no longer gets enjoyment from playing collegiate volleyball and wants to quit, but to maintain her scholarship she must remain on the team.
Attempts to justify current or anticipated future poor performance	Complaints of symptoms occur only during episodes of poor performance; when the injured area is stressed similarly but the athlete plays well, no symptoms are reported.	Statements such as "I didn't play well today because my back was hurting," or "My back is really bothering me today; I don't know if I will be 100% for the big game tomorrow."
Avoiding practice to rest for game day	Symptoms tend to "flare up" during practice days and resolve completely on game days.	A football player predictably reports symptoms each Monday (which is the practice day that involves the most contact drills).

For an in-depth review of malingering behavior, see Rotella, Ogilvie, and Perrin (1999).

pain they are reporting, even when they describe the pain as debilitating. According to Rotella, Ogilvie, and Perrin (1999), the biggest giveaway is the overexaggerated emotional response to injury. These experts believe that the greatest need is for attention and the greatest fear is getting caught.

CLINICAL TIP

The Hoover sign is a classic procedure that can be helpful in identifying malingering in individuals who complain of low back pain, because of its similarity to other legitimate special tests used during a clinical evaluation. The purpose of the Hoover sign is to determine whether a patient is actually exerting effort during a testing procedure. The patient lies supine as the examiner elevates the legs by cupping the patient's heels. The examiner then asks the patient to perform a straight leg raise on the involved side. If the patient is making a legitimate attempt to lift the leg, the examiner should feel pressure from the uninvolved leg pressing down into the hand. A positive finding occurs when no downward pressure is felt, indicating that the patient is not making an effort to perform the test (malingering). In the case of confirmed malingering, the athletic trainer should attempt to identify alternate (nonphysical) reasons for the athlete's subjective reports of pain.

It cannot be emphasized enough that malingering is not a phenomenon that should be suspected as a primary diagnosis; initially, athlete claims of injury should be believed and investigated. However, athletic trainers need to be aware of the malingering phenomenon and should consider the possibility of behaviors associated with it in scenarios similar to those seen with secondary gain. The primary determinant to distinguish the two phenomena is the motive: conscious or unconscious. Athletic trainers need to be aware of signs of both, must have developed communication skills to help determine the cause of the behavior (see Chapter 5 for a more detailed discussion of communication), and must be familiar with referral protocols to involve mental health professionals who may be able to help athletes move past these behaviors (see more on referral later in this chapter).

Emotional Disturbance Following Concussion

Considerable attention has been given throughout this textbook and within this chapter to the significant impact an injury can have on an athlete's psychological well-being. Special considerations often need to be made when dealing with concussive injuries because they are complex and can involve unique problems with respect to physical and psychological responses and recovery. In recent years, two main consensus statements have been published and widely disseminated by both the National Athletic Trainers' Association and through the International Conference on Concussions in Sport. These statements make reference to the impact that concussion can have on athletes emotionally and the importance of psychological issues in both assessment and management of a concussion. The Third International Conference on Concussions in Sport, held in Zurich, Switzerland, in 2008, culminated in a revised consensus that built off of previous statements from the First (Vienna) and Second (Prague) International Conferences. The Zurich consensus statement highlights the recognition of how quickly the science of concussion is changing and aims to formalize a consensus-based approach to dealing with concussion diagnosis, treatment, and management issues. As research and clinical evidence mounts about concussions, more knowledge is gained about the emotional distress and challenges experienced by many injured athletes.

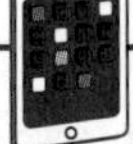

VIRTUAL FIELD TRIP

Listen to a conversation between a brother and sister discussing a recent concussion in Critical Listening Exercise #2 for this chapter.

http://davisplus.fadavis.com

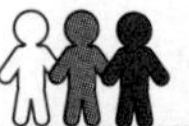

SPECIAL CONSIDERATIONS

A special population that merits particular attention is military personnel returning from active duty and integrating into an academic environment. Many have sustained concussions and other traumatic brain injuries, and may also be dealing with aspects of post-traumatic stress disorder. The complexity of dealing with these types of injuries and disorders makes it paramount that educational institutions recognize possible issues that may arise with these individuals as they adjust to civilian and student life, and make accommodations for them. Multiple symptoms associated with concussion and post-traumatic stress disorder may flare up and be exacerbated by academic stressors (e.g., exams, assignments). School administrators may need to implement special accommodations such as extensions for exams and projects because these students may continue to require rest that includes resting the mind, or ***cognitive rest***. In addition, this population may also be dealing with the consequences unique to their combat experience such as interpersonal issues, "survivor guilt," or grieving the loss of fellow soldiers, and this may hinder their ability to follow standard timelines. It is important to note, however, that with understanding, counseling, and modifications, these students can be successful.

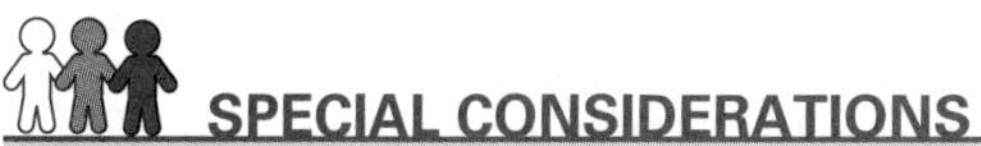

SPECIAL CONSIDERATIONS

Athletic trainers working with student–athletes who sustain concussion should be aware of the concept of cognitive rest in addition to time away from physical activity. Following concussion, it may be difficult for athletes to attend classes, focus on schoolwork, or take tests. Cognitive rest may include a temporary leave of absence from school, reduction in overall workload, and allowance for additional time to complete assignments and take tests. Athletic trainers must communicate with administrators and faculty to be sure they understand that these accommodations are legitimate and necessary to ensure full recovery following concussion (Box 4-1).

BOX 4-1 | Potential Academic Accommodations for Students Recovering from Concussion

- Reading assistance and/or extended time for tests and/or assignments
- Note takers
- Physical and/or cognitive rest during the day
- Excused absences
- Flexibility with due dates for assignments, tests, and so on
- A quiet environment (such as an alternative room) to reduce noise, light, and other potentially distracting stimuli
- Tutoring services

Source: McGrath (2010).

Although the treatment and management of concussive injuries has focused understandably on the physical aspects, it is important to note that, even within the definition of concussion forwarded in the Zurich statement, there is the recognition of the cognitive and postconcussive symptoms. It is not uncommon for concussed athletes to experience anger, depressed mood, shock, guilt, and anxiety (all of which can also be experienced by athletes with nonconcussive injuries). In addition to the physical limitations associated with many types of injuries, concussed athletes also frequently report feelings of isolation, pain, and disruption of daily life activities, which can all lead to further anxiety for athletes concerned about their athletic and cognitive future.

Concussive injuries are unique from a psychological perspective for four main reasons. First, unlike many types of other injuries, concussion is an "invisible" injury; without bruising, a cast, or crutches, it is difficult for some people to understand that the athlete is, in fact, injured. Second, concussion sometimes requires lengthy physical and cognitive rest, which can result in either real or perceived loss of fitness and exacerbate anxiety for athletes who fear losing significant aerobic capacity, combined with concerns about returning to play and potentially losing a spot on a team. Furthermore, for student–athletes, the cognitive rest may have resulted in academic challenges and cause additional distress and hardship if, for example, grades have suffered or reductions in course work have led to delays in degree progression. The third unique issue is the overlap of postconcussive symptoms with the commonly reported psychological response to injury noted earlier. It can be difficult to determine what "typical" emotional responses are and how long they may last when it can be so individual and based on so many personal and situational factors (Fig. 4-2). Because postconcussion symptoms continue for a prolonged time, it can be difficult for athletic trainers to differentiate symptoms of the "normal" healing process from ***postconcussion syndrome (PCS)***. The fourth issue relates to continued pressure on athletes from the media, pushing them to return before they are physically and psychologically ready. This is most pronounced with professional athletes; however, there is increasing media attention on injured collegiate athletes as well. The ability to aid concussed athletes in managing these unique psychological impacts may fall outside of an athletic trainer's comfort zone. As a result, athletic trainers must recognize when referral is indicated following concussion and be willing

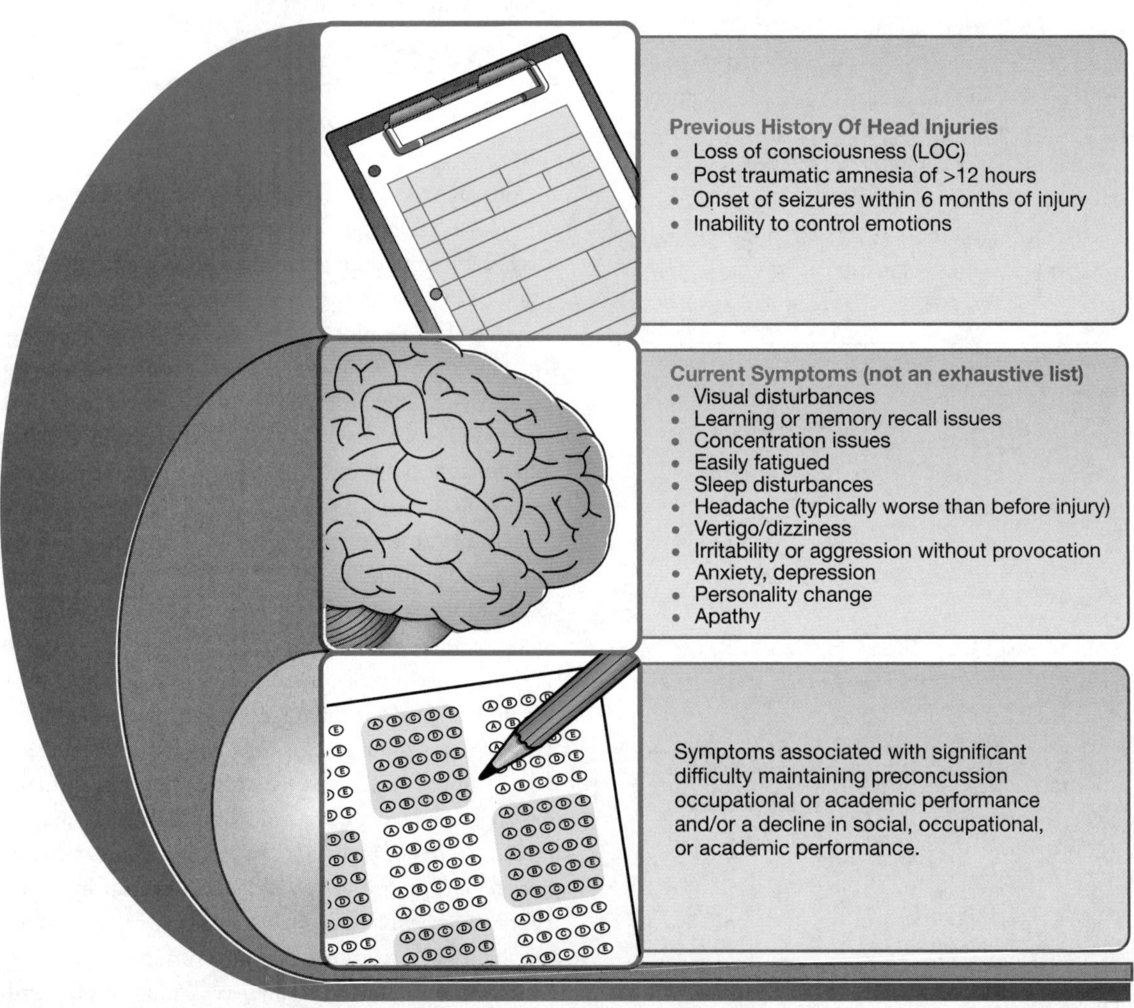

Figure 4-2 | Domains of postconcussion syndrome.

to help the athlete work through these issues with a professional who is trained to do so (learn more about referrals later in this chapter).

RED FLAG

Concussions may result in biochemical disturbances in the brain, which may put these athletes at an increased risk for suicide. Concussed athletes commonly display emotional symptoms such as depression, anxiety, anger, and confusion, and studies have shown a significant relationship between concussion and clinical depression. Many behavioral indicators of suicidal thoughts may be missed if they are considered to be characteristic of PCS. These behavioral indicators include, but are not limited to, changes in energy level, changes in academic and/or sport practice habits, sudden personality changes, and difficulty concentrating (Henderson, 2007). Athletic trainers can help prevent suicide attempts by concussed athletes by becoming aware of these red flags and being prepared to intervene on the athletes' behalf.

EVIDENCE-BASED PRACTICE

Covassin, T., Elbin, 3rd, R. J., Larson, E., et al. (2012). Sex and age differences in depression and baseline sport-related concussion neurocognitive performance and symptoms. *Clinical Journal of Sports Medicine, 22*(2), 98–104.

Description of the Study

College (n = 837) and high school (n = 779) athletes participating in a variety of competitive sports completed a baseline Immediate Post-concussion Assessment and Cognitive Test (ImPACT), symptoms inventory, and Beck Depression Inventory II. Participants were grouped based on depression scores (i.e., severe, moderate, mild, minimal), and between-group comparisons were evaluated for ImPACT composite scores (i.e., verbal memory, visual memory, reaction time, motor processing speed), total symptoms, and symptom cluster scores (i.e., sleep, cognitive, emotional, somatic/migraine).

Results of the Study

The severely depressed group scored worse on visual memory and reported more total symptoms and greater scores for each of the four symptom clusters as compared with the minimally and moderately depressed groups. Regarding Beck Depression Inventory II scores, there were no significant group differences for age or gender.

Implications for Athletic Training Practice

Just as individual differences in baseline neurocognitive performance should be expected, so should individual differences in baseline depression states. This study demonstrates that a subset of uninjured high school and collegiate athletes experiences significant depressed mood states, and that high school and college-aged athletes are equally likely to experience depression. Even in the absence of concussion, the severely depressed group demonstrated somatic symptoms that are commonly associated with mild traumatic brain injury and PCS. Athletic trainers should consider administering baseline depression assessments concurrent with baseline neurocognitive assessments in an effort to identify athletes who may be suffering with undiagnosed and unmanaged depressive mood states. The authors also discuss the difficulty of disentangling symptoms of depression from symptoms of concussion. For this reason, athletic trainers should consider screening concussed athletes for depression, because research shows depression correlates with lower ImPACT visual memory scores and increased symptom cluster scores. Treating concussed athletes for

Continued

underlying depression may result in a faster return to baseline ImPACT scores and a decrease in somatic symptoms, resulting in faster return to participation.

CLINICAL TIP

PCS is a complex disorder involving a combination of postconcussion symptoms (such as headaches and visual disturbances) that can last for weeks and sometimes months after the injury that caused the concussion. For most people, PCS symptoms generally occur within the first 7 to 10 days and go away within 2 or 3 months; however, they can persist for a year or more. Much attention has been focused on PCS in recent years because of numerous high-profile athletes in the National Hockey League (e.g., Sidney Crosby, Eric Lindros, and Pat Lafontaine) and in the National Football League (e.g., Steve Young, Troy Aikman) suffering with significant concussions and long-term issues of PCS. When one Googles "career-ending injuries due to concussion," a huge number of stories come up linking professional athletes from various sports to a shortened career because of concussion and postconcussion-related issues.

There are no specific diagnostic tests for PCS, but physicians can administer clinical assessment and neuropsychological tests to determine the presence or absence of symptoms and the extent of impairment. Three domains are involved when assessing the complexity of PCS. PCS treatments are aimed at easing specific symptoms and, based on the list of issues in Figure 4-2, can be challenging.

Catastrophic and Career-Ending Injuries

The end of an athletic career can be an emotional experience under any circumstances; however, there is an unquestionable difference in emotional response following a planned retirement as opposed to an unexpected termination caused by injury. Individuals who are coping with a catastrophic or career-ending injury may feel isolated as they grieve the loss of this important aspect of themselves. They may experience negative emotions related to their loss of career, of their identity, of their place in society, and of their social group (teammates). The inability to return to sport forces athletes into a lifestyle change from perhaps the only life they have ever known. In addition, individuals who have sustained a catastrophic injury may also be dealing with permanent loss of physical function, which can have a significant impact on athletic identity, self-concept, and general lifestyle. In what ways and to what extent the athlete grieves these losses depend on a large number of personal, situational, and social factors, including athletic identity. The purpose of rehabilitation takes on a different meaning under these circumstances: regaining everyday function versus returning to participation. When an athlete recognizes that he or she will not be returning to sport, there is a tendency to "go through the motions" of rehabilitation. Referral to a mental health professional may be necessary when athletes feel they have no sense of control (learn more about referrals later in this chapter).

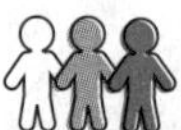

SPECIAL CONSIDERATIONS

Individuals with spinal cord injury are at particular risk for anxiety, depression, and negative impact on life satisfaction and athletic identity. Research conducted by Tasiemski and Brewer (2011) indicates that an increased amount of postinjury weekly sport participation and being able to participate in one's favorite sport are associated with higher maintenance of athletic identity and better psychological adjustment. In addition, team sport participants had greater psychological adjustment as compared with individual sport participants, which suggests that social factors are an important link between sport participation and psychological adjustment. Measures of athletic identity and life satisfaction correlate positively with each other and correlate negatively with measures of anxiety and depression. This tends to indicate that individuals who are encouraged to maintain their athletic identity by remaining engaged in their sport as much as possible are less likely to suffer from anxiety and depression postinjury.

APPLICATION AND INTEGRATION OF FACTORS THAT INFLUENCE EMOTIONAL RESPONSE AND SUBSEQUENT BEHAVIORS

Once athletes express and acknowledge their emotions, athletic trainers can help them focus on factors that are within their control. Athletes cannot change the fact that they have been injured, but they can control how they react to the injury. They could withdraw and feel sorry for themselves, or they could direct that frustration into motivation toward rehabilitation. Negative emotions lead to underadherence to rehabilitation and poor rehabilitation results, whereas positive emotions result in a more positive rehabilitation experience. Consider the scenario with Maryn, the successful women's basketball player from the Athlete Insider. She viewed injury as being threatening to her position on the team, her chances of going to college, and her overall sense of self-worth. These negative emotional responses would then likely influence her behavioral response to the injury. As presented in the scenario, it caused her to withdraw from her teammates, friends, and significant others. But what other postinjury behavioral response might it influence? Research tells us that pessimism is a characteristic that predicts underadherence to the rehabilitation program. In Maryn's case, without intervention, her negative mood state would likely cause her to neglect her rehabilitation program, which would prolong her physical recovery and result in continued negative impact on her sense of self-worth. Fortunately, there are ways to help athletes maintain their athletic identity even when they are not able to participate in their sport.

Athletic trainers can help injured athletes maintain their athletic identity by teaching them to view rehabilitation as a form of athletic performance. Many of the same skills that made the athletes successful in the sporting arena will also make them successful in rehabilitation—characteristics such as effort, motivation, and competitive spirit, as well as mental training skills. Athletic trainers should encourage injured athletes to transfer any mental skills used in their sport into the rehabilitation setting: engage them in healing and performance imagery or encourage them to use thought-stopping techniques to prevent negative thought cycles. Athletic trainers should also engage injured athletes in setting goals, working collaboratively to set meaningful goals for personal bests.

Another way to maintain athletic identity is to encourage athletes to maintain a connection with their sport, teammates, and coaches. Although it may be tempting to do so, athletic trainers should avoid scheduling rehabilitation sessions during practice; this will allow the athlete to be on the sideline with their teammates. Injured athletes should stay as involved as possible with their sport and their teammates, while also recognizing that sometimes it may be too emotionally difficult to always attend practices. This is something to be negotiated between the coach, athletic trainer, and athlete to determine the best course of action. Although it may initially be difficult for Maryn to be in the gymnasium without being on the court, her interactions with her coaches and teammates will decrease her feelings of isolation and maintain that connection to her athletic identity. Athletic trainers can also encourage coaching staff to walk through the athletic training room when athletes are rehabilitating to ask about their progress and offer encouragement (similar interactions as they would have on the court). Finally, athletic trainers should encourage athletes to develop connections with other injured athletes who are motivated to return to their sports. Athletic trainers may find it helpful to develop "rehabilitation buddies"— two individuals in similar phases of rehabilitation who are willing to work together and can challenge each other. Not only will this help maintain the athletes' athletic identities, but these individuals can serve as an important source of ***social support***.

If an athletic trainer suspects an athlete may be either intentionally or unintentionally prolonging injury, the question becomes what to do about it. Addressing the athlete directly is a sensitive process. The first step is to determine the underlying motivation (need for attention or fear of returning to sport). If attention seems to be the cause, it may be helpful to begin to decrease the attention the athletic trainer gives to the injured athlete. Begin by decreasing the frequency of in-person athletic training room treatments and encouraging athletes to self-treat (e.g., icing after practice on their own). If their behaviors are the result of fear of returning to sport, it may be helpful to use strategies similar to those suggested for maintaining athletic identity. If athletes view rehabilitation as a form of athletic performance, perceived success in rehabilitation will translate to perceived ability to succeed in returning to sport. As they achieve each new, more challenging goal, they will develop more and more confidence in the injured part. It may also be helpful to engage the injured athlete in a mental training program, including the use of positive ***self-talk*** and ***cognitive restructuring*** (see Chapter 10). It is also important to recognize when the needs of these athletes exceed your skill set and to identify athletes who may benefit from referral to someone with experience in dealing with these behaviors in athletes (see more on referral later in this chapter).

FACILITATING POSITIVE EMOTIONS AND BEHAVIORS: CHANGING TO A POSITIVE MIND-SET

Although the predominant expectation is that injury will lead to negative consequences and emotional responses, it is possible to view an injury as a positive experience. Some individuals may view the time off associated with injury as a much-needed break, or perhaps a career-ending injury may provide them with an "out" of a sport in which they no longer find enjoyment. Regardless of how and why the injury occurred and the various factors involved, disconnecting suddenly from teammates and the activity to which an athlete devoted considerable time can lead to a grieving process. Resultant appraisals and emotional reactions can have a significant impact on athlete receptiveness and adaptation to treatment and rehabilitation intervention, and can either help or hinder these processes.

The life development model (LDM) (Danish, Petitpas, & Hale, 1992) proposes that people are continually growing and developing, yet this growth is not necessarily sequential (e.g., injury could cause a downward spiral). How will athletes respond to this critical life event? They could view it as a debilitation resulting in decreased function, they could view it as causing little change at all, or they could view it as an opportunity for personal growth. Because change is inevitable in life, the central tenet of the LDM is to embrace change and look for ways to foster personal growth from it. Athletic trainers can help athletes recognize that they can use the injury situation as a way to demonstrate courage and discover inner strengths. Athletes can also be encouraged to use this time to refine other sports skills not affected by injury. The LDM suggests that we have the capability to shape, rather than simply respond to, negative events in our environment. A critical strategy in the LDM is to incorporate the life development intervention of goal setting as a way to empower athletes to gain a sense of control over their situation. Goal setting can serve many purposes, and athletic trainers are well aware of its use in sport performance. Having injured athletes focus on goals while healing from their injuries can serve to motivate them to action and to gain control over their lives, which can enhance feelings of ***self-efficacy***. This is a much more-positive perspective on injury reaction than the standard view, and can provide hope and optimism for both the injured athlete and the athletic trainer.

While not downplaying the negative impact of injury, there is potential for personal growth through the trauma of injury. A new perspective is to view the experience of injury as a possible place for growth and to transform to a positive mind-set to effectively manage emotions and better cope with the rehabilitation process. ***Posttraumatic growth (PTG)*** is a term used to describe the concept of growth occurring through trauma, and it can also apply to injured athletes. Researchers have conducted many studies on PTG with survivors of terrorist attacks, survivors of war and genocide, and in the area of psycho-oncology. These studies have explored the idea that, through trauma or life crisis, victims can discover something positive. By no means do these traumas equate to an athletic injury per se, but researchers can examine trauma victims' adjustment to adversity or life changes and apply their findings to the injury and rehabilitation setting. PTG is not something that automatically happens. A number of factors, such as personal characteristics (i.e., gender, temperament, personality traits), environmental characteristics (i.e., social support, living conditions), characteristics of the negative event (i.e., stressfulness, duration, and controllability), and the various coping resources available, lead to the potential for experiencing PTG. There are also five domains where studies demonstrate that subjects consistently experience growth (Box 4-2). Recognizing these areas can be helpful in creating an open dialogue to discuss the different aspects of athletes' lives

BOX 4-2 | Domains of Post-traumatic Growth

Social: Sense of closeness with others, having compassion for others, enhanced social resources

Cognitive: Feeling stronger and more self-assured, a better self-concept, improved problem-solving abilities

Emotional: More relaxed, less demanding as a person, greater compassion for the pain of others, better capacity to accept and express a range of affect, a feeling of self-reliance

Personal: Changed lifestyle, learning more about healthy diet and exercise

Spiritual/Philosophical: Increased appreciation of life and one's family, a change in life priorities

Source: Tedeschi and Calhoun (2004).

that represent these domains. Researchers in sport, exercise, and health psychology have identified the possibility of positive benefits of injury, and there is a growing body of literature indicating that people who are exposed to traumatic events (e.g., season-ending ski injuries and survivors of cancer) may perceive some form of growth emerging from their struggles (see Evidence-Based Practice feature). The athletic injury environment seems to be relevant to explore the potential for PTG.

CLINICAL TIP

One exercise that athletic trainers may find beneficial in helping athletes maintain a positive mind-set is to have them make two lists: one of aspects of the injury process that they can control (e.g., effort) and one of aspects they cannot control (e.g., ligament healing). They can do this either jointly with the athletic trainer or on their own. Once the two lists are made, have athletes throw away the list of uncontrollable things (a symbolic gesture) and tape the list of controllable things in a meaningful place, such as on their mirror or inside their locker.

It is common and understandable to focus on the negative aspect of suffering an injury, yet a more productive approach is to look at the positive aspect of injury and to focus on aspects that are controllable (e.g., attitude, emotional response, positive self-talk). Sometimes athletes will see the whole situation as uncontrollable; in these cases, the athletic trainer can help identify controllable aspects in an effort to empower the athlete to help themselves. Athletic trainers often talk with and promote the idea that athletes should be resilient and optimistic and display positive emotions in sport performance. They can transfer these same concepts to the injury and rehabilitation process; athletic trainers should discuss this potential for positive psychological growth with injured athletes. Interesting findings from a variety of injured athletes show perceived benefits (Box 4-3; for a review, see Wadey, Evans, Evans, & Mitchell, 2011).

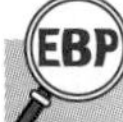

EVIDENCE-BASED PRACTICE

Burke, S., & Sabiston, C. M. (2010). The meaning of the mountain: Exploring breast cancer survivors' lived experiences of subjective well-being during a climb on Mt. Kilimanjaro. *Qualitative Research in Sport, Exercise, and Health, 2*(1), 1–16.

Description of the Study

The study examined the experiences of six breast cancer survivors during an attempt to climb Mt. Kilimanjaro. The participants had undergone a number of treatments for breast cancer including chemotherapy, radiation therapy, mastectomy, lumpectomy, and reconstructive surgeries.

Results of the Study

Researchers suggested that climbing Mt. Kilimanjaro might be a form of challenging physical activity that is rewarding for women who have completed their breast cancer treatments because it may provide an opportunity for growth and enhanced well-being and to explore the meaning of the experience.

Implications for Athletic Training Practice

This research offers unique insight into individuals who have experienced tremendous adversity

Continued

by virtue of dealing with a life-threatening illness, yet chose to adopt a positive mind-set and seek a physical challenge. The climbing of Mt. Kilimanjaro provided a unique opportunity for these women to experience PTG and to discuss the significant understanding of themselves that they gained through such a physical and emotional challenge. Research indicates that individuals who are involved in physical activity following a traumatic event may be more likely to see positive changes in their quality of life. Athletic trainers can facilitate similar benefits through the development of research partnerships; injured athletes can form a unique bond as they work together to navigate the psychosocial and physical challenges associated with injury. Embracing the recovery process in this manner can foster an attitude that leads to positive growth.

Keep in mind that facilitating positive consequences from athletic injury takes effort. Realize that reframing may not occur immediately, and acknowledge that positive consequences may extend beyond the individual athlete (hard as it may be to acknowledge, perhaps the team does better without the injured athlete). The athletic trainer must recognize different problem-solving strategies and help the athlete avoid secondary victimization (i.e., "poor me" attitudes and behaviors).

BOX 4-3 | Perceived Benefits of Sport Injury

- Increased knowledge of anatomy and risk factors of injury
- Increased ability to understand, express, and regulate emotions
- Strengthened and increased social network
- Self-discovery and self-knowledge (learned about self and about their inner strength)
- Greater ability to overcome challenges
- Motivation
- Gaining perspective
- Personal growth and development of other aspects of their lives outside of sport
- Better time-management skills

APPLICATION AND INTEGRATION OF FACILITATING POSITIVE EMOTIONS AND BEHAVIORS

Athletic trainers can play an important role in facilitating a more positive emotional response to injury. How the athlete perceives the injury is a function of changeable variables (e.g., ***trait anxiety***, self-esteem, self-motivation, coping) that can be influenced by those working with the athlete during the rehabilitation process. Athletic trainers need to recognize that emotions create anxiety and tension, which can impede rehabilitation performance, thereby negatively influencing the athlete's attitude toward rehabilitation. Athletic trainers can relieve athletes' anxiety by answering their questions, whether they verbalize them or not (learn more about postinjury communication in Chapter 5). Athletic trainers need to provide clear communication about the severity of the injury, the anticipated return to activity, and what athletes can do to help themselves. Athletic trainers can help determine whether the athlete will exaggerate the injury or realistically appraise it (and recognize that arriving at a realistic appraisal of the injury is the first step in helping the athlete cope with injury). Dealing with the emotional roller coaster one may experience following a significant injury is a process. Opening and completely expressing emotions (including grief) during this process is fundamental to rehabilitation success. Few athletes will be willing to open up right away, so athletic trainers may need to get the ball rolling a bit; however, athletic trainers should be cautious of projecting how athletes *should* feel. Most questions should be open-ended to allow athletes to express their emotions.

To apply a life development intervention/LDM method to working with athletes, athletic trainers should approach conversations with athletes in a nonjudgmental way and use ***active listening***. The goal is to empower athletes to think optimistically about rehabilitation and the personal growth potential that can stem from the experience. Athletic trainers can foster this by assisting athletes in setting realistic goals and focusing their attention on elements within their control such as their effort, thoughts, responses, and overall behavioral reactions to their situation. In addition, consider opening a dialogue to introduce the idea of PTG in a way that suggests that experiencing an injury can result in enhanced self-discovery, learning about themselves and their inner strength, recognizing that they can overcome challenges, and having an opportunity to develop other aspects of their lives outside of sport. This is a proactive alternate way of viewing the rehabilitation process.

WHEN TO REFER

Often overlooked in the injury treatment and rehabilitation processes are the emotional components and the role of the mind. Athletic trainers need to consider it within their scope of practice to help athletes cope with associated physical (e.g., loss of function) and psychological consequences of injury. As we have mentioned, common psychosocial problems associated with injury include fear and anxiety, lack of confidence, identity issues, isolation, and perhaps even depression. Consultation with a mental health specialist can assist athletes in dealing with these psychosocial issues and in coping with the temporary loss of physical function. Pain does not occur in the body without the mind reacting and contributing to the experience; therefore, emotional distress may intensify perceptions of somatic symptoms and prolong the course of physical rehabilitation. It is important that health-care professionals working with athletes identify factors related to emotional adjustment (and maladjustment) to injury. Athletic trainers are in a position to identify emotional responses and behaviors that might interfere with rehabilitation and warrant the use of psychosocial strategies or referral for psychosocial intervention.

RED FLAG

It can be difficult to determine whether athletes are experiencing a typical negative postinjury response or whether they may benefit from psychosocial intervention. Petitpas and Danish (1995) identified the following red flags as warning signs of poor adjustment to athletic injury:

- **Feelings of anger and confusion**
- **Denial; minimizing extent of injury**
- **Obsessed with when they can return to play**
- **Repeatedly coming back too soon**
- **Exaggerated bragging about past accomplishments**
- **Dwelling on minor physical complaints**
- **Feelings of guilt (letting teammates down)**
- **Withdrawal from significant others**
- **Rapid mood swings**
- **Consistent statements expressing doubt that they will ever recover**

Athletic trainers should be aware of these warnings signs and have a referral protocol in place to aid injured athletes in recovering psychologically from their injury.

Failure to address the negative emotional responses and psychosocial impact of injury influences more than the mental well-being of the individual athlete. As this chapter has discussed, emotional response to injury predicts behavioral response. In the case of athletic injury, the most common negative behavioral response is lack of adherence with the treatment and rehabilitation protocol. Researchers have identified the factors that contribute negatively to adherence to injury-rehabilitation programs, including injured athlete pessimism and unrealistic expectations regarding the effort required during rehabilitation. They also suspect other contributing factors such as fear of reinjury and pain experienced during rehabilitation. These nonadherence factors feed into a negative loop: lack of adherence leads to continued physical impairment, which leads to increased emotional disturbance and psychosocial consequences, which results in further decreases in motivation to attend rehabilitation sessions (Fig. 4-3). It is therefore in the best interest of

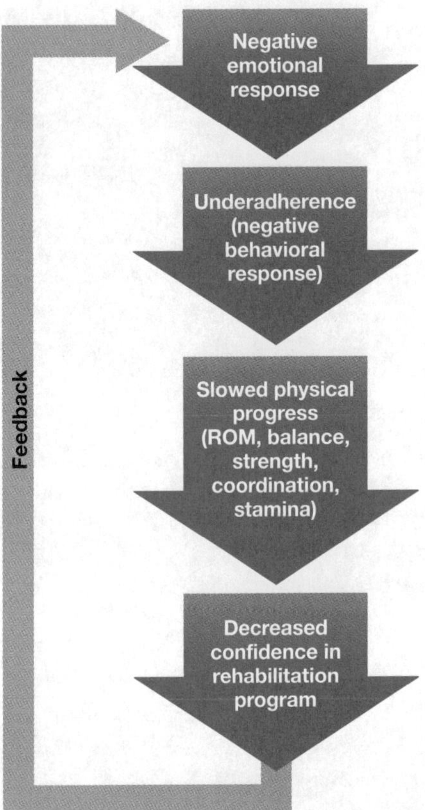

Figure 4-3 | Negative feedback loop (emotional response and rehabilitation adherence). *(Adapted from Stiller, J. L., Gould, D., Paule, A., & Ostrowski, J. A. [2006].* A preliminary investigation of certified athletic trainers' attitudes, actions, and abilities as viewed by previously injured collegiate student-athletes. *East Lansing, MI: Michigan State University.)*

athletic trainers to identify athletes who may benefit from some form of psychosocial intervention or referral—and to do so early in the postinjury process. In addition to maladaptive emotional and psychosocial response to injury, several other factors warrant special attention and consideration for referral. These are highlighted throughout this chapter and include secondary gain and malingering, emotional disturbance following concussion, and career-ending and catastrophic injuries. Information about building a referral network, developing the necessary protocols, and approaching an athlete about referral is provided in Chapter 6.

RED FLAG

Numerous studies published since 2000 have indicated that the rate of adolescent suicide is on the rise. Being a high-achieving, highly competitive athlete is not a protective factor against suicide; rather, some suggest that these individuals are most at risk due to internal and external pressures to succeed. These individuals often experience high levels of stress and, without appropriate coping skills, this stress may lead to depression and isolation. There are numerous cases of highly skilled athletes who committed suicide at what many would consider to be the peak of their athletic careers. Athletic injury may put athletes at increased risk for suicide. Smith and Millener (1994) have highlighted the following factors common to suicidal athletes:

- Surgery
- 6-week to 1-year rehabilitation process
- Depleted athletic skill
- Lack of perceived athletic competence
- Being replaced by another athlete in their sport position

Athletic trainers should pay attention to suicide threats, even if they do not believe the athlete is serious. The voicing of these threats or intentions likely provides insight into an athlete's internal thought process. Athletic trainers should not ignore athletes' "jokes" about suicide or comments indicating the perception that "no one would miss them if they were gone."

PSYCHOSOCIAL STRATEGIES

Until the 1990s, rehabilitative interventions primarily addressed physical dimensions of sports injury, focusing on helping athletes return to preinjury level of function by treating the obvious physical symptoms. The sports medicine community viewed injuries from a structural, anatomical, or physical perspective with little regard for emotional, cognitive, personal, or situational factors. Since the 1990s, this community has begun to place an emphasis on the role of psychosocial factors in the injury process; it is now realized that feelings such as pressure, tension, or anxiety can cause physiological responses that inhibit performance and healing. A goal of athletic trainers should be to facilitate positive emotional responses to injury, which, in turn, leads to behaviors that encourage rehabilitation adherence and a speedy recovery. Many of the stress-management techniques outlined in Chapter 3 can also be implemented postinjury to decrease negative emotions and to facilitate athletes' rehabilitation and return to sport participation. Various psychosocial strategies can aid in facilitating positive cognitive, emotional, and behavioral responses to injury. Strategies can aid in emotional management, maintaining appropriate focus, and increasing motivation. Athletic trainers need to relay to injured athletes that they can transfer many of the mental skills used for performance (e.g., mental imagery and focus, positive self-talk, cognitive restructuring, goal setting) to the rehabilitation environment. Sometimes athletic trainers need to remind athletes that the skills they already possess and use for successful performance will help them deal with the challenges of rehabilitation. As we discussed during the overview of cognitive appraisal models, the arrows between components (cognitive appraisal ↔ emotional response ↔ behavioral response) indicate an opportunity for intervention.

Mental Imagery

Injured athletes often feel a lack of control over the injury-and-recovery process, and this cognitive appraisal may manifest itself through failure to adhere to the rehabilitation program. This is especially evident in situations where the injury ends an athlete's season or career (such as Maryn's ACL tear in the Athlete Insider). Although limited evidence exists of a direct physical effect on healing, mental imagery has often been associated with faster recovery by providing athletes with a sense of control over their injury. In Wiese-Bjornstal and colleagues' integrated model of response to sport injury (1998), bidirectional arrows indicate that responses to injury can and will change over time, with cognitive, emotional, and behavioral responses continuously interacting to influence recovery. When athletes believe they have some measure of control over their own healing (appraisal), this results in increased confidence, motivation, and adherence to the rehabilitation program. Increased adherence to the rehabilitation program results in increased belief that healing is occurring, which then positively affects cognitive appraisal of the injury process and subsequent emotional and behavioral responses.

The use of mental imagery allows athletes to focus on aspects of injury and recovery that they can control. When working to facilitate positive emotions following injury, ***dissociative imagery*** (also known as soothing imagery or pain-management imagery) can be used as a dissociative strategy to distract the athlete from focusing on injury-related pain. Combining imagery with deep breathing or relaxation techniques can increase the effectiveness of rehabilitation and enhance athletes' perceptions of control (learn more about these techniques in Chapter 10). ***Healing imagery*** has also been associated with faster recovery times. Focusing energy on visualizing the area healing is another way to increase the athlete's perception of control over the process. Other uses of mental imagery during rehabilitation could also be to help athletes work on their "mental game"; for example, athletes who will be returning to play this season could be encouraged to study their team playbook and visualize themselves running plays in real time.

Self-Talk and Cognitive Restructuring

Athletes cannot change the fact that they have an injury, but they can control their thoughts about injury and recovery. As this chapter has covered, negative moods and a certain amount of grieving are natural parts of the postinjury process; however, it is much more productive to focus on the positive. Self-talk can have a positive impact on injured athletes' perceptions during rehabilitation and has been shown to affect injured athletes' emotions, influence self-confidence related to rehabilitation success, improve rehabilitation compliance and adherence, and reduce perception of pain. Self-talk is essentially any self-dialogue (internal or out loud), and it can be used for any number of things, ranging from giving oneself instructions to interpreting feelings. What athletes say to themselves following injury helps determine subsequent behaviors during rehabilitation (Fig. 4-4). Negative emotions (i.e., depression, anger, frustration) can lead to negative self-talk ("What's the point? I'm never going to get back on the field."), which, in turn, leads to a poor rehabilitation effort, lack of adherence to the rehabilitation program, and an overall negative rehabilitation experience. Athletes can learn skills to control inner thoughts and stop self-defeating dialogue when it occurs. Positive self-talk can lead to positive emotions. Focusing on the positive allows the athlete to channel energy into rehabilitation sessions, which, in turn, leads to improved quality of rehabilitation sessions, better adherence, and a better rehabilitation outcome.

Specific self-talk techniques that may be helpful in facilitating positive emotions include ***thought stopping***, *cognitive restructuring*, and ***countering***. Thought stopping is a technique in which the athlete develops an awareness of negative self-statements and actively terminates them, replacing negative statements with positive ones. Cognitive restructuring is a conscious shaping of thoughts into a positive format. Countering is a technique in which the athlete refutes irrational self-statements with fact and reason. Athletic trainers can encourage athletes to use these techniques. For example, athletic trainers can ask athletes how the rehabilitation session was that day, encourage them to reflect on any positive aspects, and then point out progress they have made.

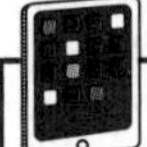

VIRTUAL FIELD TRIP

For examples of positive self-talk strategies for facilitating positive appraisal, emotions, and behaviors postinjury, go to http://davisplus.fadavis.com.

Social Support

Arriving at a realistic appraisal of the injury is the first step in helping athletes cope with injury. Part of the appraisal process is determining the amount and level of social support athletes feel is needed or available. The provision of social support for injured athletes has been extensively

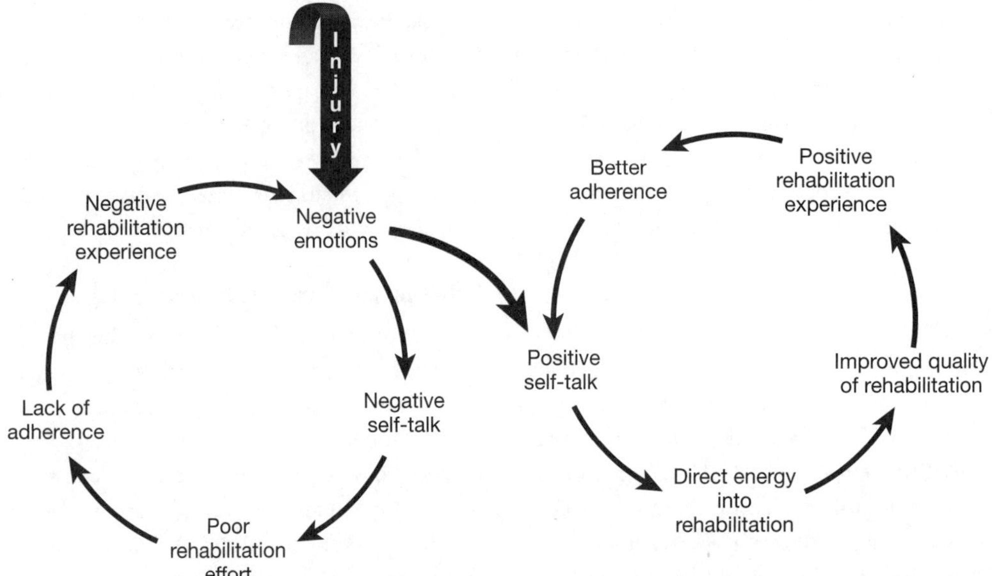

Figure 4-4 | Self-talk cycles.

researched and found to positively impact emotional reaction, stress reduction, and adherence to rehabilitation. Injured athletes often feel vulnerable and are dealing with a myriad of emotions. Actively seeking out or receiving support from various individuals can help reduce feelings of isolation and enhance confidence and motivation to proceed through the rehabilitation process. Social support is widely accepted as needed and appreciated from athletic trainers, teammates, significant others, friends, and family.

There are three major types of social support: emotional support, informational support, and tangible support (see Fig. 4-5 for definitions of each type). It is important to recognize the importance of different types of social support for athletes at various phases of the injury, rehabilitation, and return-to-participation process. Demonstrating a genuine interest in them as people and not just as athletes goes a long way in the athletic trainer–athlete relationship and may facilitate athletes' enhanced psychosocial well-being. Assisting athletes with emotional, informational, and tangible support communicates to them that the athletic trainer cares and is willing to support them in different ways (learn more about social support in Chapter 9).

Motivation

Many strategies to maintain athletic identity focus on encouraging athletes to view rehabilitation as a form of athletic performance. To this point, various creative strategies typically used to foster adherence to the rehabilitation process can also be useful to maintain motivation. Such strategies include rehabilitation partners, support groups, rehabilitation competitions (e.g., stool-scoot races, single-leg balance competitions), and goal setting. In particular, goal setting will help athletes connect the achievement of various rehabilitation "stages" to their ultimate goal of returning to activity. More detail about goal setting is provided in Chapter 10.

Athletic trainers can assist with motivation issues by suggesting injured athletes talk about dealing with rehabilitation sessions, the struggles they may be experiencing, and how to handle incorporating appointments into their lives by effectively managing their time. Athletic trainers can facilitate this by serving as a rehabilitation partner, along with other injured athletes who can partner with an athlete who has recovered from an injury. The healthy partner can offer various types of support (i.e., emotional, informational, and tangible, as discussed earlier) and is someone the injured athlete can relate to, which often results in a comfort level between the athlete and potentially a role model the injured athlete can look to for motivation to persevere through rehabilitation. Athletes can also expand this out to larger groups where those at various stages of rehabilitation meet to discuss and share issues they experience and strategies for maintaining focus and motivation in a supportive, nonthreatening environment.

Another issue not often mentioned is that of overadherence or hypermotivation. Athletes, because they are generally highly motivated, can sometimes be overzealous with respect to their rehabilitation. Whereas in sport it is often encouraged to do more than is required as a sign of true commitment (e.g., "If 10 repetitions are good, 20 must be better"), this can be counterproductive in rehabilitation. Athletic trainers sometimes need to caution injured athletes not to overdo it. Many athletes are quite accepting of the physical demands of rehabilitation and may need to be reminded that being motivated is great, but they need to apply the "Rule of Toos" and not do too much, too fast, too hard, or too soon, so as not to risk a setback (adherence is discussed in-depth in Chapter 8).

ATHLETE INSIDER CONCLUSION

Maryn's cognitive appraisal of her injury and its implications was influenced by several factors: personal (may have lost her opportunity for a college education), situational (senior year, season-ending injury), and injury context (noncontact injury may be perceived as being "her fault"), all of which influenced her emotional and behavioral responses. Her athletic trainer noticed that Maryn was consistently absent from team practices and events, and talked with her about this during rehabilitation sessions. The two discussed that what Maryn missed most about basketball was the competitive atmosphere, so her athletic trainer tried to incorporate competitions and games into the rehabilitation program whenever possible (Fig. 4-6). Her athletic trainer also encouraged Maryn to stay involved with her sport in other ways. Maryn began working with the athletic director "behind the scenes" and soon realized that she really enjoyed this aspect of

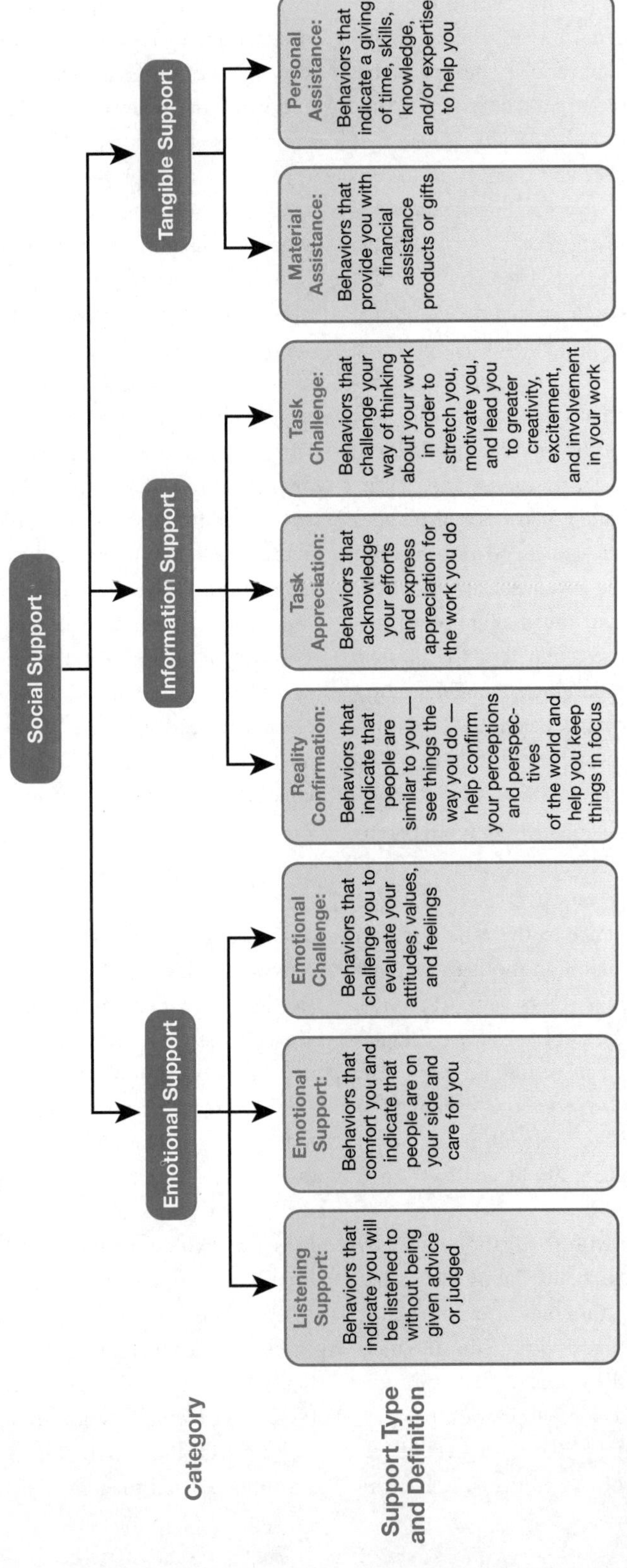

Figure 4-5 | Types of social support grouped by category.

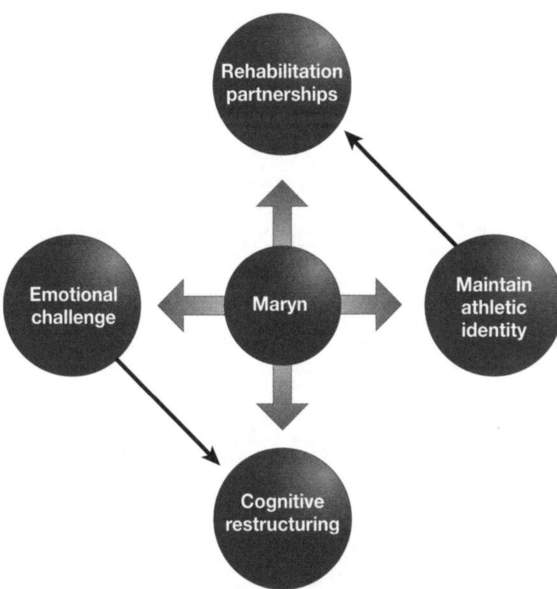

Figure 4-6 | Using psychosocial strategies with Maryn.

athletics. Although she never returned to the court during her senior year, Maryn enrolled as a Sport Management major at a local Division 3 college where she is planning to try out for the women's basketball team.

Effective Psychosocial Strategies for the Athletic Trainer to Use with Maryn

The following psychosocial strategies can be applied by the athletic trainer in working with Maryn through her injury recovery process:

1. **Strategies to help maintain athletic identity:** Maryn's athletic trainer incorporated competitions into the rehabilitation program to keep her engaged in the process and to help her see the connections between rehabilitation and athletic performance.
2. **Cognitive restructuring:** Maryn's athletic trainer helped to change her negative appraisal by encouraging her to focus on positive consequences of the injury—Maryn used time off the court to immerse herself in the administrative side of athletics, ultimately finding a career path she was interested in pursuing.
3. **Social support:** Maryn's athletic trainer provided both listening support and an emotional challenge by encouraging her to break out of her "grief cycle" and find a way to stay involved with her sport and her teammates.
4. **Motivation:** Maryn's athletic trainer partnered her with other injured athletes and engaged them in rehabilitation competitions and games. This partnership also likely worked to provide additional support through their shared experiences and emotional challenges of being injured.

CONCLUSION

Most athletes are mentally healthy individuals; therefore, mood disturbance following injury is, for them, a departure from normal. Rewards for success are significant, so athletes are prepared to go to great lengths to obtain them. They spend hours and much energy physically preparing for competition, but they are generally unprepared psychologically to handle the stress associated with an unforeseen or unexpected injury. As prudent professionals working closely with an active population, athletic trainers need to understand the emotional turmoil that is experienced following injury. Injury of any type will have an emotional impact, whether sustained by youth recreational athletes, competitive collegiate athletes, or adult recreational athletes. Although motivations to return to preinjury state and reactions to injury may be significantly different, athletic trainers must remember that injury is both a physical and an emotional loss, and that each athlete will have his or her own cognitive interpretations and emotional responses to this loss. The same factors that influenced the stress before injury (recall antecedents from Chapter 3) also influence the stress after being injured. There are also these *additional* stressors to consider: physical limitations, medical uncertainty (treatment protocol, surgical outcome), rehabilitation difficulties (slowed progress, setbacks), fear of losing fitness and/or a place on a team, financial difficulties and career worries, and a sense of missed opportunities. Athletic trainers must recognize that injury results in the loss of some aspect of self and acknowledge that athletes' reactions are normal and real. Recall that emotional responses are determined, to an extent, by how athletes perceive that others expect them to react. Athletic trainers must help athletes find the silver lining in the injury: Are there benefits of being injured or about this time away from sport? In addition, the athletic trainers treating injured athletes need to understand the emotional and cognitive repercussions of athletic injury, but more importantly, they must understand their important role in helping athletes recover both physically and psychologically from athletic injury.

There is perhaps no more rewarding experience for an athletic trainer than to see an athlete with whom they have worked make a successful return to sport. However, such a return is possible only when the athlete is both physically and emotionally prepared to reenter the athletic realm. Although the majority of athletes will handle their injury with minimal emotional disruption, many athletes will have difficulty coping with the injury itself or with the impact it has on their identity, relationships, finances, and any number of other variables. Learning to facilitate positive emotional and behavioral responses following injury is part of becoming a prudent professional, as is learning when an athlete's emotional response falls outside of an athletic trainer's scope of practice, necessitating referral for psychosocial intervention.

REFERENCES

Brewer, B. W. (1994). Review and critique of models of psychological adjustment to athletic injury. *Journal of Applied Sport Psychology, 6,* 87–100.

Brewer, B. W., Andersen, M. B., & Van Raalte, J. L. (2002). Psychological aspects of sport injury rehabilitation: toward a biopsychosocial approach. In D. L. Mostofsky & L. D. Zaichkowsky (Eds.), *Medical and Psychological Aspects of Sport and Exercise* (pp. 41–54). Morgantown, WV: Fitness Information Technology.

Brewer, B. W., Cornelius, A. E., Stephan, Y., et al. (2010). Self-protective changes in athletic identity following anterior cruciate ligament reconstruction. *Psychology of Sport and Exercise, 11*(1), 1–5.

Brewer, B. W., Van Raalte, J. L., & Linder, D. E. (1993). Athletic identity: Hercules' muscles or Achilles heel? *International Journal of Sport Psychology, 24*(2), 237–254.

Brown, T. J., & Stoudemire, A. G. (1983). Normal and pathological grief. *Journal of the American Medical Association, 250*(3), 378–382.

Burke, S., & Sabiston, C. M. (2010). The meaning of the mountain: Exploring breast cancer survivors' lived experiences of subjective well-being during a climb on Mt. Kilimanjaro. *Qualitative Research in Sport, Exercise, and Health, 2*(1), 1-16.

Covassin, T., Elbin, 3rd, R. J., Larson, E., et al. (2012). Sex and age differences in depression and baseline sport-related concussion neurocognitive performance and symptoms. *Clinical Journal of Sports Medicine, 22*(2), 98–104.

Danish, S., Petitpas, A., & Hale, B. (1992). A developmental-educational intervention model of sport psychology. *The Sport Psychologist, 6,* 403–415.

Evans, L., Mitchell, I., & Jones, S. (2006). Psychological responses to sport injury: A review of current research. In S. Hanton & S. D. Mellalieu (Eds.), *Literature Reviews in Sport Psychology* (pp. 239–319). New York: Nova Science.

Gallagher, B. V., & Gardner, F. L. (2007). An examination of the relationship between early maladaptive schemas, coping, and emotional response to athletic injury. *Journal of Clinical Sport Psychology, 1,* 47–67.

Hardy, C. J., & Crace, R. K. (1990). Dealing with injury. *Sport Psychology Training Bulletin, 1*(6), 1–8.

Hedgpeth, E. G., & Gieck, J. (2004). Psychological considerations for rehabilitation of the injured athlete. In W. E. Prentice (Ed.), *Rehabilitation Techniques for Sports Medicine and Athletic Training* (4th ed.). New York: McGraw-Hill.

Heil, J. (1993). Sport psychology, the athlete at risk and the sports medicine team. In J. Heil (Ed.), *Psychology of sport injury* (pp. 1–13). Champaign: Human Kinetics.

Henderson, J. C. (2007). Suicide in sport: Athletes at risk. In D. Pargman (Ed.), *Psychological Bases of Sport Injuries* (3rd ed.). Morgantown, WV: Fitness Information Technology Incorporated.

Kübler-Ross, E. (1970). *On Death and Dying.* London: Tavistock Publications Limited.

McGrath, N. (2010). Supporting the student-athlete's return to the classroom after a sport-related concussion. *Journal of Athletic Training, 45,* 492–498.

Morrey, M. A., Stuart, M. J., Smith, A. M., & Wiese-Bjornstal, D. M. (1999). A longitudinal examination of athletes' emotional and cognitive responses to anterior cruciate ligament injury. *Clinical Journal of Sport Medicine, 9*(2), 63–69.

Petitpas, A., & Danish, S. J. (1995). Caring for injured athletes. In S. M. Murphy (Ed.), *Sport Psychology Interventions.* Champaign, IL: Human Kinetics.

Rotella, R. J., Ogilvie, B. C., & Perrin, D. H. (1999). The malingering athlete: Psychological considerations. In D. Pargman (Ed.), *Psychological Bases of Sport Injuries* (2nd ed.). Morgantown, WV: Fitness Information Technology Incorporated.

Smith, A. M., & Millener, E. K. (1994). Injured athletes and the risk of suicide. *Journal of Athletic Training, 29*(4), 337–341.

Tasiemski, T., & Brewer, B. W. (2011). Athletic identity, sport participation, and psychological adjustment in people with spinal cord injury. *Adapted Physical Activity Quarterly, 28,* 233–250.

Tedeschi, R. G., & Calhoun, L. G. (2004). Posttraumatic growth: Conceptual foundations and empirical evidence. *Psychological Inquiry, 15*(1), 1–18.

Udry, E., Gould, D., Bridges, D., & Beck, L. (1997). Down but not out: Athletic responses to season-ending injuries. *Journal of Sport & Exercise Psychology, 19,* 229–248.

Wadey, R., Evans, L., Evans, K., & Mitchell, I. (2011). Perceived benefits following sport injury: a qualitative examination of their antecedents and underlying mechanisms. *Journal of Applied Sport Psychology, 23*(2), 142–158.

Wiese-Bjornstal, D. M., Smith A. M., Shaffer S. M., & Morrey, M. A. (1998). An integrated model of response to sport injury: Psychological and sociological dynamics. *Journal of Applied Sport Psychology, 10,* 46–69.

BOARD OF CERTIFICATION STRATEGIES AND COMPETENCIES

As the Sixth Edition Role Delineation study outlines, athletic trainers are responsible for reconditioning participants for optimal performance and function (Domain 4: Treatment and Rehabilitation). As discussed in this chapter, athletic trainers must consider the emotional impact of injury in conjunction with physical rehabilitation efforts. They must understand the theoretical background of psychosocial and emotional responses, and then apply them to athletes in varying contexts depending on their personalities, situations, and injuries. In addition, athletic trainers must learn to implement psychosocial interventions to facilitate an athlete's psychological return-to-activity needs and must be able to identify athletes who are in need of psychosocial referral. Specific to the Fifth Edition Athletic Training Education Competencies, this chapter has introduced and explained theories and models of emotional responses to injury (PS-2).

Board of Certification Style Questions

1. Intentionally prolonging recovery because of fear of returning to competition is characteristic of which phenomenon?
   a. Emotional maladjustment to injury
   b. Malingering
   c. Post-traumatic growth (PTG)
   d. Secondary gain
2. According to Wiese-Bjornstal and colleagues' (1998) integrated model of response to sport injury, which of the following would be considered to impact an athlete's cognitive appraisal of an injury? (Select all that apply.)
   a. Injury severity
   b. Coping skills
   c. Level of competition
   d. Coach/teammate influence
3. According to Hedgpeth and Gieck's (2004) progressive reactions of injured athletes based on severity of injury and length of rehabilitation model, which factors influence athlete response to injury the most?
   a. Personal and situational factors
   b. Injury severity and rehabilitation length
   c. Appraisal of injury as threatening/nonthreatening
   d. Cause of injury (accident vs. aggressive act)
4. Which of the following is NOT one of the four issues that make concussive injuries psychologically unique as compared with other athletic injuries?
   a. Concussion is considered to be an "invisible injury"
   b. Concussion requires lengthy physical and cognitive rest
   c. Clear diagnosis of post-concussion syndrome (PCS) based on lingering symptoms
   d. Pressure from the media to return to play before physically and psychologically ready
5. The domains of post-traumatic growth (PTG) include all EXCEPT which one of the following:
   a. Social
   b. Cognitive and emotional
   c. Personal
   d. Goal setting
   e. Philosophical

END-OF-CHAPTER EXERCISES

1. In considering the Athlete Insider section at the start of the chapter, make a list of the personal and situational factors that will likely influence Maryn's emotional response to injury.

2. In examining the integrated model of response to the sport injury (Wiese-Bjornstal et al., 1998), athletic trainers understand that intervention is possible to change the outcome (cognitive, emotional, behavioral response). Consider an injured athlete at your clinical site. How might you intervene to facilitate positive reactions following injury?

Factors That Affect Cognitive Appraisal	Factors That Affect Emotional Response	Factors That Affect Behavioral Response
Cognitive Intervention(s)	**Emotional Intervention(s)**	**Behavioral Intervention(s)**

3. Think back to the worst athletic injury you have ever seen (it may even be one that you experienced yourself as an athlete). What types of negative or irrational statements have you heard? Write down *specific* statements.
   a. How could you use the theory of PTG to encourage positive responses to this injury?
   b. How could you reframe these statements into realistic, positive statements?

4. "Please tell me it's not my ACL!" In cases where the diagnosis is the worst-case scenario, how should an athletic trainer respond to facilitate the most positive possible emotional reaction to the injury?

5. Read the following and describe the issues that would likely influence Matt's cognitive appraisal and emotional response to this period of forced inactivity:

   Matt is a 16-year-old lacrosse player with ambitions to play at the collegiate and professional levels someday. He has been a starting attackman for his elite club team for 3 years, and is a powerful opponent and an explosive scorer. Last month, Matt's parents' divorce was finalized, and he relocated with his mother from Massachusetts to Maryland. Matt had a hard time leaving his friends and girlfriend behind, but he was optimistic about a tryout with a local elite team that his former club coach arranged for him. As he practiced with the team this week in preparation for his game-day tryout, he realized that these players were just as skilled as he is, and many of them seemed bigger and stronger as well. He knows he needs to come out strong and play aggressively during the game to earn a spot on the team. During warm-ups, he takes stock of the opposing team; these players seem just as tough and skilled as his own potential teammates. As he heads into the locker room for the pregame talk, he overhears the head coach comment, "That new kid doesn't seem to be worth his hype." Matt is extremely anxious for the game to start; he feels his heart racing as he grips and regrips his stick throughout the National Anthem. He stands in the box and waits for his chance on the field. During the first ground ball, Matt goes hard—headfirst into an opponent. He opens his eyes to find his athletic trainer standing over him. Matt lies and says, "I'm fine; I just got the wind knocked out of me." Between periods, Matt collapses in the locker room and is taken to the hospital where he is diagnosed with a concussion. He will likely have to sit out from lacrosse for at least 2 weeks.

Cognitive	Emotional

6. Identify an injured athlete at your clinical site who you believe has a strong athletic identity. What specific strategies would you use to help him or her maintain this strong athletic identity throughout the extended rehabilitation process?

7. As an athletic trainer, what steps could you take to address suspected malingering in an athlete who complains of lower back pain?

Chapter 5

Communication and Athlete Education Skills for the Athletic Trainer

Jennifer Stiller-Ostrowski and Laura J. Kenow

CHAPTER OUTLINE

CHAPTER OUTLINE *continued*

KEY TERMS

Active listening Communication technique that requires the listener to feed back what is heard by restating or paraphrasing; to confirm what was heard and to confirm the understanding of both parties.

Affect A feeling or emotion.

Attending skills Ability to elicit information from others and listen intently to responses.

Benign pain Temporary occurrence of discomfort that is not associated with new tissue damage; characterized as dull and generalized with no swelling or localized tenderness.

Biopsychosocial perspective The view that biological, psychological (e.g., thoughts, emotions, behaviors), and social factors all play a significant role in human functioning in the context of disease or illness.

Cognitive appraisal Interpretation of a situation.

Decoding Process of interpreting meaning from the symbolic codes used to send a message.

Empathy Being sensitive to and vicariously experiencing the feelings, thoughts, or motives of another person.

Encoding Process of putting an intended message into symbolic code (e.g., words, gestures, facial expressions) that can be observed.

Feedback A verbal or nonverbal response or reaction to a message received.

Healing cycle Cycle of recovery characterized by ups, downs, plateaus, and setbacks.

Healing imagery Focusing attention on a target visual stimulus to produce a specific physiological change that can promote healing.

Injury pain Occurrence of pain that signals actual or potential tissue damage.

Listening Perception and understanding of auditory signals.

Message A thought, feeling, or idea that is conveyed to another person.

Noise Internal and external barriers that prevent effective delivery or receipt of communicated messages.

Nonverbal communication The expression of thoughts, feelings, or ideas without the use of words.

One-way communication Communication process focused exclusively on getting messages from the sender to the receiver.

Open posture An open stance in which arms and legs are not crossed in any way.

Paralanguage Vocal characteristics associated with communication.

Paraphrasing Process of restating what was understood in a message back to the sender.

Proxemics Communication expressed through the space between people as they interact.

Rapport The harmonious or synchronous relationship of two or more people who relate well to each other.

Receiver Person to whom a sender conveys a communicated message.

Reframing Changing the way one views a situation by consciously choosing to attend to different aspects of the situation.

Sender A person who wishes to convey a message to another.

Two-way communication A bidirectional sharing of information between the sender and receiver.

Verbal communication Use of written or spoken messages to convey a thought, feeling, or idea.

CHAPTER OBJECTIVES

After reading this chapter, you will be able to:

1. Identify the key components in the interpersonal communication process.
2. Identify the mechanisms of nonverbal communication.
3. Identify methods of developing rapport with athletes, both before and after injury.
4. Describe why injury education is important for healing outcomes following sport injury.
5. Describe types of relevant injury-related information that must be communicated to athletes.
6. Identify the importance of a fully developed communication skill set to provide appropriate injury-related information to injured athletes and other involved parties.
7. Recognize the importance of communication and education strategies throughout the injury process, from initial diagnosis through return to participation.
8. Recognize the need for rapport and effective communication and education skills to engage the athlete in the use of psychosocial strategies.
9. Implement communication and education strategies designed to enhance the effectiveness of other psychosocial intervention techniques.

ATHLETE INSIDER

Mike is a junior on the university's lacrosse team. He was a highly recruited, multisport athlete from a small town in Massachusetts. He had never been injured before—until he experienced shoulder pain and a loss of power with shooting and passing midway through the fall preseason of his junior year. Mike is very popular and outgoing around his teammates, and the coaches respect him for his work ethic; however, the athletic trainer knows little about him. This morning, the athletic trainer and Mike traveled to the team physician's office to review the results of his magnetic resonance imaging. Because the athletic trainer had never really spoken with him before, the car ride and the time in the waiting room were somewhat awkward. After he and the athletic trainer are called back to the office, Mike learns from the team physician that he has a significant labral tear that is causing his symptoms. As the doctor goes on about treatment options, the athletic trainer sees Mike's eyes begin to glaze over. Mike is very quiet on the return trip back to campus. As they enter the athletic training room, he looks at the athletic trainer and says, "Well, I guess I'll be spending a lot of time in here."

INTRODUCTION

This chapter focuses on the importance of communication skills and educational efforts in the daily activities of athletic trainers. The basics of interpersonal communication processes are presented and used as a foundation for discussing educational efforts with athletic trainers. This chapter discusses the development of ***rapport*** between

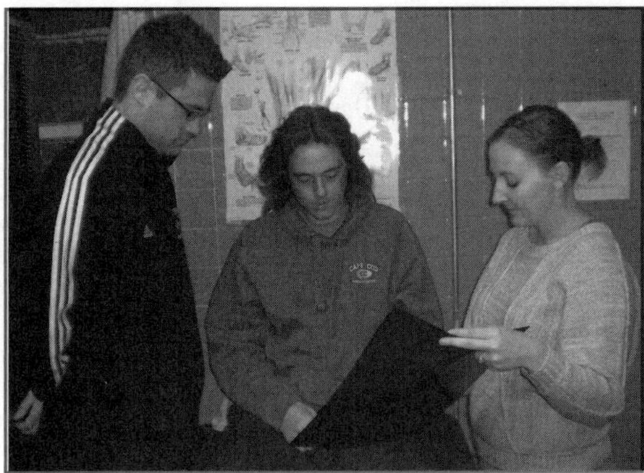

Figure 5-1 | Athlete Insider *(Courtesy of John Ostrowski)*

athletic trainers and athletes. Quite often, the first interaction athletes have with their athletic trainer is following an injury, and this presents inherent challenges for both parties. This chapter also focuses on applying communication skills when providing injury education to athletes and other stakeholders. The remainder of the chapter is dedicated to integrating communication and education skills into injury rehabilitation to facilitate holistic recovery from sports injury. This chapter emphasizes which types of information to communicate, as well as strategies and learning exercises for communicating with and educating athletes.

DEVELOPING A HOLISTICALLY TRAINED ATHLETIC TRAINER

It is essential that athletic trainers have the ability to communicate with and educate patients. They must put patients at ease, often in very scary and uncertain situations. Athletic trainers must be good listeners to help identify symptoms, and they must be excellent communicators with the ability to translate complex medical information into terms that various types of patients can understand. Because of frequent contact with injured athletes during recovery and rehabilitation, it is essential that athletic trainers be holistically trained to address the unique psychosocial consequences of injury. A holistically trained athletic trainer takes the complete athlete into consideration from a ***biopsychosocial perspective***. Although knowledge and skill in injury evaluation, therapeutic modalities, and therapeutic exercise are obviously important, the inability to effectively communicate about these assessment and treatment techniques potentially diminishes their worth. For example, athletic trainers cannot reassure athletes or facilitate positive emotional responses to injury if they cannot communicate appropriately, they cannot motivate athletes if they are unable to communicate the goals of the rehabilitation, and they cannot engage athletes in psychosocial techniques (e.g., imagery, self-talk, relaxation) if they cannot explain the benefits of the techniques in a way athletes can understand. In summary, a holistically trained athletic trainer is in the best position to facilitate optimal recovery from injury.

Teaching communication skills is an integral part of a global patient-oriented curriculum, because they are core elements of good medical practice. Clear, controlled communication is one of the primary responsibilities of athletic trainers throughout the injury-management process; in fact, athletic trainers and physiotherapists have consistently identified communication as one of the most effective strategies for facilitating psychological coping. Although there is no gold standard for good communication between the health-care provider and patient, emphasis on the patients' ideas, concerns, emotions, and needs for education are key. In athletic training, the clinician's good listening skills are essential to allow athletes to fully express themselves, to explain their injury, and to ask questions about what to expect over the course of their injury. Communication skills also enable an athletic trainer to provide effective social support to the athlete, to encourage athlete adherence with the rehabilitation program, and to engage athletes in the use of psychosocial skills.

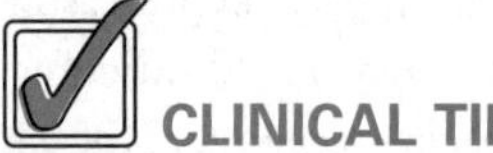

CLINICAL TIP

Evidence in the medical field has been reported that good patient–provider communication is related to better outcomes, better compliance, and higher satisfaction of both patient and provider (Brown, Stewart, & Ryan, 2003; Stewart et al., 1999). With athletic injuries, essential communication skills include establishing rapport and trust with the athletes, members of the sports medicine team, and the coaching staff; educating those same individuals about the injury process; and ongoing communication throughout the initial injury, recovery, rehabilitation, and return-to-activity phases. Athletic training students are still in the process of learning about injury pathology and rehabilitation techniques but likely already have many of the skills necessary for effective communication. Moreover, athletic training students have any number of opportunities to develop these skills. Certified athletic trainers should also strive to improve their communication skills.

EVIDENCE-BASED PRACTICE

Deveugele, M., Derese, A., De Maesschalack, S., Willems, S., Van Driel, M., & De Maeseneer, J. (2005). Teaching communication skills to medical students, a challenge in the curriculum? *Patient Education and Counseling, 58*(3), 265–270.

Description of the Study

This study reports on the implementation of a new medical communication curriculum at Ghent University (Belgium). Communication training is integrated into each year of the curriculum, beginning with basic skills and progressing to medical communication and consultation training. Miller's (1990) learning pyramid is used as a framework: knowing, knowing how, showing, and doing. The curriculum implements several different educational methods, including videotape demonstrations, paper "case studies," and role-play activities with classmates or simulated patients.

Results of the Study

Learning objectives for the 7-year curriculum are outlined; each set of learning objectives is coupled with a "real-life exercise" that allows the student to develop skill in the identified areas. Students are assessed annually by means of an objective structured clinical examination (objectives are specific for every year and build on skills from previous years). Authors reported that rehearsal each year leads to better acquisition of skills. Students who struggle with communication skills are identified early in the curriculum, and remediation is provided. Remedial training consists of extra small-group training sessions (first 3 years) and feedback following videotaped rehearsal with simulated patients (last 4 years).

Implications for Athletic Training Practice

The study highlights the disconnect between competency and performance; although students may understand the theory behind a skill, they are not able to successfully implement a technique without practicing it. Oftentimes, it is assumed that athletic training students' communication skills will develop with time and experience. In reality, the development of interpersonal skills and communication and educational techniques require deliberate training and practice. Theoretical framework should be laid early in the curriculum, with training modules and practical experience threaded throughout the curriculum.

BASICS OF COMMUNICATION

Communication is the process of sharing thoughts, ideas, and feelings with others and having those thoughts, ideas, and feelings understood by the people with whom we are communicating. The adage "say what you mean and mean what you say" makes this sound easy. However, communication is complicated and filled with opportunities for miscommunication to occur. Communication comes in two forms: ***verbal communication*** involves the use of written or spoken messages, whereas ***nonverbal communication*** involves the expression of ideas, thoughts, or feelings without the use of words. There will always be instances where communication failed or people misunderstood what was said or meant for one reason or another. However, understanding and applying the basic steps of the communication process will hopefully facilitate more effective communication efforts among athletic trainers.

The basic communication process is outlined in Figure 5-2. Communication begins when a person has

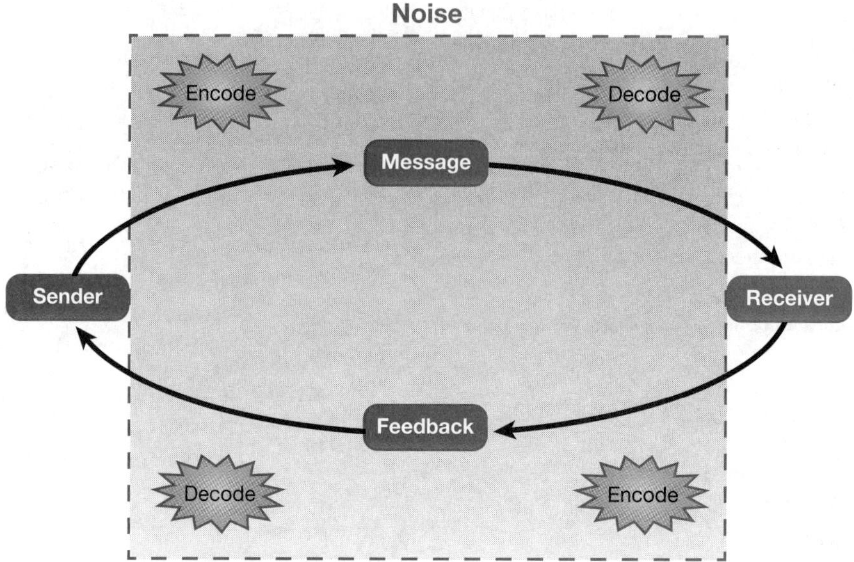

Figure 5-2 | Communication basics.

a thought or idea he or she wishes to convey. This person is the ***sender***. To get that idea, or ***message***, across to another person, it must be put into a symbolic code. ***Encoding*** refers to selecting words, actions, gestures, expressions, or some combination of all these to represent a thought, feeling, or idea. The encoded message is sent to the person with whom the sender is communicating, the ***receiver***. The receiver observes the coded communication and attempts to interpret what the coding means, a process called ***decoding***. In most communication situations, once receivers have interpreted the message, they provide ***feedback***, another message that must be encoded and decoded, to the original sender. In this way, communication is a dynamic, two-way process of information give-and-take between the sender and receiver.

Communication happens effectively when the encoding and decoding of messages are consistent. That is, the encoded thought, idea, or feeling from the sender is the same thought, idea, or feeling decoded and understood by the receiver. However, when encoding and decoding do not agree, confusion and communication pitfalls occur. For example, former FBI chief J. Edgar Hoover once corrected a memo his secretary typed by writing a note stating, "Watch the borders" (referring to the margins of the memo). Misunderstanding his intended message, she added his comment to the memo and sent it out nationwide. Instantly, all FBI agents on the Canadian and Mexican borders were placed on high alert.

Our verbal language is rife with these potential misunderstandings. Words have multiple meanings, and the cultural use of terms further complicates the process. Consider the word *bad*. Most often, this word has negative connotations; however, cultural use of the term has implied that it can also mean something emphatically good, such as a sports car described as "a bad car." Furthermore, consider the use of the terms *tonic*, *soda*, and *pop*. They are all used at times to describe soft drinks; however, use the word *tonic* to request a beverage in Colorado and seltzer will arrive. Use the same word in Boston and a cola will most likely be delivered. Cross-cultural differences further complicate communication even in countries that supposedly speak the same language. New Zealand, Australia, Great Britain, and the United States are all considered English-speaking countries, yet a jumper in the United States refers to a dress, whereas a jumper in Australia refers to a sweater.

SPECIAL CONSIDERATIONS

Athletic trainers will encounter situations where they must work with international students who do not speak English as their first language. Communication in these situations becomes even more challenging because the limited vocabulary of the international student rarely includes medical terminology. In these cases, it is extremely difficult for the international student–athlete to find the words to adequately verbalize their signs and symptoms, and athletic trainers will be challenged to find understandable terminology to effectively communicate specifics about the injury and the rehabilitation process. At that point, it may be helpful to identify interpreters, either formally or informally, with whom athletic trainers can work to assist in communicating with international student–athletes.

Verbal communication creates many challenges for athletic trainers, and yet this is only part of the communication puzzle. Nonverbal communication is equally, if not more, challenging. Nonverbal communication refers to any communication that does not involve words. It can include things such as facial expressions, gestures, and postures, among others that will be discussed shortly. Although verbal communication most often requires a conscious effort, nonverbal communication occurs at a subconscious level. People are frequently unaware of messages they are sending through their facial expressions, their degree of eye contact, or the position of their body (Table 5-1). In most communication, nonverbal messages complement verbal messages, but sometimes nonverbal expressions can produce mixed messages. Athletic trainers are often engaged in high-level multitasking during interactions with athletes. Consider how this "busy" state could affect nonverbal communication. For example, saying, "I care," but failing to look the other person in the eye raises questions about the sincerity of the verbally expressed concern. Research has demonstrated that people are more likely to believe nonverbal communication over verbal when mixed messages are present. In this case, the injured athlete may perceive that the sentiment is disingenuous. It is imperative that athletic trainers are knowledgeable about the types of subconscious nonverbal communication they may be sending. Nonverbal messages can be communicated via a number of pathways, including touch, gestures, facial expressions, body language, ***proxemics***, and ***paralanguage*** (Table 5-2).

TABLE 5-1 **Examples of Nonverbal Messages**

Nonverbal Action	Message(s) Conveyed
Crossing arms over chest	Defensiveness, boredom, disagreement, cold
Firm, positive handshake	Confidence
Smile	Happiness, warmth, acceptance
Looking at watch	Impatience, tardiness
Leaning back in chair	Relaxation, fatigue, disinterest
Leaning forward in chair	Interest, excitement
Furrowed brow	Confusion, concentration, anger
Eye contact	Interest, concern
Glazed or unfocused eyes	Overwhelm, daydreaming, fatigue
Fast, high-pitched voice	Excitement, nervousness, joy, anger
Slow, low-pitched voice	Calmness, fatigue, uncertainty

CLINICAL TIP

Because of the potential for touch to be interpreted as sexually suggestive, and the necessity of touching in the athletic training profession, athletic trainers should be cautious in their use of touch. To be on the safe side, it is advisable for athletic trainers to communicate the need for touching to the athlete before initiating contact so as not to send an unintended message.

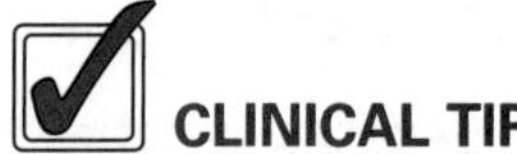

CLINICAL TIP

Athletic trainers should be cognizant of messages sent by proxemics. When communicating with injured athletes, athletic trainers should try to place themselves at a level equal to or below their athletes' level to imply equality in the communication process. Also, they should try to minimize the presence of objects such as tables or desks that could communicate a separation from injured athletes.

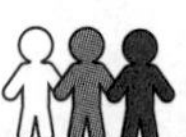

SPECIAL CONSIDERATIONS

Athletic training programs (AT programs) frequently adopt dress codes for athletic training students. Clothing can send strong nonverbal messages about personal values, attitudes, and behaviors. Professional settings call for a particular style of clothing that gives the impression of competence and quality. Deviating from expected dress codes can communicate a range of messages from ignorance to disrespect to outright rebellion. Athletic trainers should be cognizant of the messages conveyed by their daily clothing choices.

Effective communication requires the recognition and use of both verbal and nonverbal messaging skills. Using these skills to effectively convey thoughts, ideas, and feelings to others is critical; however, effective communication is a two-way street. As shown in Figure 5-3, during ***one-way communication***, information flows in only one direction. In this form, communication is treated as a manipulation of others, with one party sending out messages without any concern about whether the other person is receiving the intended message. For the receiver, this type of communication can become very frustrating, as he or she has no opportunity to ask for clarification or share personal information. However, in ***two-way communication***, information flows bidirectionally between the sender and receiver to assure that both parties share the intended message. While one person sends a message, the other engages in ***listening*** and ***attending skills***. Then the roles reverse, so the speaker engages in listening and attending while the other person is allowed to speak.

When it comes to communicating with athletes and educating them about their injury, an extremely important yet often neglected component is the *listening* aspect. Listening and attending are essential in effective communication, yet it is common to hear people comment about communication situations that "She heard me but did not really listen to what I said." Hearing implies that auditory

TABLE 5-2 **Pathways of Communicating Nonverbal Messages**

Touch. Handshakes, pats on the back, a touch on the arm, or hugs are common examples of touch used as a means of communication. The comfort level for using or receiving touch as a communication mechanism varies greatly from person to person. Depending on the style and location of touch, the individual involved, and the circumstances, touch can be perceived as reassuring, threatening, or even sexually suggestive.

Gestures. Gestures refer to physical movements used to convey a message in place of words. Examples of gestures include waving a hand to say hello or using a thumbs-up or okay sign to communicate that things are satisfactory.

Facial expressions. Emotions, or ***affect***, are often communicated through facial contortions. Emotions such as pain, anger, concern, confusion, or surprise are often easily conveyed through facial expressions.

Body language. The way communicators posture their body can send messages; however, these messages are often difficult to decode. For example, folding your arms across your chest could be interpreted as a sign of defensiveness, boredom, aggression, disagreement, or simply being physically cold. Other examples of body language include eye contact, positional leaning toward or away from a speaker, shifting body weight from foot to foot, or glancing at a watch or clock.

TABLE 5-2 Pathways of Communicating Nonverbal Messages—cont'd

Proxemics. Proxemics refers to communication through the space things occupy. This can be measured by the space or distance between people or by the arrangement of objects in a room. For example, each person has an area of comfortable personal space. Invasion of that personal space results in discomfort. On the other hand, standing or sitting far away from another person can also create uneasiness and send messages of disinterest or rejection. In relation to objects, trying to communicate across some barrier like a desk or table implies a message of detachment or a power differential. Similarly, positioning oneself above another person during communication insinuates power differences.

Paralanguage. Paralanguage refers to voice characteristics associated with communication. It includes such things as tone of voice; rate of speech; or speech volume, pitch, and rhythm. For example, expressing a verbal message in a fast, high-pitched voice can convey a message of anxiety, fear, or excitement; in contrast, speaking slowly or in a monotone voice can imply boredom or uncertainty. Although paralanguage relates to spoken messages, it is still a form of nonverbal communication because it relates to the quality of speech and not the spoken words themselves.

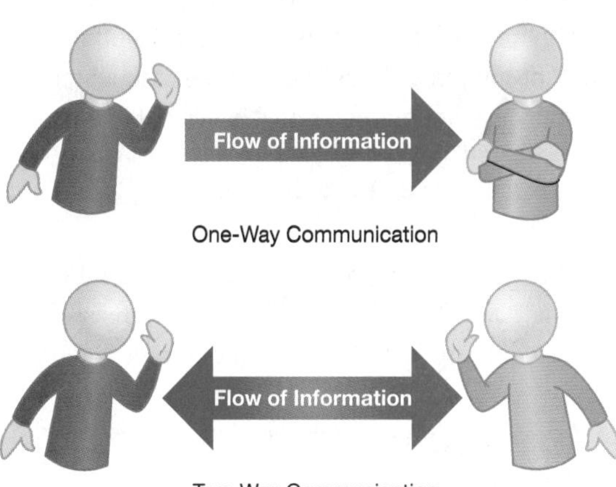

Figure 5-3 | Information flow in one-way versus two-way communication.

signals were received; however, listening requires that the auditory signals were not only received but also understood. ***Active listening*** is an oft-neglected part of the communication process because communicators become complacent. Too frequently, when people finish expressing a thought or feeling, they almost immediately begin to mentally prepare their next statement rather than truly listening or attending to the other person. A prime example of this occurs during introductions. A new person states his or her name while you are mentally preparing to say yours. As a result, seconds later you cannot remember the other person's name. Fortunately, listening and attending skills can be improved by tuning in to several key elements, as outlined in Table 5-3.

When communicating with injured athletes, it is important for athletic trainers to listen intently to the athlete's story and probe to explore their ideas, concerns, and expectations. Athletic trainers must be trained in the art of listening for several reasons: 1) to obtain information about symptoms that may be important in determining how an athlete should progress with the rehabilitation program, 2) to demonstrate an understanding of or ***empathy*** for the athlete's perspective, and 3) to identify any areas of confusion or misunderstanding regarding what will happen to them and what is expected of them. Athletic trainers often become overly concerned with communicating their knowledge and can easily lose sight of the athlete's need to be heard. In addition, true psychosocial care of the athlete requires that athletic trainers listen not only to what athletes say but also to what they *don't say*. Often, what athletes omit reflects the areas where they lack understanding or are experiencing fear or apprehension about the injury process. Attending to the athlete and ***paraphrasing*** what the athlete just said are essential communication skills, and athletic trainers should work to develop this skill set. Allowing the athlete to talk and share not only provides useful information for the athletic trainer, but talking through a situation may also help the athlete begin to cope with the injury and its repercussions. Talking through a situation with an informed listener may also help the athlete make a decision about a treatment option. When athletic

TABLE 5-3 **Methods of Improving Listening and Attending Skills**

Focus attention. When one is not sending a message, he or she should pay full attention to what the speaker is saying rather than planning his or her "next move." People who attend to their own thoughts rather than the message directed at them have poor listening habits.

Maintain good eye contact. It is important to maintain good eye contact with a speaker; however, this does not mean continual staring because this can create discomfort. On the other extreme, wandering eyes often create wandering thoughts, poor listening, and poor attending ability. A balance of eye contact, blinking, and short breaks is ideal.

Paraphrase. Paraphrasing refers to restating a message back to the speaker to ensure proper understanding. Paraphrasing often begins with "I heard you say ..." Paraphrasing enables the speaker either to confirm that the decoded message is consistent with what was intended or to provide clarification about inconsistencies with the intended message.

Ask questions. If the listener is having trouble understanding the facts being conveyed, it is important to ask for more details or clarification from the speaker.

Use empathy. Empathy refers to viewing the world through another person's eyes and accurately sensing the feelings of that person. Empathy does not mean that listeners adopt another person's feelings as their own. Rather, it implies that listeners recognize and appreciate the emotions and feelings that the other person is experiencing. The adage of "walking a mile in another person's shoes" summarizes the concept behind empathy. Expressing empathy reassures others that they are understood and it is critical to effective listening and overall communication.

trainers respond to athletes, it is important to pay attention to matching verbal and nonverbal communication to avoid sending mixed messages. For example, telling an athlete, "It will be okay," while looking concerned will not be as reassuring as the same comment matched with a smile and an optimistic nod.

Communication is a dynamic, ongoing exchange of information between a sender and a receiver. The information is exchanged through both verbal and nonverbal messages, and effective communication requires not only being an effective speaker but also an attentive listener. One final element to consider in the communication process is ***noise*** (represented by the dashed lines in Fig. 5-2). Noise refers to barriers that prevent messages from getting through effectively. It interferes with the ability to effectively encode or decode messages, or both, as well as the ease of message transmission. Many different sources of noise can compromise communication. Table 5-4 summarizes potential causes of noise and divides them into internal and external sources. Internal sources of noise originate within the individuals trying to communicate, whereas external sources of noise are barriers that exist outside of the individuals. Establishing a strong rapport with athletes can minimize some internal sources of noise. It will also minimize the times encoding and decoding differences occur.

BUILDING RAPPORT WITH ATHLETES

When an injury occurs, the relationship with the athletic trainer becomes one of the athlete's most important connections. Ideally, some form of rapport was established before injury; however, the first interaction athletes have with their athletic trainers often occurs only after they sustain an injury. Athletes are more likely to listen and adhere to what is suggested or advocated by their athletic trainer if a personal relationship has been established; whether before or after injury, development of rapport is key to ensuring optimal physical and psychosocial recovery.

Rapport is often a by-product of athletic trainers' abilities to demonstrate empathy toward athletes. As mentioned earlier, empathy is conveyed when athletic trainers demonstrate that they understand and appreciate what athletes are going through, both on and off the playing

TABLE 5-4 Sources of Noise in Communication Situations

Internal Barriers	External Barriers
• Fatigue	• Physical noise (e.g., jackhammer, automobile traffic, crowded gymnasium or athletic facility)
• Poor listening skills	• Distractions (e.g., others walking by)
• Poor attitude toward the sender	• E-mail/phone/Internet not working
• Poor attitude toward the information	• Bad phone or Skype connection
• Lack of interest in the message	• Time of the day (e.g., too early or too late in the day)
• Fear	• Language that is too technical
• Mistrust of the sender	
• Past experiences with communication in similar situations	
• Negative attitude	
• Problems at home	
• Lack of common experiences with the sender	
• Cultural expectations	
• Emotions	

field. Empathy is often reflected in the athletic trainers' nonverbal behaviors. Behaviors such as giving athletes undivided attention, looking them in the eye, sitting beside them, and maintaining an ***open posture*** all demonstrate empathic behavior during communication. In addition, athletic trainers who allow athletes to freely express their concerns and emotions in the athletic training room without judgment or criticism also demonstrate empathy. As a result of these behaviors, athletes feel supported and understood by their athletic trainer, and rapport strengthens.

Another key component in the development of rapport is mutual trust. When athletes feel supported and understood, they know they are in a safe environment, and trust quickly follows. The professional and ethical behaviors expected of all athletic trainers provide a strong basis on which to build trust. Athletic trainers are expected to demonstrate honesty and integrity, exhibit compassion and empathy, put the athletes' needs and best interests above all else, keep information shared by athletes confidential, and advocate for the athletes' needs (National Athletic Trainers' Association, 2005). Because trust is a two-way street, in return, athletic trainers should clearly tell athletes that they expect honest, direct reporting on their injuries and rehabilitation experiences. Under these conditions, athletes and athletic trainers can build strong trustworthy bonds that significantly increase rapport.

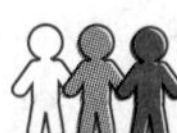

SPECIAL CONSIDERATIONS

It is important to keep in mind that injured athletes often show weakness to only two groups of people: family and athletic trainers. For example:

Athletic Trainer: "How is your shoulder feeling today?"

Athlete: "It's killing me, I think I may have done a bit too much in rehabilitation yesterday."

Coach: "How's your shoulder feeling today?"

Athlete: "Great coach, I think I can go today!"

Injured athletes are likely to tell teammates and coaching staff what they want to hear. For this reason, it is essential for athletic trainers to become excellent communicators, developing rapport with injured athletes and encouraging them to be honest about how their injury is progressing. Through this communication, athletic trainers can help to ensure that athletes are not pressured to return to play by teammates and coaches, but rather return to play only when they are ready.

VIRTUAL FIELD TRIP

To review the documents that outline the ethical and professional expectations of athletic trainers, go to http://davisplus.fadavis.com.

Establishing Rapport Before Injury

From the first day of practice, athletic trainers can begin to develop trust and rapport with their athletes. They can start by speaking to athletes on a personal level. Several appropriate topics of conversation can assist in getting to know an athlete as a person (without asking overly personal questions). For example, communicating with athletes on a personal level shows genuine interest in their lives both within and outside of the sport context. In addition, showing interest in everyday activities promotes a feeling of being cared for and supported. These conversations can occur during prepractice taping or stretching sessions, on the bus traveling to competitions, or during water breaks or downtime during practice. Asking athletes about their day, their previous sports successes, and their family, or sharing lighthearted jokes help develop an increasing sense of rapport. Athletic trainers can also share a bit of themselves with athletes, within appropriate boundaries. For example, it would be appropriate to discuss a mutual love of major league baseball teams but inappropriate to discuss details of a relationship with a significant other. Rapport will grow if athletes can see athletic trainers as people beyond their professional roles.

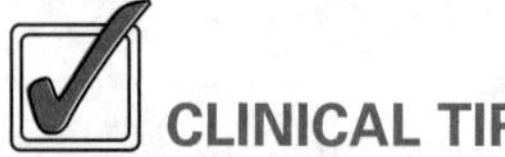

CLINICAL TIP

Athletic trainers should seek to introduce athletes to as many members of the extended sports medicine team as possible during the preseason or before injuries occur. Athletes' familiarity with the extended medical resources readily available to them should facilitate their trust and confidence in the competence of these resources.

Developing a Rapport After Injury

If an injury occurs before the athletic trainer and the athlete establish a relationship, it is essential to find common ground as a base before attempting to build a trusting relationship in rehabilitation. Even if a personal rapport was established before injury, this relationship must continue to be nurtured to provide the best care for an injured athlete. Good communication is important to help athletes cope successfully with the negative repercussions of their injury. Within the injury context, the athletic trainer must attempt to determine the types of communication that athletes prefer and respond to in order to provide clear, timely education about the healing process and to encourage adherence to the rehabilitation program.

Following injury, an easy first step to developing or increasing rapport is to listen attentively to athletes. Athletic trainers who listen nonjudgmentally and demonstrate empathic acceptance of the athlete's reaction to injury will reassure athletes who wish to or need to vent their emotions in the immediate aftermath. Athletic trainers can provide assurance that the athlete is in capable hands that will assist them in dealing with this adversity. It is important to foster the athlete's trust and communicate honestly about what is and is not known. There will be a multitude of unknowns in the immediate aftermath of injury. The goal is not to have all the answers but to reassure the athlete that the resources are in place among members of the sports medicine team to provide all the necessary answers.

Consider the scenario with Mike, our injured lacrosse player from the Athlete Insider section at the beginning of the chapter. Mike and his athletic trainer had clearly not established a rapport before injury; however, the athletic trainer will now take on an extremely important role in Mike's life as they work together toward the common goal of returning him to the lacrosse field. To communicate effectively through this process and provide Mike with the information needed to make a treatment decision, his athletic trainer will have to find a way to earn Mike's trust and confidence in their ability to move him successfully through this process.

EVIDENCE-BASED PRACTICE

Stiller, J. L., & Ostrowski, J. A. (2007). Tricks of the trade: Enhancing interpersonal skills. *Athletic Therapy Today, 12*(6), 33–35.

Description of the Study

This article outlines attributes of athletic trainers perceived by injured athletes to have excellent interpersonal skills. This report comes from an unpublished research study that involved in-depth interviews with nine injured collegiate athletes.

Results of the Study

Athletes respond best to athletic trainers who demonstrate empathy, who seem interested in them as people (outside of sport), who listen intently, and who model a positive attitude toward recovery. A table in the report designates positive and negative traits of athletic trainers, as reported by injured athletes. The report highlights the importance of developing an appropriate personal relationship and rapport with the injured athlete, indicating that athletes are more likely to adhere to the rehabilitation program if they have a rapport with their athletic trainers. Injured athletes' confidence in the knowledge and ability of their athletic trainers is strengthened when athletic trainers are willing to admit when they do not know the answer to a question; searching for answers and following up with athletes was viewed as a way that athletic trainers demonstrated commitment to the athlete's recovery.

Implications for Athletic Training Practice

The majority of traits perceived as being negative by injured athletes center on the athletic trainer's poor communication and interpersonal skills. Positive traits centered on the ability to relate to athletes on a personal level, and to explain injuries and treatments in language that athletes could understand. Athletic trainers should also not be afraid to admit they don't know the answer to an athlete's question; rather, honesty about one's own lack of knowledge, followed up with a search for answers, aids in the development of a trusting relationship. Developing a rapport and appropriate personal relationships with athletes during the rehabilitation process can be helpful in ensuring adherence to the rehabilitation program; athletes are less likely to skip rehabilitation sessions if they have a personal relationship with their athletic trainer because they feel more accountable and committed.

COMMUNICATION SKILLS USED TO EDUCATE INJURED ATHLETES

Although the development of rapport is important to forge a "bond" between two individuals and open the lines of communication, it is only the foundation on which effective injury education will occur. The verbal and nonverbal communication skills discussed previously are critically important to delivering efficient and effective educational information to athletes following injury. Anyone who has sat through good versus bad academic class lectures can attest to the important relationship between communication skills and effective education. Educating injured athletes will require athletic trainers to engage in two-way communication, solicit information from injured athletes, encourage paraphrasing to ensure comprehension, remain mindful of nonverbal messages, and engage in listening as well as speaking.

Why Injury Education Is Important

When athletes sustain injury, they often have a great deal to learn. It is common for them to have a great deal of uncertainty about what happened, what they need to do to heal, and how quickly all this will take place so that they can return to sport participation. Even if athletes have previously sustained a similar injury, they may be uncertain whether this new injury experience will be any different from their first one. As discussed in Chapter 4, uncertainty produces psychological consequences for injured athletes that can interfere with the healing process. The athletic trainer must educate injured athletes about all aspects of their injury and the recovery that lies ahead.

Injury education is important for several reasons. Facilitating an accurate understanding of the injury and its associated consequences has a direct effect on athletes' ***cognitive appraisal*** processes, and consequently their emotional and behavioral reactions following injury. As mentioned in Chapter 4, following injury, athletes engage in repeated cognitive appraisals of their situation and generate a perceived ability to meet current demands. Athletes who are uncertain or lack an understanding of their injury will often make inaccurate appraisals of both the demands of the injury situation and their available resources. This can result in psychosocial and emotional challenges, and negative behavioral consequences. For example, athletes who do not understand a diagnosis of a tibial stress fracture may assume they will need to be casted (like most other fractures would). This mistaken perception may lead to increased anxiety as they reflect on the impact to their training program. Once an athlete realizes that casting is not required, continued lack of understanding of the treatment process may manifest itself through the lack of adherence with the rehabilitation program. Educating injured athletes enables them to have more realistic appraisals of their situation, often resulting in more positive psychosocial and emotional reactions.

Quality education of injured athletes is also important because of its relationship to motivation. People in general have a difficult time giving optimal effort to something they do not fully understand. For example, if people are told to jump out of a second-floor window, they will most likely hesitate to do so. However, if they are informed that they need to jump out of the window because the building is on fire and will explode at any second, they are more likely to make the jump. The same is true when working with injured athletes. If athletes can understand the "why" behind all of the rehabilitation activities they will be asked to do and how these activities directly relate to achieving the long-term goal of returning to play as quickly as possible, they are more motivated to adhere to the rehabilitation program and exert strong effort along the way. It is important to keep in mind that education is truly a process, extending from initial injury through the end of the rehabilitation process. Athletes will need frequent educational "reminders," because they are likely overwhelmed by the amount of new injury-related information they are constantly being asked to process.

What to Include in Injury Education

Depending on athletes' injury history and their familiarity with human anatomy, they will have varying degrees of knowledge about what has happened to them and what needs to occur to recover from injury. However, in all cases, there is a great deal they need to know. Box 5-1 summarizes many of the items that athletic trainers should include in injury education discussions with athletes. This list is long and will obviously take a great deal of time to address. However, this time should be considered an investment that will produce dividends in the long run. The returns on invested time to educate injured athletes include more accurate cognitive appraisals of the injury situation, more realistic expectations about the recovery process, increased confidence in the ability to heal and return to play, enhanced adherence and motivation during rehabilitation, and decreased anxiety and frustration. Together, these benefits will more than offset the time dedicated to the education process at the start.

How to Deliver the Educational Information

Break the Educational Information Into Manageable Doses

Because of the extensive amount of information that needs to be shared with injured athletes, a major challenge is to educate athletes without overloading them. There is no way that athletic trainers can deliver all the information in Box 5-1 in one or even a few discussions with injured athletes. The human attention span is limited in how much information can be perceived, processed, and stored at one time. As a result, the more information that is delivered in one dose, the greater the chances that some of it will not be attended to or stored. In addition, injured athletes are likely to experience increased levels of stress because of their injury that may compromise their ability to maintain focus and retain information. Thus, athletic trainers should break up the required information into small, manageable bites spread across the injury-recovery process. Certain pieces of information—such as options for surgical repair—will be more relevant and important at specific points in the

BOX 5-1 | Potential Content for Injury Education Discussions

- Anatomical structure of the injured body part (use of models, diagrams, books)
- Description of how the injury changes athlete's mobility or activity limits
- Guidelines for use of independent modalities, braces, and/or crutches
- Guidelines for use of medications (include purposes and negative side effects)
- Options for repairing the injury
- Explanation of diagnostic (e.g., x-ray, bone scan, magnetic resonance imaging) or surgical procedures
- Anticipated timeline for rehabilitation and recovery
- Rationale for activity restrictions during rehabilitation and healing
- Description of how rehabilitation exercises and modalities work
- Purpose for rehabilitation exercises and how they tie to recovery goals
- Guidelines for distinguishing "good" pain versus "bad" pain
- Explanation that plateaus in treatment progress should be anticipated
- Importance of athlete maintaining a positive attitude and outlook
- Description of how readiness to return will be determined
- Emphasis that rehabilitation will be cooperative effort between athlete and sports medicine team
- Resources available to assist with physical and psychosocial challenges

Source: Adapted from Heil (1993).

rehabilitation process. However, other topics will need to be addressed numerous times throughout the recovery process, such as the rationale for activity limits or the purposes for rehabilitation activities. Athletic trainers need to choose the most important and relevant information for athletes at any particular time in the rehabilitation process and provide that information first (see Table 5-5 for suggestions on ordering of information delivery). Once athletic trainers deliver the key, time-sensitive pieces, they can provide additional information as athletes demonstrate understanding of the initial, basic information.

When athletes have reached their limits of comprehension, they will most likely send nonverbal messages indicating overload. These messages can include the loss of eye contact or a "glazed" look, fidgeting or frequently shifting positions, increased distractibility by the people or things around them, yawning, or providing decreased levels of feedback. Consider the scenario with Mike, the injured lacrosse player in the Athlete Insider section at the beginning of the chapter. As the physician delivered the treatment options, his athletic trainer watched Mike for nonverbal cues that indicated the information was not being received (in this case, the athletic trainer noticed Mike's eyes begin to glaze over as the physician went on about treatment options). Thus, his athletic trainer knew what to follow up on and reinforce during a subsequent information session. Athletic trainers must remain vigilant in observing athletes' body language and eye contact for signs that it is time to stop an information session for the day. At the end of each session, the athletic trainer should ask athletes if they have any questions or concerns about the material that was discussed. These questions and concerns will highlight areas that were inadequately covered or where additional education is needed.

Use Language That Athletes Can Understand

As mentioned earlier, injured athletes will have varying degrees of familiarity with anatomical terminology and experience with injury. When communicating with athletes who have a great deal of experience with injury or who are knowledgeable about anatomical structures,

TABLE 5-5 **Integration of Communication and Education Strategies in the Injury Recovery Process**

Injury Recovery Phase	Communication Suggestions	Education Suggestions
Immediate postinjury period	• Use a calm, reassuring tone of voice. • Control nonverbal messages (keep a poker face if the injury is severe). • Minimize external noise. • Listen to the athlete's description of signs and symptoms. • Maintain eye contact. • Use proxemics and body language that express empathy. • Speak slowly and clearly when providing instruction.	• Provide instructions for ice/elevation. • Write down important instructions. • Explain use of needed crutches, braces, and slings. • Educate (with permission) the athlete's support network (family, coaches, teammates).
Initial injury evaluation	• Use proxemics and body language that express empathy. • Ask athletes to paraphrase what they have learned. • Ask about athletes' concerns and paraphrase them for clarity.	• Use models, diagrams, and pictures to help clarify anatomical details. • Give important points first. • Give possible timeline for rehabilitation scenarios. • Provide rationale for rest, ice, compression, elevation, medications, and activity limits. • Describe options for treatment. • Discuss surgical options (if needed). • Repeat important points at the end.
Surgical decision-making	• Use verbal and nonverbal (touch, eye contact, proxemics, etc.) messages to provide reassurance. • Ask athletes about their concerns. • Listen attentively and empathically.	• Discuss what athletes can expect regarding pain. • Review surgical procedural options (use diagrams or anatomical models to help clarify). • Discuss options for anesthesia if offered to the athlete.
During rehabilitation	• Build trust through solid education efforts and rehabilitation progressions. • Build rapport through conversations during rehabilitation activities. • Listen to and paraphrase athletes' concerns. • Convey empathy through nonverbal communication (proxemics, body language, eye contact, etc.) and active listening. • Observe athletes' nonverbal messages and listen to their verbal	• Continually educate athletes about what they should expect during the healing process. • Teach them how to perform rehabilitation activities properly. • Discuss why they are performing certain rehabilitation exercises or using therapeutic modalities. • Describe how exercises and modalities link to the long-term goal of returning to play.

TABLE 5-5 **Integration of Communication and Education Strategies in the Injury Recovery Process—cont'd**

Injury Recovery Phase	Communication Suggestions	Education Suggestions
	messages for signs of psychosocial or emotional distress. • Communicate verbally with athletes about what is happening to their body during rehabilitation and encourage them to paraphrase what they have learned. • Use proxemics and body language that signal an openness to receive questions. • Check in frequently and ask athletes about their motivation and satisfaction with rehabilitation sessions and overall recovery; listen closely to what is said and what is left unsaid. • Provide frequent verbal and nonverbal encouragement and feedback about rehabilitation progress. • Reassure athletes about their recovered abilities.	• Continue to use simple language (models, drawings, analogies, etc.) to discuss the anatomical changes that occur during recovery. • Discuss rationale for activity limits. • Explain the likelihood of recovery plateaus and the chance of setbacks. • Teach athletes coping techniques for frustration, boredom, and/or anxiety that they may experience. • Continually update athletes on the timeline for rehabilitation progressions. • Keep coaches and family members updated on the recovery progress and timeline. • Reinforce the differences between "good" and "bad" pain.
Return to play	• Directly question athletes about their concerns and listen attentively. • Show empathy for their feelings of uncertainty. • Discuss the mutual trust developed in your relationship and encourage athletes to trust in their rehabilitation efforts. • Communicate before, during, and after the first return to practice. • Observe nonverbal signs of discomfort or apprehension during their return and discuss those concerns. • Use appropriate proxemics by sitting next to athletes, making eye contact, and displaying body language that invites them to share concerns with you. • Normalize the apprehension that athletes may experience.	• Teach athletes relaxation techniques they can use to reduce anxiety. • Discuss what athletes should expect when returning to play regarding game fitness and feelings of uneasiness. • Educate athletes on the functional testing that will be used to determine physical readiness. • Revisit how to distinguish "good" pain from "bad" pain. • Educate coaches on signs or symptoms that would necessitate removing athletes from practice.

athletic trainers can use medical terms to describe the injury and the healing process. However, in most cases, injured athletes will have limited or no familiarity with medical language. In these instances, it is critical that athletic trainers use whatever means possible to help athletes understand their injury. Analogies or metaphoric descriptions of anatomical structures, such as describing a sprained ligament as a rubber band that has been stretched or torn, may help athletes unfamiliar with anatomy. Table 5-6 provides examples of some analogies that may help athletic trainers explain injury anatomy, modality functions, or rehabilitation purposes. In addition, athletic trainers can use pictures, diagrams, or anatomical models to give injured athletes a mental picture of what has happened during injury or what needs to happen during recovery. Injured athletes' ability to "see" their injury and the recovery process may also facilitate the use of mental imagery intervention techniques (see Psychosocial Strategies section later in this chapter).

Use Written Material to Complement Verbal Communication

It is highly unlikely that injured athletes will recall all the details of an educational session even if the athletic trainer presents limited information. To facilitate recall, athletic trainers may want to write down important instructions for injured athletes (e.g., at-home exercises, instructions for icing, athletic trainer contact numbers). Many athletic trainers already use this technique with concussion-management instructions, but it could be expanded for use with any injury. Another use for written materials is to enable injured athletes to learn more about their injury, possible surgical techniques, or rehabilitation exercises outside of their interactions with athletic trainers. These materials could include references to outside sources such as books, pamphlets, videos, or websites, or could be developed by athletic trainers to cover frequently discussed issues.

Maintain Two-Way Communication in the Educational Process

As shown in Figure 5-3, when communication is a two-way street, information flows back and forth between the communicators. It is essential during injury education that there is a bidirectional flow of information between the athletic trainer and the injured athlete. The athletic trainer will have a great deal of information to share with the injured athlete; however, the injured athlete must be encouraged to actively participate in the conversation. Athletic trainers should encourage athletes to ask questions about their situation and provide information that their athletic trainer may need to know. Sometimes injured athletes will feel so overwhelmed that they have no idea what questions to ask or what information to share. In these situations, the athletic trainer can facilitate two-way communication by asking athletes about their major concerns; these areas of concern will most likely highlight areas where additional education is needed. Athletic trainers can paraphrase athletes' concerns to make sure they are understood before attempting to provide additional information. Similarly, injured athletes should be encouraged to paraphrase what they have learned during education discussions to assure that there are no misunderstandings or needs for further clarification. Table 5-7 offers guidance to athletic trainers in providing effective injury education in digestible doses to injured athletes.

SPECIAL CONSIDERATIONS

It is worth noting that an athlete's self-presentation style may influence the attention and education provided by athletic trainers. In other words, athletic trainers may provide more or less information to certain athletes based on certain behavioral cues. For example, athletes who ask many questions when they do not understand are excellent prospects for education by athletic trainers. However, athletes who give the impression that they already know everything about their injury or who constantly complain about difficulties and only focus on the negative aspects of injury and rehabilitation may cause athletic trainers to feel inadequate in their ability to help. It is important to realize that these outward appearances do not necessarily reflect internal thoughts or needs for information; therefore, athletic trainers should learn to recognize introverted styles and probe to determine whether a need exists below this exterior. Do you communicate effectively with injured athletes? Take the communication "self-check" in Figure 5-4 to find out.

TABLE 5-6 **Examples of Analogies to Simplify Anatomical or Therapeutic Information**

Ligament	A rubber band that helps hold the bones together at a joint
Sprain	A rubber band that gets stretched too far and either partially or fully tears
Bursa	An empty paper sack or empty balloon, which, when it gets irritated, fills up with fluid
Nonthermal ultrasound	Sound waves that act like a mini-massage, vibrating the tissue
Thermal ultrasound	Sounds waves that penetrate deep into the tissue as a healing glow
Nonsteroidal anti-inflammatory medications	Medicines that act like sponges absorbing local tissue irritants
Articular cartilage	Like a Teflon surface on a fry pan that permits smooth movement

TABLE 5-7 **Tips for Providing Injury Education Information**

Give the most important instructions first.	The primacy effect suggests that information given first is remembered more readily.
Repeat important points at the end.	The recency effect suggests that information presented late is also more readily remembered.
Write down instructions.	The stresses of injury may compromise athletes' ability to retain information. Having written instructions can offset this challenge.
Use language that athletes can understand.	Analogies, drawings, diagrams, models, and charts can all enhance athletes' ability to gain a mental picture of what is happening to them and what needs to happen during the recovery process.
Ask athletes to paraphrase key points.	If injured athletes can repeat important information back to the athletic trainer, they obviously understand it. Inability to effectively paraphrase information reveals the need for further education.
Ask about athletes' concerns after every education session.	Expressed concerns reveal areas where athletes need additional education. Their questions should assist athletic trainers in fine-tuning the content of education discussions.

INTEGRATING COMMUNICATION AND EDUCATION AT SIGNIFICANT REHABILITATION POINTS

Communication skills and the ability to educate the injured athlete are essential elements for athletic trainers. However, several critical events deserve special attention on how to integrate communication and education to produce positive outcomes. These events include delivering the diagnosis, discussing pain expectations, outlining rehabilitation expectations and effort, and confronting the return-to-play process (see Fig. 5-5 for a quick reference to fundamentals of effective injury communication).

Delivering the Diagnosis: Facilitating a Positive Coping Response

When delivering injury information, it is important to send very informative messages (regarding diagnosis, prognosis, treatment options, etc.). Athletic trainers must help athletes accept their injuries. Educating them about the injury soon after it is sustained is often the first step in coping with it. Athletic trainers should use understandable language when explaining mechanisms of injury, diagnosis, and treatment options, and focus on delivering information in a clear and concise way so that athletes can understand and remember key points. They should give athletes relevant information, including the anticipated severity of the injury, prognosis,

Never	Almost Never	Seldom	Occasionally	About Half The Time	Often	Frequently	Almost Always	Always
1	2	3	4	5	6	7	8	9

How often are you able to do these things with your injured athletes?	Score
I am able to develop a rapport (carry on a conversation) with most of my athletes.	
I am able to explain to my athletes how the exercises they are doing will help them return to their sport more quickly.	
I explain to athletes the progression they can expect during rehabilitation.	
I make sure that my athletes know what to expect during the course of their injury (pain, range of motion, function, etc.).	
I explain the purpose of the exercise or treatments that I am having my athletes do.	
I explain treatments and exercises in terms and language that my athletes can understand.	
I explain the purpose of the modality that I am using with my athletes.	

Figure 5-4 | Communication self-check. *(Adapted from Stiller, J. L. [2008].* An evaluation of an educational intervention in psychology of injury for athletic training students. *Doctoral Dissertation, Michigan State University, East Lansing, MI.)*

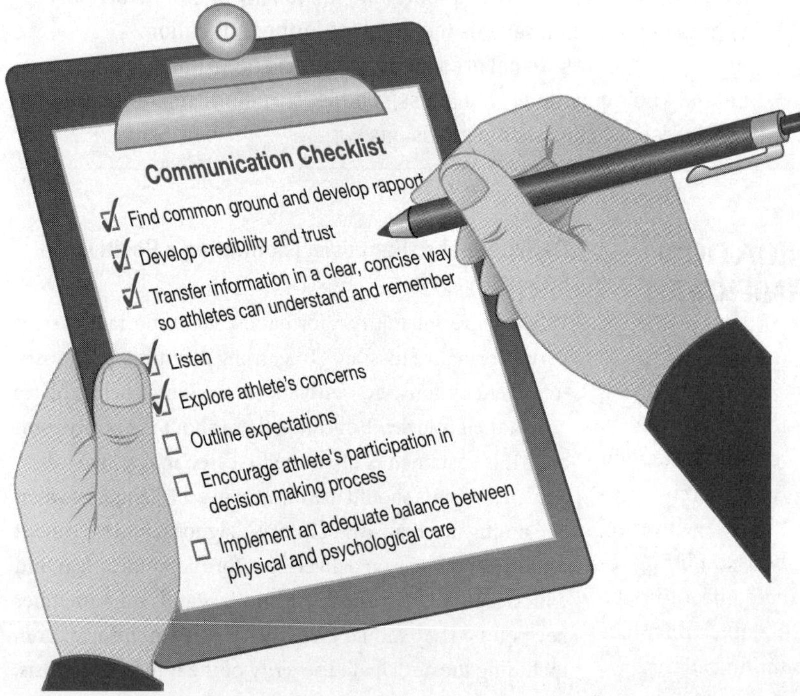

Figure 5-5 | Fundamentals of effective injury communication. *(Adapted from Stiller, J. L. [2008].* An evaluation of an educational intervention in psychology of injury for athletic training students. *Doctoral Dissertation, Michigan State University, East Lansing, MI.)*

and return-to-activity time frame. Education should take place throughout all stages of rehabilitation. Athletic trainers who provide candid information, use terminology that athletes can understand, and encourage athletes to discuss matters of concern will improve athletes' cognitive appraisal of the injury event.

When sharing injury-related information with athletes, it is helpful to communicate using a positive approach. As discussed in Chapter 4, although injuries are generally perceived to be negative, there can also be positive consequences of injury. Communication should express a positive regard for injured athletes and their thoughts and feelings, helping them feel that the athletic trainer realizes this is an emotionally challenging time and wants to try to understand what they are dealing with and how they are feeling about the event. Athletic trainers should display a positive attitude in verbal and nonverbal communication, promote a positive attitude toward recovery, and encourage the athlete to think and behave in a positive manner. Recall from Chapter 4 that an athlete's emotional response and subsequent behaviors are influenced by their cognitive perception of the meaning of the injury. Whenever possible, athletic trainers should emphasize any "upside" to the injury. ***Reframing***, or rephrasing the problem, can help break free of immobilizing perceptions and help athletes search for meaning in their injury experience. Honest information communicated in a positive manner provides reassurance to injured athletes and promotes a positive attitude toward recovery. Factual positive information delivery also aids in the development of trust and social support between the athletic trainer and the injured athlete (learn more about social support in Chapter 9).

Educating Athletes About Pain Expectations

Injured athletes need to be realistic about the likelihood of pain, both during the "injury" phase and during the recovery phase. Athletic trainers may think that forewarning an athlete about pain will make the process worse; however, fear of the unknown could potentially be worse than knowing what to expect and preparing for it. Proper communication can aid in shaping the athlete's perception of the meaning of pain. For example, athletic trainers may explain that the sensations the athlete will likely experience are a natural response to being injured and discuss which pain sensations to expect at various stages of injury. Educating the athlete about the healing process may help them to interpret "painful" sensations as temporary discomforts or as necessary evils moving them toward recovery.

One of the most important communication goals during the injury and recovery processes is assisting athletes in the interpretation of pain. For example, they must understand both good pain and bad pain, and the level of pain that indicates they should stop an exercise because of tissue damage. If athletes can differentiate between certain types of pain, pain will be a source of information to adjust and monitor their recovery. Athletes must recognize that pain is a normal part of the healing process; an understanding of this ***benign pain*** will prevent the athlete from backing off from rehabilitation and may actually become a positive, motivating factor. Athletes must learn to differentiate this benign pain from ***injury pain***, which signals that continued activity could result in additional injury and delay recovery. Recognition of harmful pain can actually help to speed recovery; listening to the body and knowing when to decrease intensity of rehabilitation or increase recovery time between rehabilitation sessions may prevent the onset of ***healing cycles*** (learn more about benign and harmful pain in Chapter 7 and the use of a pain continuum in Chapters 2 and 7).

Communicating About Rehabilitation Expectations and Effort Required

Injury recovery and rehabilitation should not be a mystery to the athlete and certainly not to the athletic trainer. Providing information about what should be expected serves to decrease athlete anxiety and to answer those often unasked questions, like "What is an ACL anyway?" Some athletes may find it helpful to see an outline of the entire rehabilitation protocol at the beginning of rehabilitation so that they can relate the early-stage exercises to their ultimate goal of returning to activity. Other athletes may find such an overview overwhelming, preferring to learn about each stage of rehabilitation as they progress through it. Regardless of the athlete's preference, the athletic trainer should provide a clear explanation of the rehabilitation regimen and involve the athlete in the process of goal setting. Ultimately, athletic trainers need to communicate the expectation that athletes are responsible for their own treatment and recovery. It may be helpful to discuss the athletes' responsibilities at the start of any long-term rehabilitation program so they realize that they are expected to play an active role in their own recovery. Enabling and encouraging athletes to share in decision making and goal setting aids in the development of self-confidence and self-reliance. Athletic trainers should educate athletes about what they can do to help themselves and communicate the message that hard work will aid their recovery.

CLINICAL TIP

Athletic trainers can use the following analogy to encourage injured athletes to actively participate in communication regarding their injury process: Athletes can be encouraged to be in the driver's seat, not the passenger seat, in their recovery. Being in the driver's seat does not imply that the injured athlete doesn't follow a map (most likely drawn by the athletic trainer) to navigate his or her way through the rehabilitation process, nor does it imply that, if the injured athlete feels lost, he or she doesn't stop and ask for directions to get back on the proper path. It does, however, suggest that injured athletes should play an active role in their healing and be the ones driving the recovery vehicle.

CLINICAL TIP

Athletic trainers may find it helpful to make athletes aware of the commitment of both time and effort during rehabilitation. Athletic trainers should not assume that an athlete knows how long a typical rehabilitation session lasts. Rehabilitation sessions longer than 30 minutes are not a deterrent to adherence unless the length was unexpected (Fisher & Hoisington, 1993). Injured athletes also need to understand the effort that will be required during rehabilitation and must learn to accurately appraise how hard they are actually working during individual rehabilitation sessions. Athletic trainers should educate injured athletes about how the healing process works and that sometimes the body needs some time to rest and recover before continued improvements can be realized. Making athletes aware of expected highs, lows, and plateaus over the course of rehabilitation and explaining that temporary setbacks are a normal part of rehabilitation will assist in maintaining a positive, productive rehabilitation environment.

Challenges of Nonadherence

The rehabilitation process can often be lengthy, and decreases in rehabilitation vigor, effort, and adherence are to be expected in even the most motivated athlete. However, not all injured athletes have the same level of motivation to return to their sport; of those who are motivated, not all "buy into" the athletic trainer's ideas about how the rehabilitation process should progress. It can be extremely frustrating to work with athletes who do not seem invested in their own recovery and whose attendance at rehabilitation sessions is spotty. Athletic trainers often report an athlete's rehabilitation nonadherence to the coaching staff; however, doing so seriously undermines the developing relationship between the athletic trainer and the injured athlete. When working with nonadherent athletes who are still able to participate in their sport, it may be helpful to provide choices and consequences.

When dealing with a pessimistic athlete, try to ignore attention-seeking comments and complaints. Instead, reinforce any positive comments (no matter how small). Recall the concept of operant conditioning from your psychology courses—reinforcing desirable behaviors leads to increased frequency of the behavior! Pessimistic attitudes and undesirable behaviors will not change overnight, but they will improve with consistent positive reinforcement. It may also be helpful to engage athletes in rehabilitation programming by soliciting suggestions from them about how their treatment should progress. Athletic trainers might say, for example, "Since you know your knee best, what do you think will help you?" Being an effective athletic trainer is not always about knowing the answers or about being right; it is about developing strategies to engage the athlete in the rehabilitation process and move them toward their ultimate goal of recovery and returning to participation.

Athletic trainers may be surprised at how insightful some athletes are and at the types of rehabilitation exercises they come up with. Chapter 8 will provide more information about strategies to ensure athlete adherence to the rehabilitation program; however, it is important to recognize that effective communication skills are the foundation for ensuring adherence and for implementing motivational strategies. It is also extremely important for athletic trainers to be consistent in how they communicate with injured athletes, regarding both communicating with different athletes and with individual athletes. Athletic trainers must be mindful of subconscious preferences or prejudices toward certain athletes. They must be fair and consistent in how they respond to different athletes in similar situations (how they handle a missed rehabilitation appointment, for example). When necessary, they should criticize behaviors, not athletes.

Communication During the Return-to-Activity Process

As injured athletes prepare to return to their sport, they may fear reinjury or worry about not regaining their preinjury skill level. It is important to communicate with athletes about any physical or psychological recovery concerns when entering the final stages of rehabilitation. The decision to conclude rehabilitation and return to sport should not be underestimated (see later Special Considerations feature). The athletic trainer should communicate with athletes about their feelings regarding returning to play with the goals of identifying and addressing any concerns they may express. Common return-to-play concerns to discuss before the athlete's initial return to sport include anxiety, loss of confidence, and unrealistic performance expectations. It is especially important for the athletic trainer to assist athletes in developing realistic expectations about their physical abilities as they prepare to return to sport; failure to do so may cause athletes to view this stage as a setback. Another concern during this stage is athletes pushing themselves too hard too soon, which could lead to compensatory injuries and further delay their return to sport. It is advisable to structure a plan with coaches to temper this transition. Psychosocial aspects of return-to-participation are discussed in-depth in Chapter 11.

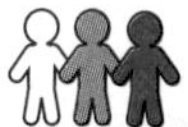

SPECIAL CONSIDERATIONS

Is the athlete feeling internal or external pressure to return "too soon"? These types of pressures are especially prominent in scholarship and professional athletes who may perceive that their opportunity to earn an education or a living is dependent on them returning to the athletic arena as quickly as possible. Psychological preparedness to return to sport is as important as physical readiness. Athletes who are overly anxious about their return to participation may be at a greater risk for reinjury (recall stress response from Chapter 3). As athletes progress toward return to sport, it is important for athletic trainers to communicate with them about any outside pressures or concerns they are experiencing, to ensure they are mentally prepared for the challenges of returning to their sport. For athletes who feel financial pressures to return to play, it is essential to educate them on the cost–benefits of returning early, highlighting the potential financial consequences if they sustain reinjury because of an early return.

As an athlete prepares to return to competition, fear of reinjury may appear, often as the result of time and distance away from their sport. Athletes may have a distorted perception of the probability of injury occurring again, particularly if they find themselves in a situation similar to that which caused the initial injury. Athletic trainers should use their communication skills to discuss the athlete's feelings, expectations, and concerns. Athletic trainers can help athletes understand that doubt and fear are normal, and that these feelings will usually pass as they learn to trust their own body again. It may be helpful to provide the athlete with relevant information that counters the fear. For example, an athletic trainer may say, "Your surgeon wouldn't have cleared you if he didn't believe that you were ready" (example of a *spoken* verbal communication tactic). Or the athletic trainer may provide direct evidence that the injured area can sustain the demand (e.g., "Your isokinetic test results prove that your injured knee is just as strong as your uninjured side"—an example of a *written* verbal communication tactic). Athletic trainers should remind athletes that their rehabilitation provided regular chances to "test" the injured area, and redirect their focus onto positive aspects of competition (learn strategies to address fear of reinjury in the Psychosocial Strategies section later in this chapter).

USING COMMUNICATION AND EDUCATION WITH OTHER INVOLVED PARTIES

In addition to communication and education efforts directed toward injured athletes, athletic trainers will also need communication and education skills when interacting with other individuals surrounding the injured athlete, such as other medical providers and members of the athlete's support network. Communication skills and educational efforts are of critical importance in these interactions to prevent misunderstandings among caregivers and to prevent athletes from getting conflicting advice or messages from their support network. In all these situations, it is essential that athletic trainers clearly define for athletes the confidentiality of interactions and what types of information will be shared with coaches, other members of the sports medicine team, and parents or other family members, so as not to compromise the trust developed in the relationships. Remember that although injury reports are critical pieces of information, they are medical reports that contain private health information. Injury information should be shared only with the athlete's permission, and information should be shared only with those who have a legitimate need.

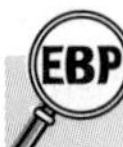

EVIDENCE-BASED PRACTICE

Stiller-Ostrowski, J. L., & Ostrowski, J. A. (2009). Recently certified athletic trainers' undergraduate educational preparation in psychosocial intervention and referral. *Journal of Athletic Training, 44*(1), 67–75.

Description of the Study

Semistructured focus group interviews were conducted with 11 recently certified athletic trainers (mean = 2.7 years) who graduated from AT programs across a range of geographic locations and NCAA athletic divisions, and who currently practiced in a variety of employment settings. The purpose of the study was to explore the educational preparation of these athletic trainers with regard to content within the psychosocial intervention and referral content area (specifically, communication skills, motivation strategies, and intervention and referral). Questions related to communication skills centered on ability to communicate with coaches, physicians, and parents. Participants were also asked to rank the level to which their AT program prepared them to handle each set of issues (scale: 1–10, with 1 being *completely unprepared* and 10 being *completely prepared*).

Results of the Study

On all issues related to communication, the average preparedness ranking was 6.7 (range: 2.0–8.5); preparation related specifically to communicating with physicians averaged 6.7, with coaches averaged 6.1, and with parents averaged 4.3. AT programs that best prepared their students transitioned athletic training students in their interactions with coaches, ultimately having students assume the primary role in informing coaches about injury status updates. Regarding communication with physicians, the highest ranked AT programs allowed athletic training students to present athletes' cases to physicians and required them to be the liaison between the physician and the injured athlete. Regarding communication with parents, participants in this study recalled being educated about what information can and cannot be legally shared with parents but had no opportunity to interact with parents regarding athlete injuries in their role as athletic training students.

Implications for Athletic Training Practice

The results of this study imply that athletic training students must have experience in handling communication with other parties involved in the care of injured athletes, because these skill sets are essential in the professional realm. AT programs should be making concerted efforts to allow athletic training students to practice communicating with these involved parties and should craft a system whereby students progress incrementally until they are prepared to assume a primary role in communicating injury-related information with all parties involved in the care of the injured athlete.

Physicians

Communication among members of the sports medicine team is essential to quality care for injured athletes. Athletic trainers may need to communicate with physicians or surgeons for a number of reasons: 1) to consult on patient care, 2) to make a referral for diagnosis, 3) to follow up on the results of athletes' office visits, or 4) to get consensus on treatment plans or return-to-participation timelines. In all these interactions, the principles of two-way communication are critical. Verbal and nonverbal messages must be sent clearly and concisely, and paraphrasing is essential to assure that intended messages are received and understood.

Because information about injured athletes must be shared among members of the sports medicine team, it is critical that, before the season, athletic trainers disclose to athletes the extent to which information will be shared. Athletes must understand what types of information will be passed among sports medicine team members and under what conditions information will be shared to avoid misunderstandings that could potentially compromise trust and rapport between athletes and their care providers. Consent forms should be used to clarify the boundaries of confidentiality for all parties involved.

Athletic trainers may find they need to act as interpreters to assist athletes in understanding information provided by physicians, surgeons, or other members of the sports medicine team. To facilitate clear understanding, it is ideal if athletic trainers can accompany athletes to their visits with physicians to hear firsthand what is shared at these appointments. As discussed earlier, athletes may not know what questions to ask physicians or may feel intimidated to ask questions when meeting a physician with whom they do not have an established rapport. Again, consider Mike in the Athlete Insider section. Mike failed to ask questions at the doctor's office or during the drive back to campus. It is likely that Mike was suffering from "information overload" at this point and likely did not know where to begin with regard to asking questions. Athletic trainers can serve as a facilitator of two-way communication in these situations. When they cannot accompany athletes to physician appointments, it is common for athletes to have questions regarding what all the medical information they received at those appointments really means. This is not a criticism of physicians' communication abilities, but rather is indicative of the demands of their office schedules, which often prevent them from spending as much time as they would like with patients on education and answering questions. In these situations, athletic trainers can help athletes "fill in the blanks"; however, it is critical that they not guess at what physicians may have communicated. Rather, they should make phone calls to the attending physicians to discuss the full details of the appointment so they can accurately translate information for athletes.

Parents or Family Members

Although communication and education with injured athletes are important, it is equally important that members of the injured athlete's support network be educated in all aspects of the injury situation. The athletes' parents and family members are most likely trusted advisors to whom they will turn following injury. It is essential that these parties understand as much about the injury process as athletes to minimize sending potential conflicting messages to athletes about the best choices for injury treatment or care.

The age of the athlete is a very important consideration when communicating with parents or family members. For minors, communication with parents is essential, as they will most likely be significant players in treatment decisions. Therefore, parents will need the same information about all aspects of the injury situation as the athlete. However, if injured athletes are legal adults, communication with their parents or family members cannot occur without the athlete's consent. This potentially places athletic trainers in a challenging position if athletes wish to maintain confidentiality regarding their condition or progress. In these situations, athletic trainers are obligated to inform family members that all information regarding the injury or treatment, or both, must come directly from their son or daughter.

Coaching Staff

Communication with and injury education for the coaching staff are also important. As mentioned earlier regarding communication with physicians, athletic trainers need to proactively disclose to athletes what medical information will be passed along to members of the coaching staff and under what conditions it will be shared. This will prevent feelings of betrayal of the trust or rapport previously established with the athlete.

Coaches have various philosophies about injury and athletes playing through pain. Some will exhibit great caution and encourage athletes to fully heal before attempting a return to play, whereas others espouse a win-at-all-costs mentality that can pressure or coerce athletes to return to play before they are physically or psychologically ready. It is essential that athletic trainers actively engage in behaviors that establish trust and rapport with coaches because this can facilitate better cooperation when athletes are injured. Regardless of coaches' injury-management philosophies, they need to be educated about the injuries their athletes sustain, the limits injured athletes have, the rationale for those limits, and the consequences if the limits are not followed. Athletic trainers need to be willing to intervene on behalf of the athlete if they feel pressured by coaches to do more than they feel they can during the injury recovery process. In most cases, coaches have genuine concern for the long-term health and well-being of their athletes and will cooperate with athletic trainers to do what is best, but athletic trainers need to be prepared in situations where this is not the case. Educating coaches on all aspects of their athletes' injuries and developing positive rapport and trust with coaches will likely increase the coaches' willingness to cooperate with athletic trainers' advice and decisions.

CLINICAL TIP

In addition to communicating with coaches about athletes' return-to-play status, athletic trainers should continue to educate athletes about what to expect during this period. Informing athletes about the difference between benign and harmful pain can prevent them from pushing their bodies too far or having exaggerated expectations of their abilities during this initial return-to-play phase.

Athletic trainers should make daily efforts to keep coaches abreast of the injury status of all their players. Injury report forms can help facilitate communication with coaches but are not a substitute for face-to-face communication and education. When coaches and athletic trainers communicate face-to-face, two-way communication skills (discussed earlier in this chapter) can be used to minimize confusion and misunderstandings. Paraphrasing needs to be an essential component of these communication efforts. Coaches should be encouraged to ask questions and communicate concerns they have about their athletes' health. Athletic trainers need to listen with empathy to these concerns while maintaining focus on athletes' overall health and well-being as the driving factor behind how recovery must proceed. Good rapport and trust will enable coaches to work collaboratively with athletic trainers to assure athletes are competing in a healthy playing environment.

CLINICAL TIP

Athletic trainers should avoid asking athletes to tell their coaches about their injury status and practice limitations. Just as in the game of "telephone", messages can easily become convoluted as they pass through multiple recipients. In addition, athletes may not be entirely truthful in their representation of their situation if they think it may slow their return to participation or compromise their playing time. It is essential that the athletic trainer speak directly to the coach regarding an injured athlete's status.

PSYCHOSOCIAL STRATEGIES

Communication and education skills can be applied throughout the injury recovery process to assist injured athletes (refer to Table 5-5). The rest of this section focuses first on specific ways athletic trainers can facilitate their communication and educational efforts with injured athletes, and illustrates how communication and education serve as a foundation for the successful implementation of specific psychosocial intervention techniques.

Develop a Library of Materials to Complement Verbal Communication and Education

The first part of this chapter discussed the possibility of overloading injured athletes with extensive amounts of information about their injury or rehabilitation. One technique to counteract the possibility of overload is to develop a library of written or video materials to give to athletes to complement the verbal information or education they receive. These materials can include handouts, pamphlets, lists of credible websites, educational podcasts and vodcasts, and videotaped interviews of previously injured athletes. Athletes can refer to these materials on their own to confirm what they thought they heard verbally or to educate themselves further about their injury or rehabilitation program.

In addition, athletic trainers may struggle to adequately explain the injury and healing process to athletes who have limited or no understanding of anatomy. In this case, athletic trainers may want to develop a collection of anatomical models, charts, and diagrams that help simplify and clarify complex medical information. These instructional aids will help give athletes a clear picture of what has happened to them during injury and what must happen during the recovery process (Fig. 5-6). These items should be readily available and accessible to both athletic trainers and injured athletes. Examples of topics for such written and instructional material include, but are not limited to:

- Anatomical models, charts, diagrams
- Information and diagrams that discuss common sport injuries
- Handouts highlighting the needed at-home care for the first night following injury
- Podcasts/vodcasts or descriptions and diagrams of at-home exercises
- Podcasts/vodcasts or descriptions and diagrams of various surgical procedures
- Instructions for postconcussion care

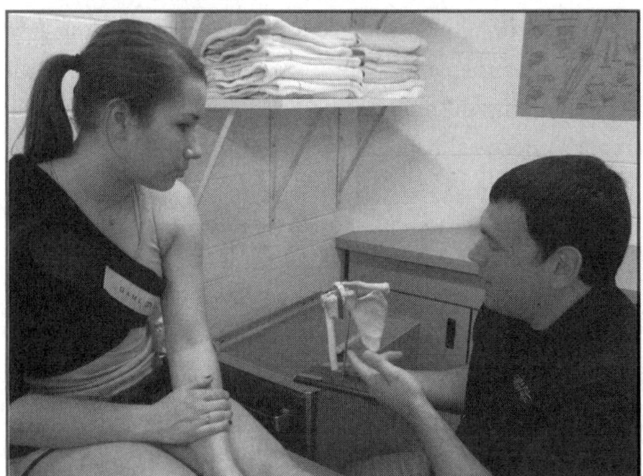

Figure 5-6 | Athletic trainer using anatomical model to assist injury education.

This list is certainly not an exhaustive one; the content for a potential library is limited only by athletic trainers' creativity. Topics that athletic trainers find themselves repeating frequently are prime areas for developing written information materials. Another benefit of a library of materials is that it allows athletes to educate themselves when athletic trainers are pressed for time. Most athletic trainers struggle to find sufficient time to counsel and educate every athlete. These libraries can assist them in delivering information to athletes expeditiously.

Vodcasting interviews with previously injured athletes as they discuss their injury and rehabilitation experiences enables athletic trainers to easily develop a modeling library. The vodcasts of these interviews are invaluable in educating currently injured athletes about the overall rehabilitation process, obstacles they may encounter during healing, and strategies for overcoming obstacles or setbacks. Injured athletes gain knowledge and confidence as they learn from the experience of others who have been in their position and successfully returned to sport. A modeling vodcast library enables injured athletes to self-acquire information about their injury, which is a time-saver for athletic trainers. In addition, vodcast modeling on various educational topics allows injured athletes to engage in multiple viewings of desired content to increase their understanding or reinforce positive psychological outcomes, such as increased confidence and motivation.

Communication and Education as Foundations for Effective Implementation of Psychosocial Interventions

The following section highlights how communication and education are the foundational groundwork for successful implementation of many psychosocial interventions, including goal setting, relaxation, mental imagery, and cognitive restructuring. The specifics of each of these intervention techniques are discussed in detail in Chapter 10. This section focuses instead on how communication and education facilitate the effective implementation of these techniques.

Goal Setting

Communication and education are important elements in facilitating effective goal setting with injured athletes. As mentioned earlier, injured athletes need to play an active role in their rehabilitation planning and progress. Collaborative goal setting with injured athletes is much preferred over athletic trainers engaging in one-way communication about what athletes will do each day in rehabilitation. For athletes to be active participants in this collaborative process, they must first be educated about the progressions required in an effective rehabilitation program, as well as the guidelines they need to follow in setting "good" and realistic goals. Once educated, injured athletes can effectively engage in two-way communication with their athletic trainers to collaboratively develop goals for their rehabilitation progression. After goals are established, communication again becomes a critical component in that these goals need to be communicated to coaches and other stakeholders in the athletes' healing progress. In addition, athletic trainers must constantly provide feedback to athletes and other stakeholders about athletes' progress toward achieving these goals. (Learn more about goal setting in Chapter 10.)

Relaxation Techniques

As discussed in Chapters 3 and 10, athletes can use relaxation interventions in many ways to prevent injury, help reduce pain, and enhance the recovery process. Athletes need to learn how relaxation techniques can contribute to these outcomes. In addition, they need education about how and when to implement relaxation techniques to achieve the desired results. Communication skills are critical in this education process and also as athletic trainers implement relaxation interventions with athletes. For example, nonverbal communication skills such as proxemics and/or paralanguage are vitally important in calming athletes immediately following injury, guiding athletes through relaxation exercises during their rehabilitation, or creating prerecorded relaxation scripts for athletes' independent use. In these ways, communication skills and education enhance the effectiveness of relaxation interventions.

Mental Imagery

Oftentimes, athletes already have strong mental imagery skills. For example, basketball players may close their eyes and visualize a free throw going in before they shoot, or a golfer will visualize sinking a putt. Lacrosse, hockey, and basketball players may visualize running plays given different reactions by the defense. Gymnasts or divers may visualize their routine during quiet preparation time before their event. If athletes are already engaging in sport-specific mental imagery, they likely know the benefits of this technique. The role of athletic trainers working with injured athletes is to encourage them to transfer these imagery skills into the rehabilitation setting by educating them about their use and application during the recovery and return-to-play process.

As discussed in Chapter 10, imagery can be used for relaxation, pain relief, visualizing the healing process, rehabilitation rehearsal, performance rehearsal when physical practice is not possible, or visualizing successful return to sport. In each of these instances, athletic trainers may first have to educate and assist athletes in developing appropriate images to use for each of these purposes. For example, the use of anatomical models, pictures, and diagrams in educating athletes about their injury will facilitate athletes' ability to envision the internal processes and anatomical healing that take place during recovery, and thus select appropriate images to use in ***healing imagery***. For example, a hockey player may relate to a metaphor of tissue remodeling by imaging how the ice looks at the end of a period: torn up, scratched, and disorganized—until the Zamboni comes out and scrapes off the damaged layer, leaving a smooth path behind (other ideas of possible images to develop are in Table 5-6). As discussed earlier in the Goal Setting section, collaboration with athletes in developing appropriate images is preferred over athletic trainers engaging in one-way communication about what images to use. In healing imagery, athletes will also need to learn about the timing of and need for modifying their choice of image as healing progresses so the image accurately depicts the physical healing occurring. For athletes unfamiliar with using imagery, or using imagery in a novel manner, athletic trainers will have to educate athletes regarding the suggested guidelines and principles for creating effective imagery (covered in Chapter 10).

VIRTUAL FIELD TRIP

Sometimes it is not clear whether an athlete is a good candidate for mental imagery techniques. The Davis*Plus* website (http://davisplus.fadavis.com) describes an activity that helps evaluate an injured athlete's receptivity to the use of mental imagery during the rehabilitation process.

Self-Talk and Cognitive Restructuring

Communication skills will be of vital importance when working with injured athletes on their self-talk and cognitive patterns. Athletic trainers must diligently engage in active listening while working with injured athletes to help identify nonproductive thought and self-talk patterns. When they identify these patterns, athletic trainers should seek to educate athletes on how negative self-talk or unrealistic expectations can compromise the healing process. By using the two-way communication skills discussed earlier, athletic trainers can collaborate with athletes on developing more productive and realistic patterns of thinking and self-talk. For example, an athlete who experiences pain or discomfort during rehabilitation may react negatively and withdraw from the activity if he or she views this discomfort negatively. However, athletes who have been educated by their athletic trainers about various types of pain (benign pain vs. injury pain) may be helped by cognitive restructuring techniques that allow them to "work through" benign pain if it is viewed as a signal that the body is working hard and building strength. Basically, athletes learn to change their view of pain from a negative ("I can't believe how much this hurts; I have to stop.") to a positive ("It hurts, but I know the pain is not dangerous and is a sign that I'm getting stronger.") through the use of cognitive restructuring and self-talk.

As discussed earlier, athletic trainers should be aware that nonverbal messages conveyed by injured athletes are just as important in reflecting their thinking as what they express verbally. Take, for example, the athlete who verbally responds to inquiries as to how he's doing with "I'm fine," but his nonverbal messages expressed through body language contradict this. Athletic trainers can use their knowledge of communication skills to more accurately assess athletes' needs for self-talk or cognitive-restructuring interventions.

ATHLETE INSIDER CONCLUSION

After much discussion with the sports medicine team and his parents, Mike opted for surgery to repair his torn labrum. The time spent away from the lacrosse field was difficult for Mike, and he struggled with losing connections with teammates and worrying about maintaining his fitness and sport-specific skills. His athletic trainer recognized these struggles and empathized with his situation—sharing stories about being an injured athlete himself. Initially, Mike was noncompliant in using his sling, and teammates commonly reported seeing him around campus without it. The athletic trainer spoke to Mike about his decision and educated him about the importance of immobilization and its impact on protecting the repair site, showing Mike his operative scans and explaining the healing process. As the two got to know each other better, the athletic trainer learned which types of communication Mike responded to best and began to recognize nonverbal cues indicating that he was confused. Mike worked closely with his athletic trainer to learn about his injury and about the rehabilitation process (Fig. 5-7). As his anticipated return-to-play date neared, his athletic trainer communicated with the coaching staff about his practice limitations and helped Mike develop realistic expectations regarding his physical abilities. Mike returned to lacrosse after missing only 2 weeks of his junior season and quickly reclaimed his place on the team.

Effective Psychosocial Strategies for the Athletic Trainer to Use with Mike

The following psychosocial strategies can be used with Mike as he recovers from his injury:

1. Upon returning to campus following Mike's physician visit, use diagrams, models, or pictures to help interpret the information the physician shared with him.
2. Discuss available written, video, or online information sources that Mike could consult to learn more about his injury, surgical options and outcomes, or the rehabilitation process.
3. Communicate with Mike regarding the rationale for limitations to prevent him from engaging in actions that may hinder the healing process.
4. Educate Mike about what healing has to occur and develop healing imagery scripts and "mini-images" to increase his sense of control over the healing process.
5. Encourage Mike to use cognitive restructuring techniques to change his interpretation of "pain" during

Educate Mike about rehabilitation progression and engage him in collaborative goal setting
Educate Mike with anatomical models to provide a foundation for healing imagery
Use verbal and nonverbal communication skills to calm Mike and guide him through relaxation exercises

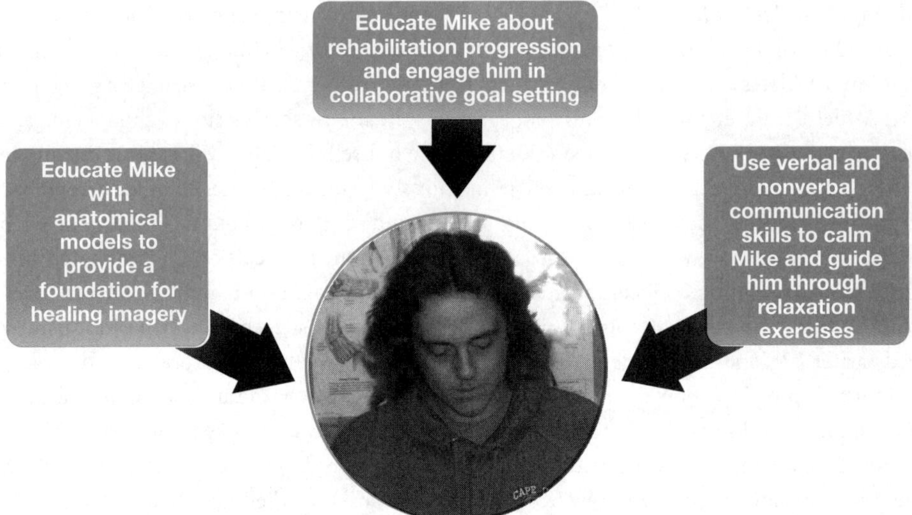

Figure 5-7 | Using psychosocial strategies with Mike.

his initial return to play, viewing it instead as discomfort that is the result of structures being (safely) stressed in ways that they have not been for several months.

6. Communicate about any fears of reinjury and engage Mike in return-to-play imagery to increase his confidence in his ability to return to sport successfully.

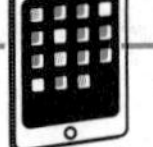

VIRTUAL FIELD TRIP

For an example of a return-to-play imagery script, go to http://davisplus.fadavis.com.

CONCLUSION

Strong communication skills provide a firm foundation on which athletic trainers can establish rapport and engage in effective educational efforts for all individuals affected by sport injury. This chapter gave an overview of the keys to effective verbal and nonverbal communication, and highlighted how these skills affect the ability of athletic trainers to demonstrate empathy, build trust and rapport, and effectively educate athletes and others about injury. Young professional athletic trainers often lack confidence in their communication skills; therefore, this chapter intentionally highlighted this content and offered practical application and integration advice that athletic trainers can rely on in their educational and professional pursuits. Whether athletic trainers continue onto graduate school or immediately enter the workforce, they will need a fully developed communication skill set from their first day on the job to facilitate holistic recovery from athletic injury.

REFERENCES

Brown, J. B., Stewart, M., & Ryan, B. L. (2003). Outcomes of patient-provider interaction. In T. L. Thompson, A. M. Dorsey, K. I. Miller, R. Parrott (Eds.), *Handbook of Health Communication* (pp. 141–161). New York: Routledge.

Deveugele, M., Derese, A., De Maesschalack, S., Willems, S., Van Driel, M., & De Maeseneer, J. (2005). Teaching communication skills to medical students, a challenge in the curriculum? *Patient Education and Counseling, 58*(3), 265–270.

Fisher, A. C., & Hoisington, L. L. (1993). Injured athletes' attitudes and judgments toward rehabilitation adherence. *Journal of Athletic Training, 28*(1), 48–54.

Heil, J. (1993). *Psychology of sport injury*. Champaign, IL: Human Kinetics.

Miller, G. E. (1990). The assessment of clinical skills/competence/performance. *Academic Medicine, 65*(1), 63–67.

National Athletic Trainers' Association. (2005). *NATA code of ethics*. Retrieved May 8, 2012, from http://www.nata.org/codeofethics.

Stewart, M., Brown, J.B., Boon, H., Galajda, J., Meredith, L., & Sangster, M. (1999). Evidence on patient-doctor communication. *Cancer Prevention and Control, 3*(1), 25–30.

Stiller, J. L., & Ostrowski, J. A. (2007). Tricks of the trade: Enhancing interpersonal skills. *Athletic Therapy Today, 12*(6), 33–35.

Stiller-Ostrowski, J. L., & Ostrowski, J. A. (2009). Recently certified athletic trainers' undergraduate educational preparation in psychosocial intervention and referral. *Journal of Athletic Training, 44*(1), 67–75.

BOARD OF CERTIFICATION STRATEGIES AND COMPETENCIES

As the Sixth Edition Role Delineation Study outlines, athletic trainers are involved in all aspects of injury, from clinical evaluation and diagnosis (Domain 2) through treatment and rehabilitation (Domain 4). Threaded throughout these domains is specific application of several of the Fifth Edition Athletic Training Education Competencies related to communication and education. Athletic trainers must understand the basic processes of effective interpersonal communication, including how cultural differences can create noise that potentially compromises effective communication (PS-4, PS-5, PS-6). It is also essential to recognize how appropriate communication and injury education impacts athletes' cognitive-appraisal processes, their motivation to be an active participant in the process of recovery, and their overall psychosocial and emotional well-being (PS-4, PS-5, PS-6). Where appropriate, athletic trainers must educate those within the athlete's support network regarding the injury and recovery process while maintaining necessary confidentiality (PS-4, PS-6, PS-18). Athletic trainers must also recognize the importance of establishing rapport and developing communication skills to engage injured athletes in various psychosocial strategies that may facilitate a positive and expedient recovery process (PS-4, PS-5).

Board of Certification Style Questions

1. Effective injury education has the ability to influence which of the following (select all that apply):
   a. Injured athletes' cognitive appraisals of the injury situation
   b. Coaches' reactions to activity limits imposed on their athletes
   c. Injured athletes' motivation during rehabilitation
   d. Parents' communication with their child following injury
2. The communication process involves which of the following components? (Select all that apply.)
   a. Sender
   b. Feedback
   c. Noise
   d. Decoding
3. Restating a message back to the sender to ensure proper understanding describes which communication process?
   a. Empathy
   b. Paraphrasing
   c. Rapport
   d. Trust
4. In communication, sources of noise include (select all that apply):
   a. Cultural differences
   b. Fatigue
   c. Crowded gymnasium
   d. Emotions of the communicators
   e. Poor listening skills
5. Education of the injured athlete should include (select all that apply):
   a. Rationale for limits on healing
   b. Departure date for the team bus
   c. Anatomy of the involved area
   d. Mechanisms by which rehabilitation exercises work
6. Nonverbal messages can be communicated through which of the following pathways? (Select all that apply.)
   a. Proxemics
   b. Paraphrasing
   c. Eye contact
   d. Facial expressions
   e. Body language

END-OF-CHAPTER EXERCISES

1. Choose two athletes at your clinical site whom you do not yet know. Introduce yourself to these athletes and engage them in conversation to attempt to find some common ground. Reflect on the following:
   - How did you initiate the conversation?
   - What were the challenges in doing so?
   - Was the second time easier than the first?
2. A component of coping with a diagnosis is developing an understanding of the repercussions and impact of the injury. Once the initial shock of the diagnosis has worn off, most athletes will want information regarding when they will be able to return to their sport. The athletic trainer's response is crucial for developing a foundation for understanding the rehabilitation process, engaging the athlete in psychosocial skills, and facilitating a positive attitude toward the rehabilitation process. How should an athletic trainer respond to the question, "How long am I going to be out?"
3. Psychological readiness to return to sport is as important as physical readiness, and athletic trainers need to identify athletes' concerns and address them accordingly. Consider an athlete you have worked with who was preparing to conclude the rehabilitation process. What types of concerns did this athlete have? How should you address these concerns?
4. Providing information and clarifying expectations during rehabilitation serves several important purposes; please list two such purposes.
5. Consider a nonadherent athlete with whom you have worked at one of your clinical sites. Of the communication strategies presented in this chapter, which do you think may be effective at enhancing this athlete's adherence to or investment in the rehabilitation process?
6. An essential communication skill for athletic trainers is the ability to effectively educate injured athletes about what has happened to them and what they are now facing as a result of their injury. Role-play with a fellow classmate (one playing the role of an injured athlete, the other playing an athletic trainer) on how you would educate an athlete in one of the following scenarios:
   a. An athlete has just sustained a possible ACL rupture
   b. A football player has sustained a second-degree acromioclavicular separation
   c. A volleyball or baseball athlete is suffering from impingement syndrome
   d. A cross-country runner is suffering from medial tibial stress syndrome
   e. An athlete has postconcussive symptoms 24 hours after the injury.

   In the role-play, include *what* needs to be said to the athlete, *how* best to say it, and the *medium* through which you will get your message across (remember very few athletes understand anatomical terms).
7. Take an hour *outside of your clinical experience time* to observe and critique the nonverbal communication in your athletic training facility. During the hour, take notes on the types of nonverbal messages exchanged between athletic trainers and the athletes with whom they work. Make notes on the types of effective and ineffective nonverbal messages you observe. Share your observations with your classmates and fellow athletic training students, and discuss how to improve nonverbal communication.
8. Brainstorm with your classmates on specific ways that athletic trainers can communicate empathy to their athletes. Be sure to include both verbal and nonverbal communication techniques.

9. An important way to facilitate injured athletes' comprehension of information is to use written materials to complement verbal communication. Develop an informational handout or pamphlet that could be given to injured athletes as a way to complement verbal communication. The written work could focus on information about a specific injury or on instructions to follow during a specific period during the recovery process (e.g., the first night after injury).

10. Develop a comprehensive list of credible websites that injured athletes could visit to obtain additional information about specific injuries.

Chapter 6

Identification of Psychosocial Distress and Referral

Megan D. Granquist and Laura J. Kenow

CHAPTER OUTLINE

KEY TERMS

Arousal Psychological or physiological state of being alert.

Depersonalization Being detached from oneself.

Derealization Feelings of unreality.

Empathy Being sensitive to and vicariously experiencing the feelings, thoughts, or motives of another person.

Holistic Related to healing; a holistic approach includes all parts of the healing system—the mind and the body—in the healing process.

Mood Emotional state (e.g., happy, sad).

Paresthesias Numbness or tingling sensations.

Proactively Acting in advance to deal with an expected difficulty; anticipatory.

KEY TERMS *continued*

Proxemics Communication expressed through the space between two people as they interact.

Rapport The harmonious or synchronous relationship of two or more people who relate well to each other.

Subclinical The early stages or a very mild form of a condition.

Suicidal ideation Serious thoughts about committing suicide.

Tolerance Reaction to a drug is progressively reduced thereby requiring an increase in concentration to achieve the desired effect.

Withdrawal Symptoms that occur due to the decrease or discontinuation in intake of drugs.

CHAPTER OBJECTIVES

After reading this chapter, you will be able to:

1. Describe the role and scope of practice of the athletic trainer in the referral process.
2. Identify professionals within a mental health referral network.
3. Establish a mental health referral network.
4. Identify signs and symptoms of distress and mental disorders that warrant referral.
5. Describe the mental health referral process.

ATHLETE INSIDER

Amelia is a sophomore collegiate volleyball player who has sustained a severe sprain of her ankle. Amelia is currently beginning rehabilitation, and her athletic trainer recognizes that she may be having difficulty adjusting to the injury. During one of the rehabilitation sessions, the athletic trainer mentions to Amelia that she seems to lack energy and appears to be distracted. Amelia does, in fact, feel lethargic and is thankful that her athletic trainer noticed. Because of the rapport that the athletic trainer has built with Amelia over the season, Amelia feels comfortable confiding in the athletic trainer. Amelia shares that she is not sleeping well and is constantly worrying about how the injury is going to influence her athletic career; this is affecting her ability to attend class, and when she does attend, it is difficult for her to concentrate. Amelia also shares that she feels like she is no longer an athlete because she is not able to participate in her sport. The athletic trainer recognizes that Amelia's injury situation is interfering with her daily functioning and understands that Amelia could be in need of a mental health referral.

INTRODUCTION

This chapter focuses on the athletic trainer's role and scope of practice in the identification and management of psychosocial distress in athletes with whom they work. The athletic trainer's role as part of a multidisciplinary sports medicine team is emphasized. Although it is clearly beyond the scope of practice for athletic trainers to diagnose mental health conditions (e.g., depression, anxiety), "Athletic trainers must be able to recognize clients/patients exhibiting abnormal social, emotional, and mental behaviors" (National Athletic Trainers' Association [NATA], 2011, p. 27) and make referrals appropriately. This chapter explains the process of developing a psychosocial referral network and identifying signs and symptoms of psychosocial distress in injured athletes. This chapter provides a framework to guide athletic trainers through the psychosocial consultation and referral process.

Athletic Trainers' Role in the Holistic Care of Athletes

Athletic trainers, relative to other members of the sports medicine team, have a unique relationship with athletes.

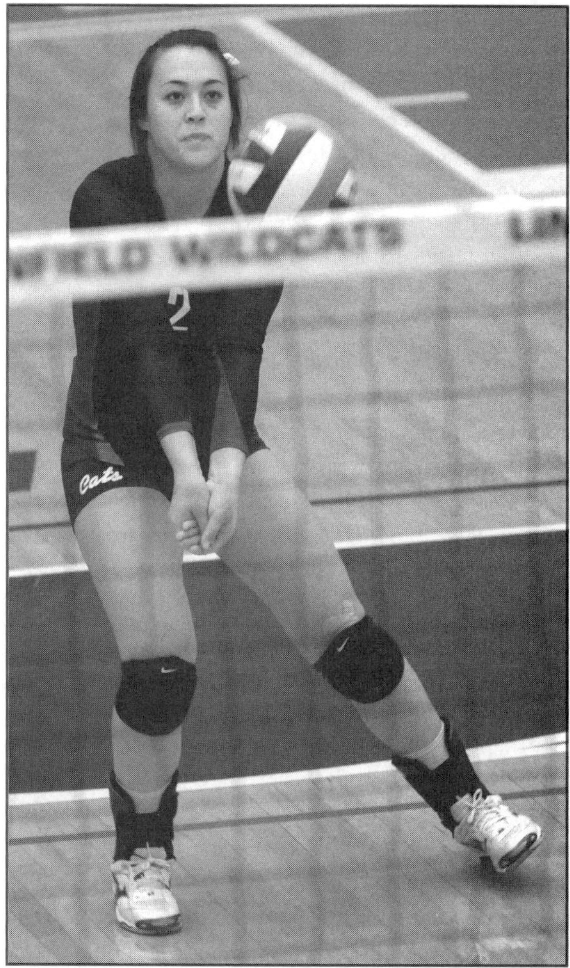

Figure 6-1 | Athlete Insider *(Courtesy of Stephen Bricher)*

Athletic trainers in traditional settings interact with athletes on a daily basis following injury but also before injuries ever occur. Before the season even begins, athletic trainers are often involved with athletes through preseason health screening and assessment, as well as conditioning and training programs. Once the season begins, athletic trainers are involved daily with athletes during preparation for (e.g., taping and stretching) and coverage of practices. Athletic trainers are often present at each home competition and in some instances will travel with the team to away competitions. As a result, athletic trainers are frequently onsite when injuries occur or are the first to respond and provide the immediate first aid, both physically and psychologically. After injuries occur, athletic trainers work daily with athletes throughout the rehabilitation and recovery process. This degree of contact between athletic trainers and athletes far exceeds what most other members of the sports medicine team encounter.

As mentioned in Chapter 5, through all these interactions, athletic trainers proactively work to develop solid ***rapport*** and trust with athletes, coaches, and teams. As a result, athletic trainers are often accepted into the inner circle and considered to be an integral and trusted part of the athletes' sport network. In this position, athletic trainers are privy to information and experiences that other sports medicine team members may never encounter. The trust and rapport athletic trainers actively foster with athletes create a safe and comfortable environment in which athletes feel free to express their feelings and share personal experiences.

Consequently, athletic trainers often serve in an advisor-like or counselor-like role to athletes in a number of ways. For instance, athletes frequently ask for advice from athletic trainers about seemingly inconsequential, nonathletic matters related to life situations (e.g., where to take their car for service, what advice the athletic trainer would offer about taking a certain class from a certain instructor). These discussions are often informal conversations that develop during taping or rehabilitation sessions, on bus trips to and from contests, or even during water breaks at practices.

Other times, athletic trainers counsel athletes on more germane, health-related matters, such as how often to ice following injury, what to include in a quality pregame meal, when to begin a workout taper, or the pros and cons of using a certain type of graft in an anterior cruciate ligament reconstruction. Athletic trainers also comfort athletes in the immediate aftermath of injury, offering initial emotional support and challenge; attentively listening to the concerns of athletes, coaches, and parents; and discussing various treatment options. During the arduous process of rehabilitation, athletic trainers also frequently advise athletes on what to expect in terms of pain and dysfunction, how to control pain and discomfort, and how to remain motivated through the monotony of long-term rehabilitation.

Athletic trainers often overhear conversations or observe behaviors of athletes simply because of the physical proximity they have to the athletes, and athletic trainers also encounter information on any number of topics from conversations shared and interactions among athletes in the athletic training room, at practices and games, and on bus rides (Table 6-1). The physical design of most athletic training rooms with treatment tables spaced close together makes it easy for athletic trainers to overhear conversations as they administer treatments or move from table to table during rehabilitation sessions. Prepractice taping or stretching sessions are often times where athletes catch up with one another and update each other on their day. Athletic trainers may hear about how Jake did on his anatomy exam or learn that Kim and Katie are going grocery shopping after practice. The presence of athletic trainers is often discounted or ignored by athletes as they engage in these conversations. Postevent icing or treatment creates further situations where athletic trainers are exposed to athletes' reflections on what occurred at practices or games. For instance, athletic trainers may observe Chris in tears after a particularly disappointing game or hear teammates complimenting Scott on an exceptionally good save in practice.

As mentioned earlier, sometimes athletic trainers' observation skills result in conversations that, when initiated, seem casual, but that may become a cause for concern as they progress. For example, an athletic trainer while taping an athlete before practice may notice he or she seems unusually tired and may casually make a comment like, "Gosh, you sure look wiped out today." The athlete may respond by telling the athletic trainer he or she hasn't been sleeping well due to any number of issues such as a death in the family, personal relationship problems, stress over grades or finances, or being in a funk that he or she just can't shake. The athletic trainer can show obvious concern and ***empathy*** for the athlete by asking, "Wow, how are you handling that?" The athlete's response should be assessed against the athletic trainer's internal barometer of concern to decide on the next and most appropriate course of action to take. We discuss this in greater detail later in this chapter.

Athletic trainers may also encounter instances where athletes feel safe and free to disclose personal information that they may not disclose to other sports medicine personnel, their coaches, family members, or teammates. This tendency is often a result of the close and consistent contact athletic trainers have with athletes, and the trust and rapport that athletic trainers have actively fostered. Sometimes athletes bring not only their own personal concerns but also concerns over the behaviors, attitudes, or actions of others. For instance, athletes may confide to athletic trainers that a teammate isn't eating much during the day or escapes to the rest room immediately after each team meal. In one real-life situation, an athletic trainer had concerned teammates bring up the fact that they noticed cut-like marks on a teammate's forearms that weren't there the day before.

In summary, athletic trainers are privy to a great deal of information given to them intentionally through athlete disclosure or unintentionally through observed conversations and interactions. Much of this information is part of the normal daily activities of athletes; however, on occasion, as mentioned earlier, athletic trainers will hear or observe something that raises a red flag regarding athletes' physical and/or psychological health and well-being. In these cases, more formal counseling by experts with greater training may be required, and athletic trainers become the first line of defense in identifying issues of concern and the need for potential referral.

Fortunately, athletic trainers in traditional settings probably know their athletes well. They may see them in

TABLE 6-1 **Examples of Conversation Topics Often Encountered by Athletic Trainers**

Relationship issues
Social activities
Dissention and satisfaction among teammates
Concerns about teammates' activities
Level of satisfaction with coaches
Frustrations
Status of fantasy-league teams
Academic successes and frustrations
Team dynamics issues
Jokes

classes or on campus in addition to their daily practice interactions and be familiar with how athletes typically behave. As a result, athletic trainers learn what is normal or customary behavior in their athletes and what is out of the ordinary. When something out of the ordinary occurs, athletic trainers are ready to recognize and respond accordingly.

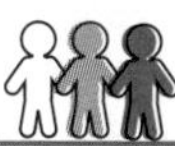

SPECIAL CONSIDERATIONS

Not all athletic trainers work in traditional settings that grant them daily contact with their patients. Athletic trainers working in clinical settings, industrial settings, or with military or emergency personnel may not enjoy the luxury of daily contact. In fact, they may encounter their patients no more frequently than physicians or physical therapists. In these settings, identifying typical behavior for patients is more challenging, and efforts to establish rapport may have to be more intentional.

Scope of Practice of the Athletic Trainer

Determining the best course of action for responding to athletes' mental health needs is based on athletic trainers understanding the scope of their training and preparation to deal with such issues. Table 6-2 lists the documents that help define athletic trainers' scope of practice in such cases. The Board of Certification (BOC) Role Delineation Study (2010) outlines the areas of professional practice critical for an entry-level athletic training practitioner and serves as a basis for the BOC examination. The NATA *Athletic Training Educational Competencies, Fifth Edition* (2011) provides educational programs and other personnel with the knowledge, skills, and clinical abilities to be mastered by students enrolled in accredited athletic training programs. Collectively, these documents can be considered a gauge for the entry-level athletic trainers' scope of practice. Table 6-3 summarizes the knowledge and skills these documents declare athletic trainers should have relative to identifying psychosocial distress and making appropriate referrals.

TABLE 6-2 Documents Defining Athletic Trainers' Scope of Practice

National Athletic Trainers' Association	Board of Certification
NATA Code of Ethics (2005)	BOC Standards of Professional Practice (2006)
NATA Athletic Training Educational Competencies (5th ed.) (2011)	BOC Role Delineation Study (6th ed.) (2010)

The NATA Code of Ethics states that athletic trainers shall "be committed to providing competent care" and shall "provide only those services for which they are qualified through education or experience and which are allowed by their practice acts and other pertinent regulation" (NATA, 2005). As part of their academic preparation and/or continued education, athletic trainers are required to have knowledge of and skill in the areas outlined in Table 6-3, and it should be noted that some athletic trainers may have acquired additional continuing education. Providing casual advice, listening to athletes' concerns, and providing initial emotional support in the immediate aftermath of injury or during the rigors of prolonged rehabilitation all probably fall safely within the scope of most athletic trainers' expertise. However, as mentioned earlier, there will be times when athletic trainers encounter situations that seem beyond their level of training. There are no concrete lines drawn in the sand as to when this will occur, and athletic trainers must trust their judgment and honest appraisal of their level of skill and training in these cases. Competent care stipulates that athletic trainers not having education and experience sufficient to the demands of the situation are ethically bound to refer those athletes to other qualified members of the sports medicine team. Athletic trainers can rely upon three basic guiding principles to help them govern what falls within their scope of practice:

- Do what you've been trained to do.
- Don't do what you haven't been trained to do.
- When in doubt, refer it out!

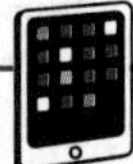

VIRTUAL FIELD TRIP

Go to http://davisplus.fadavis.com to find links to the following documents that guide athletic trainers' scope of ethical practice:

- NATA Code of Ethics
- BOC Standards of Professional Practice
- BOC Role Delineation Study (6th ed.)
- NATA Athletic Training Educational Competencies (5th ed.)

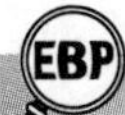

EVIDENCE-BASED PRACTICE

Newcomer, R., & Perna, F. M. (2003). Features of posttraumatic distress among adolescent athletes. *Journal of Athletic Training, 38*(2), 163.

Description of the Study

The purpose of the study was to explore posttraumatic distress among adolescent athletes. Athletes (age range: 13–18 years; mean age: 16.7 years; *n* = 283; 140 girls, 143 boys) representing the sports of football, girls' soccer, basketball, and volleyball participated in the study. Participants were classified according to injury occurrence in the past 12 months; 43 participants reported a loss of playing time due to injury and were classified into the Injury History group, and 240 participants were in the No Injury History group. Intrusive thoughts and avoidance behaviors were self-reported on the Impact of Events Scale at the beginning of the competitive season.

Results of the Study

Participants in the Injury History group reported significantly greater frequency of intrusive thoughts and avoidance behaviors compared with participants in the No Injury History group.

Implications for Athletic Training Practice

Adolescent athletes who have experienced injury may have increased distress and maladaptive coping behaviors. Athletic trainers should therefore take athletes' age into consideration. In addition, adolescent athletes may demonstrate greater injury-related distress than mature athletes.

ESTABLISHING A REFERRAL NETWORK

When referral is needed, it is critical that athletic trainers have an established and trusted referral network in place. This network is built by ***proactively*** identifying qualified providers who have the requisite training and expertise to address all aspects of athletes' health care, including medicine, nutrition, mental health, wellness and health promotion, and even possibly legal counsel (Fig. 6-2, pg. 153). Athletic trainers are typically very good at proactively establishing a comprehensive referral network to address the physical needs of injured athletes. They research competent and experienced medical personnel who may be able and willing to assist with the variety of conditions (e.g., dermatology, neurology, internal medicine, orthopedics) associated with athletic participation. However, athletic trainers may be less thorough in developing other specialties in the referral network (e.g., nutritionist/dietitian, psychologist, substance abuse counselor, social workers, lawyers). Ask athletic trainers to provide the name of a good orthopedic surgeon for an athlete with an injured shoulder and they will most likely provide several; however, ask athletic trainers to provide the name of a good psychologist for a clinically depressed athlete and they may hesitate or struggle to provide that information.

Unfortunately, mental health professionals are too frequently identified as a reaction to conditions athletic trainers encounter with their athletes, rather than a forethought before necessity arises. There are several problems with this approach. First, it may be difficult to locate, adequately screen, and identify ideal mental health professionals for referral networks when there is an issue of time urgency. Just as some physicians are more suitable as referral resources because of their

TABLE 6-3 **Knowledge and Skills Required of Entry-Level Certified Athletic Trainers**

Knowledge of:	Skill in:
• Predisposing factors for nutritional and stress-related disorders • Nutritional disorders, inactivity-related diseases, overtraining issues, and stress-related disorders • Usage patterns, general effects, and short- and long-term adverse effects of commonly used/misused dietary supplements, performance-enhancing drugs, and recreational drugs • Therapeutic drugs, supplements, and performance-enhancing substances banned by sport and workplace organizations • Professional resources for addictions, stress management, and behavior modification • Psychosocial dysfunction associated with injuries, illnesses, catastrophic events, and health-related conditions • Indications for referral • Role and scope of practice of various mental health-care professionals • Using appropriate counseling techniques	• Identifying and describing the signs, symptoms, and physiological and psychological responses of individuals with disordered eating or eating disorders, mental health disorders, substance misuse/abuse, and personal/social conflict • Communicating with appropriate professionals regarding referral • Recognizing signs and symptoms of nutritional, addiction, and stress-related disorders • Directing a referral to the appropriate professionals • Providing guidance/counseling for the individual during the treatment, rehabilitation, and reconditioning process

expertise in sports medicine, their knowledge of the sport culture, or their willingness to expedite appointment scheduling for athletes, mental health professionals should be screened and evaluated on the same criteria to find ideal matches with the athletic trainers' care network. This can be successfully accomplished only when athletic trainers work in a proactive manner. Table 6-4 describes mental health professionals who may be part of the referral network.

Second, when mental health professionals are identified in a reactive manner, it makes a referral to their care seem unnatural—as if this is an odd or unforeseen need in sports medicine. To the contrary, mental health professionals should be presented to coaches and athletes as normal components of a ***holistic*** sports medicine referral network. Often, athletes perceive a stigma surrounding referral to mental health professionals. They may perceive referral to mental health professionals as indicative of weakness or mental instability.

CLINICAL TIP

It is advisable to introduce mental health professionals to coaches and athletes at the same time athletic trainers introduce team physicians. For instance, at preseason team meetings, athletic trainers can either personally introduce the sports medicine team, or at least inform athletes and coaches that, for example, "this is our team physician, Dr. Smith, and this is our team psychologist, Dr. Jones." This will go a long way in making the mental health professionals appear similar to any other member of the sports medicine team.

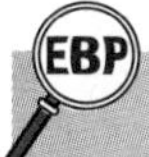

EVIDENCE-BASED PRACTICE

Concannon, M., & Pringle, B. (2012). Psychology in sports injury rehabilitation. *British Journal of Nursing, 21*(8), 484–490.

Continued

Description of the Study

The article presents evidence for adopting a multidisciplinary team approach to the treatment and rehabilitation of sport injury. The case study presents James, an elite 18-year-old track athlete who has been selected to take part in the national trials for the British track and field team for the International Association of Athletics Federation World Championships. Diagnosed with Sever's disease at 12 years of age, James has struggled with chronic, recurrent Achilles tendon problems that are becoming more frequent and, in James's opinion, more severe. His ongoing physical health issues have James questioning the accuracy of his diagnosis, experiencing anxiety and uncertainty about his ability to adequately prepare for the national trials, and suffering doubts about his long-term health and well-being.

Results of the Study

James's initial health-care network consisted of his general practitioner, a physiotherapist (similar to an athletic trainer), and his coach. He was initially treated with anti-inflammatory medication, ultrasound therapy, and at-home stretching exercises. Although these steps partially resolved his symptoms, they did not lead to full recovery. During a repeat visit to his general practitioner for further advice and treatment, it becomes apparent that James's holistic well-being is being affected by the fact that he is suffering from an ongoing condition that has reduced his confidence in obtaining a full recovery. The decision is made to refer James to a podiatrist and a sports psychologist for further consultations on the physical and psychological effects of his injury. As a result, James's treatment plan was altered significantly to address both his physical and his psychological needs. Specifically, the contributions of the sports psychologist allowed James to establish positive short- and long-term goals, gain proficiency in thought stoppage and positive self-talk, and effectively use performance imagery. The combined efforts of James's expanded health-care network provided an accurate diagnosis of his condition, appropriate and effective rehabilitation and prophylaxis, education about the injury and recovery processes, and specific psychological coping skills that resulted in a successful recovery.

Implications for Athletic Training Practice

It is important for athletic trainers to collaborate with all relevant health-care professionals to provide the best possible holistic care for athletes sustaining and recovering from sports injuries. The role of more nontraditional referral resources, and mental health professionals specifically, should not be discounted. It is essential that athletic trainers proactively incorporate these areas into their comprehensive referral network.

Even when athletes perceive referral to mental health experts as useful, researchers (Etzel, Zizzi, Newcomer-Appeneal, Ferrante, & Perna, 2007) have identified the following barriers to attaining psychological services:

- **High visibility of student–athletes on campus:** The high profile of many student–athletes on campus makes it difficult for them to enter counseling centers (especially those on campus) without being recognized. To avoid being identified by others on campus, they may avoid those places.
- **Time demands:** Student–athletes' schedules are already a balancing act of academic, sports, and personal obligations. Adding counseling appointments to an already packed schedule is often difficult.
- **Misconceptions about student–athletes:** Student–athletes are often already viewed as a privileged group

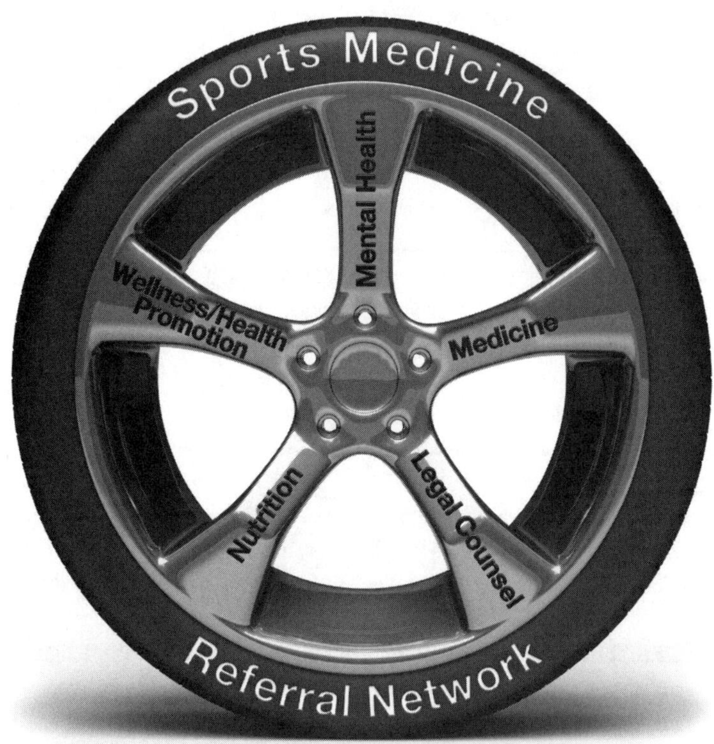

Figure 6-2 | Holistic sports medicine referral network.

on campuses, with all their needs met by the athletic department. Counseling centers may not see any need to reach out to an already "spoiled" group.

- **Restrictive environments:** Athletic departments or coaches may see mental health professionals as "outsiders" and not trust the care or advice that could be provided.
- **Student–athlete attributes:** Student–athletes by nature are often self-sufficient, self-motivated, and independent—traits that have made them successful

TABLE 6-4 Mental Health Professionals

Professional	Description	Common Degree
Clinical psychologist	Works with patients in diagnosing and treating mental disorders; regulated by the American Psychological Association	PhD, PsyD, EdD
Psychiatrist	Medical doctor who works with patients in diagnosing and treating mental disorders; allowed to prescribe medication	MD, DO
Licensed counselor	Provides mental health care; also known as licensed clinical professional counselors or licensed mental health counselors	LPC, LCPC, LMHC
Clinical social worker	Licensed mental health professional	MA, MS, MSW, MSSW, DSW, PhD

in athletics. However, these same attributes may inhibit athletes' willingness to seek assistance or to view mental health difficulties as a betrayal of their independent nature.

CLINICAL TIP

Athletic trainers working at an educational institution that provides mental health services to students should proactively make contact with mental health providers to establish a referral protocol for student–athletes. Using onsite mental health services may reduce the barriers of access and cost of services.

Because of the stigma often attached to using psychological services and the barriers listed earlier, it is important for athletic trainers to "normalize" the psychosocial referral network as just another part of the sports medicine team. Athletes need to be convinced that, just as they are readily open to seeking expert advice for physical difficulties in injury (e.g., consulting an orthopedic surgeon on how to best care for their torn anterior cruciate ligament), seeking expert advice from a mental health professional regarding issues such as adjustment issues to injury, disordered eating, or substance abuse is no different. In fact, seeking such advice is a sign of taking control of their situation and actively pursuing assistance for optimal care.

CLINICAL TIP

It may be helpful for athletic trainers to go into referral discussions with more than one referral possibility in mind. For example, if an athlete responds to your suggestion for a referral with, "There's no way I'm going to see a shrink!" you may ask the athlete what type of professional he or she may be most comfortable seeing. Well-trained professionals in most fields will make appropriate referrals to other professionals (e.g., your sports medicine physician may be able to make a referral to a licensed psychologist for depression or disordered eating), making the athlete more receptive to the athletic trainer's initial referral, but accomplishing the same end result.

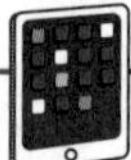

VIRTUAL FIELD TRIP

View the NATA Consensus Statement on "Developing a Plan for Recognition and Referral of Student-Athletes with Psychological Concerns at the Collegiate Level" (Neal et al., 2013) (link available at http://davisplus.fadavis.com).

RECOGNIZING THE NEED FOR REFERRAL

Athletic trainers are expected to identify the signs and symptoms associated with general distress, as well as with specific mental health conditions, and help the athlete seek support through referral. Fortunately, conditions of psychological or psychosocial distress often present with unique signs and symptoms, just as physical impairments do, as discussed later. As stated earlier, although it is not within the scope of athletic trainers' practice to diagnose mental health conditions, athletic trainers are expected to recognize the signs and symptoms of distress and refer appropriately.

Identifying Signs and Symptoms of Concern

There are several ways to identify these signs and symptoms and the modes of gathering information, including:

- Athlete's self-report
- Direct observation of athlete's behavior
- Indirect report/observation of athlete from others (e.g., teammates, coaches)

Athletic trainers should be aware of athletes who are experiencing psychological or psychosocial issues caused by injury and rehabilitation or other impaired functioning related to athletics, school, family, or other relationships. The athlete may also present with specific signs and symptoms that are indicative of a mental health condition. The next section discusses specific conditions that warrant referral.

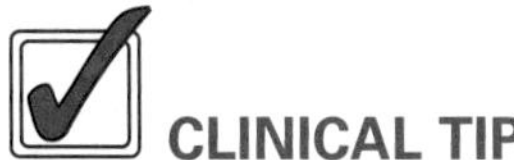

CLINICAL TIP

Athletic trainers can use a SOAP-note approach when assessing athletes on psychosocial factors.

S = Subjective: what the athlete says is going on (e.g., athlete reports difficulty sleeping)

O = Objective: what the athletic trainer observes (e.g., athlete seems sad)

A = Assessment: what the athletic trainer thinks is going on with the athlete (e.g., athlete might be feeling discouraged with lack of progress in rehabilitation)

P = Plan of action: what the athletic trainer plans to do (e.g., psychosocial strategies that can be used or whether referral is warranted at the current time)

CLINICAL TIP

Referral should be considered for any athletes who experience psychosocial distress symptoms that interfere with their activities of daily living. Athletic trainers are sometimes uncertain how severe symptoms need to be before referring. This guideline can provide a comfortable barometer.

Conditions That Warrant Referral

It is not the role of athletic trainers to diagnose conditions, but they must be able to identify the signs and symptoms of these conditions and refer appropriately. Although this is not an exhaustive list, described in this section are conditions that warrant referral, including depression, anxiety, post-traumatic stress disorder (PTSD), panic attack, eating disorders, and substance dependence and abuse. Based on the presented signs and symptoms, as well as the athletic trainer's best judgment of the athlete and situation, the athletic trainer should identify athletes for whom referral is warranted. The conditions described in this section are based in part on the clinical diagnoses set forth in *Diagnostic and Statistical Manual of Mental Disorders*, Fourth Edition (DSM-IV-TR) (American Psychiatric Association [APA], 2000). Although this section discusses clinical signs and symptoms, it is important for athletic trainers to recognize that athletes may present with ***subclinical*** signs and symptoms that should be identified as potential red flags for referral.

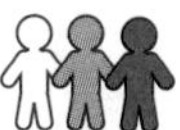

SPECIAL CONSIDERATIONS

Culture and gender can influence how athletes experience depression and how they describe and share the symptoms of depression (APA, 2000).

Depression

Clinical depression is considered a ***mood*** disorder and may be demonstrated as a "major depressive episode" (APA, 2000). Depressed mood or loss of interest in normal activities over a 2-week period with changes in areas such as sleep, appetite, energy, thinking, ***suicidal ideation***, plans, or attempts exemplify a major depressive episode (APA, 2000).

The following signs and symptoms are used to classify a major depressive episode (APA, 2000):

- Depressed mood
- Decreased interest in pleasurable activities
- Weight loss or decreased appetite
- Insomnia or hypersomnia
- Psychomotor agitation
- Fatigue or loss of energy
- Worthlessness or guilt
- Cognitive disruption
- Suicidal ideation, suicide plan, or suicide attempt

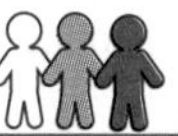

SPECIAL CONSIDERATIONS

Children and adolescents with depression may exhibit an irritable, rather than depressed, mood (APA, 2000).

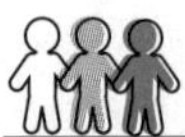

SPECIAL CONSIDERATIONS

Risk factors for suicide include family history, neurobiology (e.g., serotonin levels), existing psychological disorders (e.g., depression, drug abuse), and stressful life events (Barlow & Durand, 2005).

Anxiety

Anxiety is a mood state with excessive worry, and it has psychological, physiological, and behavioral responses. Anxiety and depression may be coupled together or may present as separate conditions.

Signs and symptoms of anxiety may include (Barlow & Durand, 2005):

- Apprehension
- Tension
- Edginess
- Trembling
- Excessive worry
- Nightmares

Post-traumatic Stress Disorder

PTSD is an anxiety disorder that DSM-IV-TR describes as "symptoms following exposure to an extreme traumatic stressor involving direct personal experience of an event that involves actual or threatened death or serious injury or other threat to one's physical integrity; or witnessing an event that involves death, injury, or a threat to the physical integrity of another person; or learning about unexpected or violent death, serious harm, or threat of death or injury experienced by a family member or other close associate" (APA, 2000, p. 463). PTSD may be acute (symptoms last less than 3 months), chronic (symptoms last 3 months or longer), or delayed onset (symptoms occur at least 6 months after the event) (APA, 2000).

PTSD is characterized by the following signs and symptoms, and may cause impairment in social, occupational, or other functioning (APA, 2000):

- Intense fear, helplessness, or horror
- Persistent re-experiencing of the event
- Persistent avoidance of associated stimuli
- Numbing of general responsiveness
- Persistent increased ***arousal***

SPECIAL CONSIDERATIONS

Catastrophic events such as death to teammates or coaches, or even accidents during team travel can precipitate signs and symptoms indicative of referral.

Panic Attack

A panic attack may fall under the general category of anxiety, but it may also be associated with other mental disorders such as mood and substance-related disorders, as well as other general medical conditions such as cardiorespiratory or gastrointestinal conditions (APA, 2000). DSM-IV-TR describes it as "a discrete period in which there is the sudden onset of intense apprehension, fearfulness, or terror, often associated with feelings of impending doom" (APA, 2000, p. 429). These psychological symptoms are accompanied by physical signs and symptoms.

Panic attacks may be unexpected/uncued in which the attack occurs spontaneously, situationally bound, in which the attack occurs in response to a trigger, or situationally predisposed, in which an attack is similar to a situationally bound attack but does not have a specific trigger (APA, 2000). For example, athletes may have a spontaneous panic attack in the cafeteria that they cannot associate with a cue or trigger (unexpected/uncued), or they may have an attack on entering the bus to go to a competition (situationally bound), or the bus may be a trigger for them, but they may or may not have an attack associated specifically with the trigger (situationally predisposed).

Panic attacks are characterized by the following signs and symptoms (APA, 2000):

- Palpitations, pounding heart, or accelerated heart rate
- Sweating
- Shaking
- Shortness of breath or feelings of smothering
- Feeling of choking
- Chest pain/discomfort

- Nausea
- Dizziness, light-headedness, or fainting
- ***Derealization*** or ***depersonalization***
- Fear of losing control or going crazy
- Fear of death
- ***Paresthesias***
- Chills or hot flashes

Disordered Eating and Eating Disorders

As was mentioned at the beginning of this section, the signs and symptoms discussed within this area are clinical in nature. This continues to hold true with eating disorders, in that an athlete may engage in a pattern of disordered eating behaviors but may not present with an eating disorder. An example of disordered eating in athletics is a wrestler trying to "make weight" for a match, in which the athlete may participate in unhealthy caloric restriction, purging behaviors (e.g., vomiting, laxatives, diuretics, diet pills) and excessive exercise; however, these behaviors may be at subclinical levels and, therefore, would not be classified as an eating disorder. Two specific eating disorders are anorexia nervosa and bulimia nervosa.

Signs and symptoms of anorexia nervosa include (APA, 2000):

- Refusal to maintain weight at a minimally normal weight for age and height
- Severe fear of gaining weight or becoming fat (although underweight)
- Amenorrhea (in postmenarchal women)

Similarly, signs and symptoms of bulimia nervosa include (APA, 2000):

- Recurrent episodes of binge eating
- Recurrent inappropriate compensatory behaviors to prevent weight gain (i.e., purging)
- Binging and purging on average two times a week for 3 months
- Self-evaluation overly influenced by body shape and weight
- Signs and symptoms do not occur exclusively during episodes of anorexia nervosa

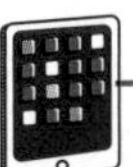

VIRTUAL FIELD TRIP

View the NATA Position Statement on "Preventing, Detecting, and Managing Disordered Eating in Athletes" (Bonci et al., 2008) (link available at http://davisplus.fadavis.com).

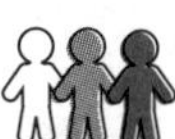

SPECIAL CONSIDERATIONS

Most cases (approximately 90%) of anorexia nervosa are diagnosed in female individuals (APA, 2000), but athletic trainers should be aware of male athletes who present with signs and symptoms.

Substance Dependence and Abuse

A substance includes "a drug of abuse, a medication [prescribed and over-the-counter], or a toxin" (APA, 2000, p. 191). Substance dependence is a "maladaptive pattern of substance use, leading to clinically significant impairment or distress" (APA, 2000, p. 197). Substance dependence may cause athletes to increase their ***tolerance*** and to experience ***withdrawal***.

Substance dependence includes three or more of the following within a 12-month time frame (APA, 2000):

- Tolerance
- Withdrawal
- Taking either larger quantities or for a longer time than intended
- Desire or inability to decrease use
- Increased time spent in drug-related activities
- Interference with social, occupational, or recreational activities
- Use in spite of physical or psychological harm

Substance abuse is "a maladaptive pattern of substance use manifested by recurrent and significant adverse consequences related to the repeated use of substances" (APA, 2000, p. 198). Substance abuse includes one or more of the following within a 12-month time frame and has not met the criteria for substance dependence (APA, 2000):

- Failure to uphold major obligations because of substance use
- Engagement in physically dangerous situations because of substance use
- Legal issues caused by substance use
- Social issues caused by substance use

Athletic trainers who suspect that an athlete may have issues related to a substance dependence or substance abuse should refer the athlete to a qualified professional. It is important to recognize, however, that athletes do not have to have a substance use disorder to misuse substances. The following medications are commonly used by athletes and may be drugs on which athletes become dependent or abuse (including but not limited to): anesthetic and analgesic medications, corticosteroids, and nonsteroidal anti-inflammatory medications. Other drugs, including but not limited to alcohol, amphetamines, cannabis, cocaine, hallucinogens, inhalants, nicotine, opioids, and sedatives, may also be the source of dependence or abuse by athletes.

SPECIAL CONSIDERATIONS

Individuals in their late teens and early 20s may have a particularly high rate of substance use and dependence; although it can be developed at any age, it usually begins in the range of 20 to 40 years of age (APA, 2000). Therefore, athletic trainers who work with athletes in this age range should:

- be vigilant in educating athletes on the negative effects of drugs, including alcohol.
- provide athletes with resources to assist if they believe they may need assistance with substance use.
- refer athletes to qualified professionals if they suspect issues related to substance use.

SPECIAL CONSIDERATIONS

Athletic trainers should be aware of the sport culture surrounding drinking and the use of other drugs, and how this culture may influence athletes to engage in unhealthy behaviors. When athletes perceive drinking or use of other drugs to be a team or sport norm, they may be more likely to engage in those behaviors to keep up (e.g., think of Lance Armstrong and the cycling culture), fit in with teammates, or enhance team cohesiveness.

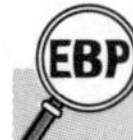

EVIDENCE-BASED PRACTICE

Storch, E. A., Storch, J. B., Killiany, E. M., & Roberti, J. W. (2005). Self-reported psychopathology in athletes: A comparison of intercollegiate student-athletes and non-athletes. *Journal of Sport Behavior, 28*(1), 86–97.

Description of the Study

The study compared the psychosocial adjustment of a sample of intercollegiate student–athletes with a sample of their nonathlete peers. Participants were 398 undergraduate students (133 males, 265 females), 105 of whom were intercollegiate athletes (54 males, 51 females). Participants completed the Social Anxiety Scale for Adolescents and the Personality Assessment Inventory, which measured depression, alcohol problems, and social support.

Results of the Study

Female athletes reported greater social anxiety and depressive symptoms, and lower scores of social support than male athletes and nonathletes. Although there were no clinically significant differences with alcohol problems, depression, or social anxiety between male and female athletes or between athletes and nonathletes, it was noted that clinical levels of alcohol use and depression were reported in all participant groups.

Implications for Athletic Training Practice

Although this study is limited in that participants were from a single public university in the southeastern United States, athletic trainers should recognize that student–athletes experience clinical levels of psychopathology (specifically alcohol use and depression). In addition, athletic trainers should be aware that female athletes may experience less social support, and greater anxiety and depressive symptoms than their male peers.

REFERRAL PROCESS

Once the athletic trainer recognizes the signs and symptoms of an athlete experiencing distress or of a mental health condition, the referral may take one of two forms: spontaneous or planned. In a spontaneous referral, the situation is severe enough that it warrants immediate referral. For example, in an extreme case, the athlete may mention to the athletic trainer that he or she plans to do physical self-harm (referred to as nonsuicidal self-injury). Also in a spontaneous referral, the situation may be more organic in that referral seems like a natural step, and the rapport between the athletic trainer and athlete is such that referral seems like a natural extension of the care process. For example, the athletic trainer may be talking to the athlete about an upcoming exam and the athlete mentions other stresses. The athletic trainer then suggests to the athlete to look into several stress-management groups offered at the campus counseling center.

If the referral is planned, the athletic trainer should take several things into consideration (Fig. 6-3).

Athletic trainers should role-play scenarios in which referral is warranted and keep in mind the strategies discussed within this section. Specific to place and timing, for example, a busy athletic training room may not be an appropriate place to initiate a referral because of confidentiality concerns; therefore, the athletic trainer should plan a different place to initiate a conversation with the athlete about referral. Right before a game or practice may not be an appropriate time to initiate a referral. In addition, looking for objective signs of mental health distress and asking open-ended questions (as discussed in Chapter 5 with communication skills) are important in the referral conversation (Fig. 6-4).

How to do it?
When to do it?
What to ask?
What to look for?
Where to do it?
Where to refer?
Referral

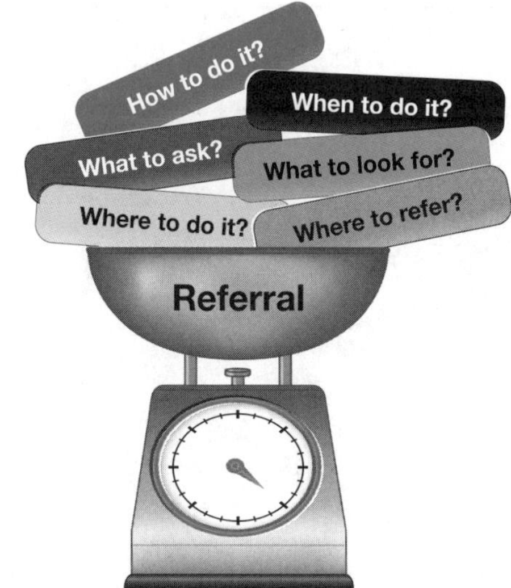

Figure 6-3 | Referral considerations.

Both the actual process of referral and to whom the athlete will be referred greatly depend on the athlete and the situation, but the athletic trainer should have this planned before initiating the referral conversation. Timing of a referral will be based on the following factors (Brewer, Petipas, & Van Raalte, 1999):

- Severity of signs and symptoms
- Coping resources of the athlete
- Skills training of the athletic trainer
- Relationship between the athlete and athletic trainer
- Relationship between the athletic trainer and mental health professional
- Immediate situational and environmental factors

RED FLAG

Destructive behavior of an athlete toward others or the intent to harm others should be reported immediately to the appropriate authority based on the athletic trainer's institutional setup (e.g., counseling center, campus safety).

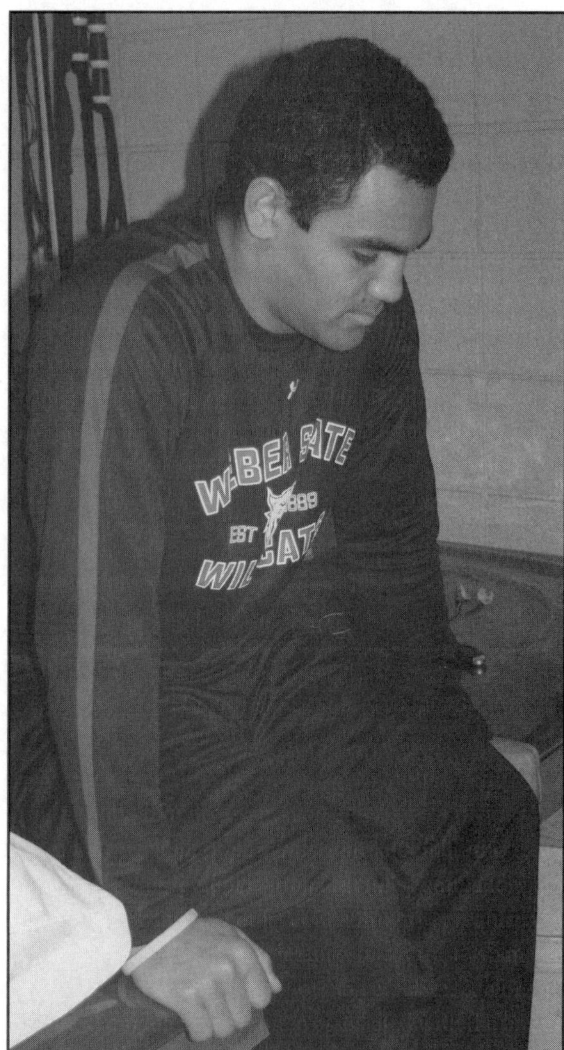

Figure 6-4 | Identifying athlete distress.

How to Refer

A five-phase process of referral includes (Brewer et al., 1999):

- Assessment
- Consultation
- Trial intervention
- Referral
- Follow-up

During the assessment phase, the athletic trainer uses athletes' signs and symptoms to evaluate them to determine their potential mental health needs. During the consultation phase, the athletic trainer contacts a mental health professional within the already identified referral network to discuss the athlete based on the athletic trainer's assessment. When talking with a mental health professional, the athletic trainer can gain guidance as to the appropriate immediacy of referral and potential intervention steps the athletic trainer can take toward helping the athlete. If a trial intervention is advised, the athletic trainer works with the athletes to assist them with the suggested coping and management strategies aimed at decreasing their distress. Depending on the athlete and the situation, and the efficacy of the trial intervention, referral to a mental health professional may be warranted. During the referral phase, the athletic trainer initiates the referral process with the athlete. As stated earlier in the chapter, during this time, it is important for the athletic trainer to normalize the process. For example, the athletic trainer may say, "Just as you would seek assistance from a physician for a broken bone, you would seek assistance from a professional for the stress that you're experiencing." The athletic trainer can also discuss the physical and performance implications that the athlete's stress may be causing. If the athlete agrees to referral, the athletic trainer should help with the process of setting an appointment and, similar to other referrals for physical conditions, may even accompany the athlete to the referral site. If the athlete does not agree to referral, the athletic trainer should continue to monitor the athlete and initiate another trial intervention and referral at a later time. Finally, during the follow-up phase, the athletic trainer communicates with the athlete and mental health professional (with a waiver of confidentiality from the athlete). This communication may be as simple as the mental health professional reporting to the athletic trainer that the athlete has been seen for referral, or it may include suggested actions the athletic trainer can take to further assist the athlete.

A possible challenge in making mental health referrals is the fact that athletes sometimes do not perceive that they have a problem. Although athletes occasionally deny physical injuries, physical injuries often produce readily perceptible impairments on athletes' physical abilities. In contrast, athletes may be less aware of the deleterious effects of psychosocial conditions (e.g., disordered eating, substance misuse/abuse, depression, anxiety) on physical performance, or be unwilling to admit that such conditions are sport performance concerns. A strategy that the athletic trainer can use when approaching the topic of mental health issues is to discuss these psychosocial conditions in relation to the athlete's sport performance. For example, when working with an athlete who shows signs of disordered eating, the athletic trainer may discuss the role of proper caloric intake related to optimal performance.

The referral process is dynamic and dependent on a variety of factors. Just as athletic trainers use their best clinical knowledge and professional judgment to determine referral for a physical condition, so must they use their best clinical knowledge and professional judgment to determine the need for a mental health referral. The athletic trainer's clinical skills are important in the mental health referral process, and similar to the practice of physical assessment, the practice of mental health referral protocols should be rehearsed and role-played so that athletic trainers are comfortable referring when the need arises.

PSYCHOSOCIAL STRATEGIES

Social support, and more specifically satisfaction with social support, may be important in the mental health of athletes. As discussed in Chapter 9, the athletic trainer can help athletes identify individuals within their social support network. By identifying this social support network, athletes may see that different individuals are able to provide different types of social support (e.g., emotional, informational, tangible).

Communication skills are critical in making a referral suggestion. As discussed in Chapter 5, the athletic trainer needs to make proper application of ***proxemics***, eye contact, body language, and vocal tone to make the referral conversation comfortable and nonthreatening to the athlete. Two-way communication allowing the athlete to verbalize concerns and questions will further increase the likelihood of positive outcomes.

Stress is part of the human experience, and athletes have many demands placed on them (e.g., sport, school, work, social). As discussed in Chapter 3, stress-management techniques such as cognitive or somatic relaxation can be incorporated into the athletes' treatment. Ideally, this would be a proactive approach, such that stress-management techniques are used before distress occurs. However, they may also be incorporated into the rehabilitation program or used as a trial intervention before referral.

ATHLETE INSIDER CONCLUSION

Based on the five phases of referral (assessment, consultation, trial intervention, referral, follow-up; Brewer et al., 1999), the athletic trainer has assessed that Amelia's response to injury is interfering with her daily functioning and seeks consultation with a psychologist in the university's counseling center. In consultation with the psychologist, a trial intervention of assisting Amelia in identifying coping resources (e.g., social support) and the use of a relaxation script for assistance with falling asleep will be implemented by the athletic trainer. The athletic trainer suggests these strategies to Amelia, and she is open to trying them. After approximately a week, Amelia reports to the athletic trainer that, although she has been listening to the relaxation script and has been trying to talk more with her friends, she is still feeling lost and is worried about the future. At this point, the athletic trainer decides to suggest to Amelia that she talk with a professional in the counseling center about her situation and the stress that she is experiencing. The athletic trainer shares that other athletes have worked with the counseling center, and they have had positive outcomes. Amelia agrees to set up an appointment. The athletic trainer does a follow-up with the psychologist to ensure that Amelia attends the appointment (Amelia has given written permission for the follow-up), continues to work with Amelia in rehabilitation, and lets her know that he will periodically check in with her to ensure the counseling is going well. The athletic trainer also lets Amelia know that he is always available if Amelia would like to share her experience.

Effective Psychosocial Strategies for the Athletic Trainer to Use with Amelia

The athletic trainer can implement the following psychosocial strategies with Amelia during rehabilitation and return to participation:

1. Identify coping resources. These resources may include identification of individuals within Amelia's social support network (as discussed in Chapter 9 with social support).

2. Introduce the use of a relaxation script for Amelia to use to assist with sleep.
3. Initiate collaborative goal setting, with Amelia taking an active role in the setting of goals, to give her more ownership in the process and help her see the steps to return to volleyball participation.
4. Coordinate a conversation between Amelia and her coach to discuss and hopefully minimize Amelia's concerns about her injury's impact on her career.

CONCLUSION

This chapter has discussed the athletic trainer's role and scope of practice in the identification and management of distress and mental health disorders. The importance of both a multidisciplinary sports medicine team and a mental health referral network was emphasized. This chapter provided a framework to help guide athletic trainers through the psychosocial consultation and referral process. This chapter also emphasized the importance of athletic trainers practicing referral situations so that they are comfortable in the referral process when the need arises.

REFERENCES

American Psychiatric Association (APA). (2000). *Diagnostic and Statistical Manual of Mental Disorders* (DSM-IV-TR, 4th ed., Text Revision). Arlington, VA: APA.

Barlow, D. H., & Durand, V. M. (2005). *Abnormal Psychology: An Integrative Approach* (4th ed.). Belmont, CA: Thomson Wadsworth.

Board of Certification. (2006). *BOC Standards of Professional Practice.* Retrieved October 22, 2012, from www.bocatc.org/index.php?option=com_content&view=article&id=188&Itemid=190

Board of Certification. (2010). *The 2009 Athletic Trainer Role Delineation Study.* Omaha, NE: Stephen B. Johnson.

Bonci, C. M., Bonci, L. J., Granger, L. R., Johnson, C. L., Malina, R. M., Milne, L. W., Ryan R.R., & Vanderbunt, E. M. (2008). National Athletic Trainers' Association position statement: Preventing, detecting, and managing disordered eating in athletes. In: *NATA Position, Consensus, Official and Support Statements.* Dallas, TX: National Athletic Trainers' Association.

Brewer, B. W., Petitpas, A. J., & Van Raalte, J. L. (1999). Referral of injured athletes for counseling and psychotherapy. In: R. Ray & D. M. Wiese-Bjornstal (Eds.), *Counseling in Sports Medicine* (pp. 127–141). Champaign, IL: Human Kinetics.

Concannon, M., & Pringle, B. (2012). Psychology in sports injury rehabilitation. *British Journal of Nursing, 21*(8), 484–490.

Etzel, E. F., Zizzi, S., Newcomer-Appeneal, R. R., Ferrante, A. P., & Perna, F. M. (2007). Providing psychological assistance to college student-athletes with injuries and disabilities. In: Pargman, D. (Ed.), *Psychological Bases of Sport Injuries* (3rd ed., pp. 151–169). Morgantown, WV: Fitness Information Technology.

National Athletic Trainers' Association. (2005). *NATA Code of Ethics.* Retrieved October 2, 2012, from www.nata.org/insets/about_NATA/index.htm.

National Athletic Trainers' Association. (2011). *Athletic Training Educational Competencies* (5th ed.). Retrieved October 5, 2012, from www.nata.org/education/competencies.

Neal, T. L., Diamond, A. B., Goldman, S., Klossner, D., Morse, E. D., Pajak, D. E., ...Wallack, C. (2013). *Inter-Association recommendations in developing a plan for recognition and referral of student-athletes with psychological concerns at the collegiate level: A consensus statement.* Retrieved from http://www.nata.org/consensus-statements.

Newcomer, R., & Perna, F. M. (2003). Features of posttraumatic distress among adolescent athletes. *Journal of Athletic Training, 38*(2), 163.

Storch, E. A., Storch, J. B., Killiany, E. M., & Roberti, J. W. (2005). Self-reported psychopathology in athletes: A comparison of intercollegiate student-athletes and non-athletes. *Journal of Sport Behavior, 28*(1), 86–97.

BOARD OF CERTIFICATION STRATEGIES AND COMPETENCIES

As the Sixth Edition of the BOC's Role Delineation Study outlines, athletic trainers are involved in the prevention and care of athletic injury (Domain 1). The Fifth Edition Athletic Training Education Competencies content area of Psychosocial Strategies and Referral (PS) contains eight competencies specific to "Mental Health and Referral." These include describing the role of mental health-care providers who are part of the referral network (PS-11), identifying and describing the signs and symptoms of mental conditions that warrant referral to a mental health professional (PS-12, PS-13), and educating the athlete and ensuring appropriate privacy (PS-18). Recognizing the need for and initiating a referral for athletes with suspected eating disorders and substance abuse issues is also included in this content area (PS-14, PS-15, PS-16). When catastrophic events occur, recognizing the need for psychological intervention and a referral for those affected by the event is included in this content area (PS-17). In addition, one of the Clinical Integration Proficiencies (CIP-8) specifically addresses the ability to develop a mental health referral plan, as well as recognize and refer individuals who are in need to a mental health professional. Beyond the PS content area but still within the Fifth Edition Athletic Training Education Competencies, content within the area of Prevention and Health Promotion (PHP) includes referral by addressing appropriate management and referral for athletes with eating disorders (PHP-47), and the content area of Professional Development and Responsibility (PD) includes referral by formulating and implementing strategies to facilitate referral (PD-9).

Board of Certification Style Questions

1. Which of the following is (are) examples of athletic trainers' role as advisor to the athlete? (Select all that apply.)
   a. How many times to ice the evening after injury
   b. The pros and cons of surgery immediately versus waiting until the season is over
   c. Providing clinical diagnosis of depression
   d. Listening to an injured athlete's concerns about return to play following injury

2. What barriers often impact athletes' receptivity to referral for mental health services? (Select all that apply.)
   a. Concerns of appearing weak
   b. High visibility of student–athletes on campus
   c. Lack of independence
   d. Time demands of typical student–athletes' schedules

3. Potential referral sources should be screened on what criteria? (Select all that apply.)
   a. Professional credentials
   b. Expertise in sports medicine
   c. Knowledge or understanding of the sport culture
   d. Willingness to expedite appointments for student–athletes

4. Which of the following documents assist in defining the scope of practice for athletic trainers in terms of psychosocial intervention and referral? (Select all that apply.)
   a. NATA Code of Ethics
   b. BOC Standards of Professional Practice
   c. BOC Role Delineation Study
   d. NATA Athletic Training Educational Competencies

5. Comprehensive referral networks should include experts in which of the following? (Select all that apply.)
   a. Medicine
   b. Insurance fraud
   c. Mental health
   d. Nutrition

6. Which knowledge and/or skills should all athletic trainers have relative to psychosocial strategies and referral? (Select all that apply.)
   a. Clinical counseling skills
   b. Recognizing signs and symptoms of nutritional disorders
   c. Understanding the role and scope of practice of various mental health-care professionals
   d. Recognizing indications for referral

7. Which of the following documents outlines the knowledge, skills, and clinical abilities to be mastered by students in professional athletic training programs? (Select all that apply.)
   a. NATA Athletic Training Educational Competencies
   b. BOC Role Delineation Study
   c. NATA Code of Ethics
   d. BOC Standards of Professional Practice

END-OF-CHAPTER EXERCISES

1. Develop a list of screening questions that could be used to interview a potential mental health professional regarding becoming a member of your sports medicine network.
2. Describe the role of various mental health providers (e.g., psychologist, psychiatrist, counselor) who may comprise a mental health referral network.
3. Use available resources to identify and compile a list of available mental health professionals (include their credentials) on campus or in the greater community that could potentially serve as mental health referral resources.
4. Interview a mental health professional on campus or in the community regarding that person's interest in or qualifications to work as a referral resource in your sports medicine network.
5. List the signs and symptoms of the following clinical disorders:
   a. Depression
   b. Anxiety, post-traumatic stress disorder, panic attack
   c. Anorexia nervosa
   d. Bulimia nervosa
   e. Substance abuse
6. Read the NATA Position Statement on "Preventing, Detecting, and Managing Disordered Eating in Athletes" (Bonci et al., 2008). Discuss the important points of this statement and describe how you can use it to guide your clinical practice.
7. Describe the five phases of referral (Brewer et al., 1999).
8. Read the following case study involving Brad.
   a. As the athletic trainer, what will you do?
   b. What indications do you recognize that warrant your plan?
   c. Role-play the conversation of suggesting referral. Have others observe this role-play and provide feedback on what went well and offer suggestions on how to improve.

CASE STUDY

Brad is a junior baseball player with a good chance of being drafted at the end of the year. He was the #2 starter this season until he sustained a torn rotator cuff muscle 2 weeks ago. Doctors have told him that his season is over and that he will need surgery to repair the damage. Brad has decided to wait until the summer to have the surgery. You overhear Brad's teammates talking at practice one day about the "funk" that Brad is in. When you ask them about it, they tell you that Brad is really down about his injury. He is concerned that his chances for a professional baseball career are gone. His teammates tell you that he hasn't gone to classes or attended practice for the past week. They say, "All he wants to do is sit in his room alone. He won't go to meals with us; he won't go out with us. He just sits there all day. . . . I don't even think he's taken a shower for the past week. Yesterday, he even talked about dropping out of school and not coming back for his senior year."

Chapter 7

Introduction and Overview of Pain

Megan D. Granquist and Jennifer Stiller-Ostrowski

CHAPTER OUTLINE

KEY TERMS

Acute pain Pain of recent and sudden onset; typically high-intensity pain localized at or near the site of injury.

Allodynia Extreme sensitivity to an innocuous stimulus (such as light touch or cold); pain from sunburn is a common example.

Anterior cingulate cortex Frontal part of cingulate cortex in the brain; plays a role in cognitive functions such as reward anticipation, decision making, empathy, and emotion.

Benign pain Temporary occurrence of discomfort that is not associated with new tissue damage; characterized as dull and generalized with no swelling or localized tenderness.

Cerebral cortex A part of the brain that plays a key role in memory, attention, perceptual awareness, thought, language, and consciousness.

Chronic pain Pain that persists beyond the normal time expected for healing (typically a minimum of 3–6 months).

Extrovert Manifested in outgoing, talkative, energetic behavior.

Hyperalgesia Heightened sensation response to noxious stimulus.

Hypothalamus A part of the brain responsible for certain metabolic processes and other activities of the autonomic nervous system (including body temperature, hunger, thirst, fatigue, sleep, and circadian cycles).

Injury pain Occurrence of pain that signals actual or potential tissue damage.

Introvert Manifested in more reserved, quiet, shy behavior.

Limbic system A complex set of brain structures that lies on both sides of the thalamus; supports a variety of functions including emotion, behavior, and long-term memory.

Nociception The process of pain sensation by the nociceptors.

Nociceptors Sensory neurons that respond to potentially damaging stimuli by sending nerve signals to the spinal cord and brain.

Noxious An actually or potentially tissue-damaging event; may be mechanical, chemical, or thermal.

Pain perception Conscious interpretation of nociceptive stimulus as pain.

Pain sensation Stimulus is received by the nervous system (via nociceptors).

Pain-spasm cycle Pain that causes vasoconstriction and muscle spasm, which, in turn, causes more pain, which, in turn, exacerbates the cycle; sometimes referred to as the pain-spasm-pain cycle.

Pain threshold Point at which pain begins to be felt; an entirely subjective phenomenon.

Pain tolerance The ability of the patient to withstand pain or painful stimuli for a period of time.

Periaqueductal gray A role in the descending modulation of pain.

Persistent pain Pain that meets the time frame defined as chronic but is actually a symptom of a treatable condition.

Sensation Stimulus is received by the nervous system (via nociceptors).

Somatic Of the body; relating to the body; bodily illness.

Somatosensory cortex The main sensory receptive area for the sense of touch.

Stress-induced analgesia A reduction in pain sensitivity during stress conditions.

Thalamus A part of the brain that relays sensory and motor signals to the cerebral cortex and regulates consciousness, sleep, and alertness.

CHAPTER OBJECTIVES

After reading this chapter, you will be able to:

1. Describe the process of pain sensation and perception.
2. Describe the psychosocial factors that affect persistent pain sensation and perception.
3. Differentiate between types of pain, such as acute, chronic, persistent, injury, and performance.
4. Identify physiological and psychosocial contributions to chronic pain.
5. Differentiate between pain threshold and pain tolerance.
6. Identify personal, cultural, and gender factors that influence an individual's perception of pain and pain tolerance.
7. Describe ascending and descending pain-control theories, and the role of the mind in pain interpretation and modulation.
8. Select and integrate nonpharmacological pain-management techniques that should be used during interactions with injured athletes.
9. Identify multidisciplinary approaches for assisting patients with persistent pain.

ATHLETE INSIDER

Jayda is a collegiate soccer player finishing her junior year. She has continued pain in her lower leg. She has a history of ankle sprains, with her longest ankle rehabilitation being approximately 3 months. She had bilateral compartment syndrome release 2 years ago and then sustained a fracture of her tibia and fibula during a match a year ago last spring. She had surgery to place a rod in her tibia and began rehabilitation and eventually walking last summer. During this past fall season, she continued to rehabilitate but had sustained ongoing pain. She was then diagnosed with nonfusion of the fibula and had surgery to implant a plate on the fibula. In December, she began running again, but she continues to have pain in her leg. The orthopedic surgeon and team physician have assured her she is fully cleared to play; however, she is hesitant to play due to her pain. She describes this pain as "shooting" pain upon her foot contacting the ground while running; the pain is also worse when it is cold or the season changes. The team began spring practice in February, and she is currently working on agility drills. Her goal is to play again next fall during her senior year, but she has some fear of reinjury. She describes seeing herself in her mind getting

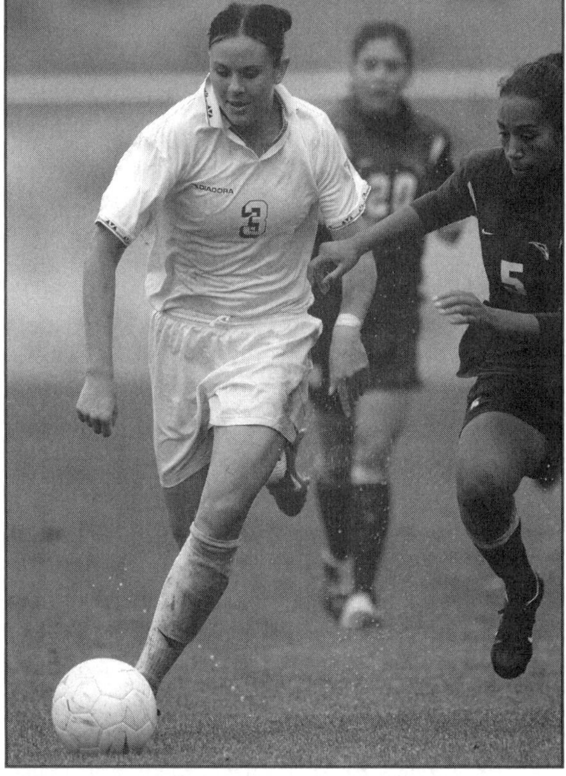

Figure 7-1 | Athlete Insider *(Courtesy of Weber State University Athletics)*

injured again. She has good family and team support but describes herself as currently personally exhausted.

INTRODUCTION

This chapter introduces the concept of pain as not just a physiological experience, but as one with both cognitive and emotional contributions. With an overview of the physiology of pain, this chapter discusses basic concepts of pain that pertain to the athletic training setting. It will further help to shape the athletic trainer's view of athlete pain as being important information about internal processes and guide the athletic trainer in educating the athlete about pain and its role throughout the rehabilitation process. Specifically, performance pain (benign discomfort that should be pushed through) will be differentiated from injury pain (harmful pain that signals an athlete needs to scale back), and acute pain will be differentiated from chronic pain. The role of pain throughout the injury process is overviewed, with special attention on nonadaptive behaviors following injury. Finally, this chapter overviews nonpharmacological pain management, such as psychological strategies, and teaches the athletic trainer how these techniques can be applied to each stage of the rehabilitation process to aid in the athlete's interpretation and modulation of pain.

OVERVIEW OF PAIN

It is very important to remember that pain is both a sensory *and* an emotional experience. Pain is complex. Pain has been described as "an unpleasant sensory and emotional experience associated with actual or potential tissue damage, or described in terms of such damage" (Merskey et al, 1979). Consider, however, that pain is completely subjective and cannot be directly measured. As a result, it is difficult to objectively determine how much pain an athlete is in and what levels of pain management are appropriate. Athletic trainers and other allied health-care providers often attempt to have patients quantify pain or discomfort. Such practice not only provides information to the athletic trainer, but also benefits the injured athlete. A quantifiable assessment of pain helps the athlete recognize and discriminate between different levels of pain, identifies in what situations and why pain occurs, provides feedback about the effectiveness of various pain-management strategies, and contributes to a greater sense of control by making pain more tangible. The most straightforward quantifiable, albeit subjective, measurement of pain is on a 0 to 10 scale, where 0 represents no pain and 10 represents the worst pain possible (Fig. 7-2). (Note: It may be helpful to inquire what the athlete's worst pain to date has been.) Pain-measurement methods are discussed in detail later in this chapter.

Pain does not occur in the body without the mind reacting and contributing to the experience. Take, for example, the experience of stubbing your toe. Under any circumstance, this can be regarded as a painful experience; however, the amount of pain will be subjectively evaluated based on the individual's emotional state at the time. Consider the following:

- **Example 1:** You are having a good day, racing around the house getting ready for a highly anticipated second date when you stub your toe. Ouch! But you move on quickly, not focusing on the pain for long.
- **Example 2:** Your day is not starting off so well—you overslept and are late for a test in your class. As you race around the house getting what you need for class, you stub your toe. Ouch! Ever notice that the pain is that much worse when you are already having a bad day?

This is perhaps one of the simplest examples of how emotional distress can intensify perception of ***somatic*** symptoms (Fig. 7-3). When significant emotional distress follows injury, this may negatively impact recovery and may actually prolong physical rehabilitation. Let us begin our overview of pain with a review of the purpose and physiology of pain.

CLINICAL TIP

When working with athletes, athletic trainers should keep these key points in mind:

- Pain is sensory *and* emotional.
- Pain is sensed and perceived (e.g., interpreted) (perception ≠ sensation).
- Injury may not produce pain, and pain may not be caused by an injury (injury ≠ pain).
- Pain sensitization may become increased by repeated stimulation.

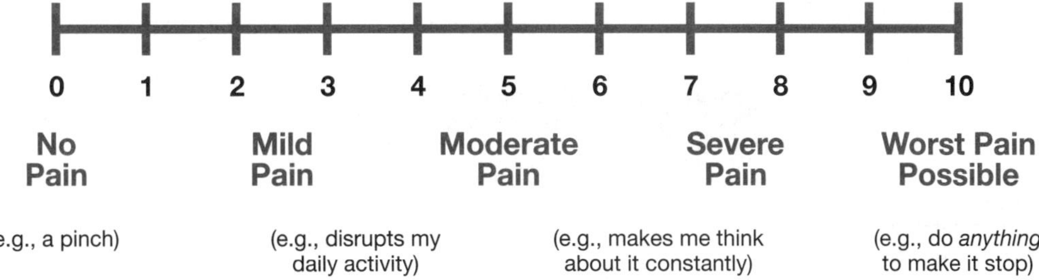

Figure 7-2 | Pain continuum.

PURPOSE AND PHYSIOLOGY OF PAIN

Although unpleasant, pain actually serves a useful purpose in that it warns us that something is wrong internally. Pain often occurs before tissue injury is sustained, which allows the individual time to react or provoke a withdrawal response to prevent injury from occurring. Pain also cues muscle spasm, which serves to guard or protect the injured part. However, we know that this spasm can persist after it is no longer useful and can promote additional dysfunction. Pain can even be perceived in the absence of tissue damage (a headache, for example). Consider also that emotional distress and/or stress can actually *cause* somatic symptoms (Fig. 7-4). Individuals may feel nauseous and even vomit after getting bad news. An argument with a significant other can lead to stomach pains or cramping. Stress leading into finals week can cause muscle pains or migraine headaches. However, not all unpleasant or abnormal experiences should be called pain; athletes need to be educated about pain versus discomfort and about ***benign pain*** (performance) versus ***injury pain*** (harmful) (see discussion later in this chapter).

Physiology of Pain

Physical pain is caused by activation of ***nociceptors***, which transmit sensory information to the brain via the spinal cord; this process is known as ***nociception***. Nociceptors can be mechanical (response to distension or stretch), thermal (response to temperatures), or chemical (activated by the presence of proinflammatory mediators or neurotransmitters). The stimulation of nociceptors by chemical stimuli explains why pain is felt even after the injurious force has been removed. As part of the acute inflammatory process, chemical mediators appear in damaged tissues. As long as these chemicals are present, we feel residual pain from the original injury. In addition, because nociceptors become more sensitive to the presence of ongoing stimulation, the

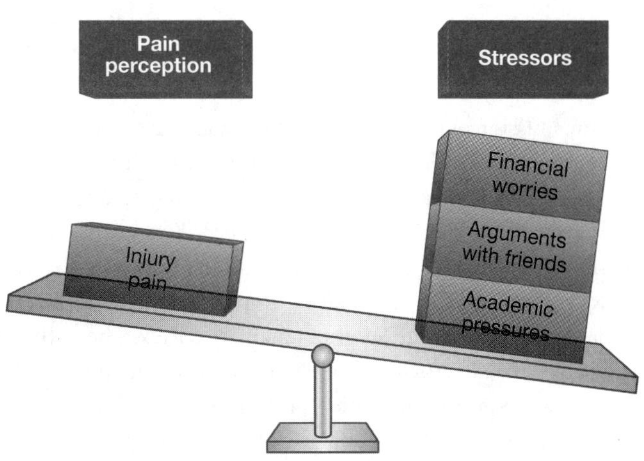

Figure 7-3 | Impact of emotional distress on pain perception.

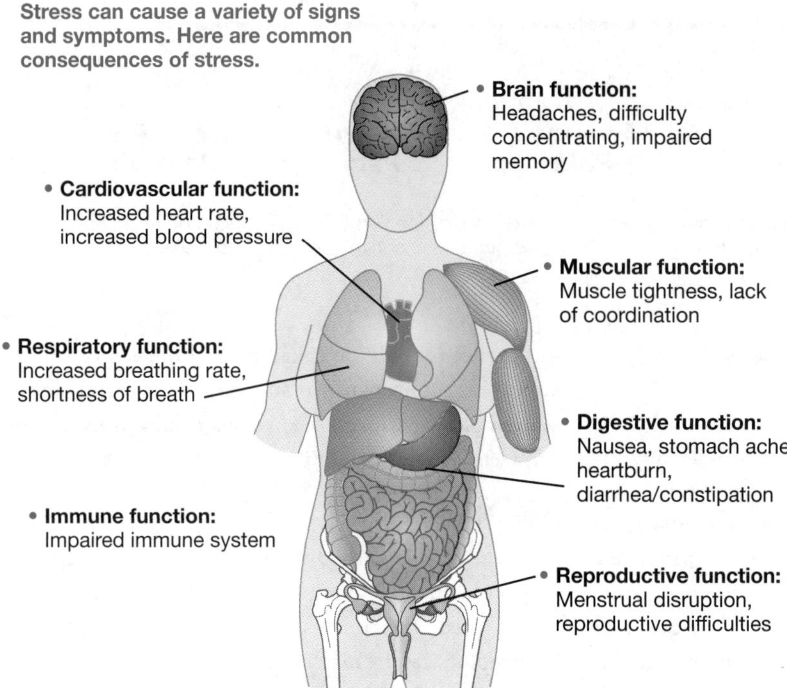

Figure 7-4 | Consequences of stress.

injured athlete may actually experience increased sensitivity to noxious stimuli (***hyperalgesia***). Once nociceptors have been stimulated (via mechanical, thermal, or chemical stimuli), they carry information to the dorsal horn within the spinal cord. From here, pain information continues up to the brain. Specific brain structures involved in processing pain information include the ***thalamus*** and ***hypothalamus***, the ***periaqueductal gray*** within the brainstem, the ***limbic system***, and the ***cerebral cortex*** (including the ***anterior cingulate cortex*** and the ***somatosensory cortex***; see Fig. 7-5).

Transmission of pain information through the hypothalamus explains the autonomic changes associated with pain (pallor, sweating, dilated pupils, and increased heart rate, blood pressure, and pulse rate). However, possibly of greatest interest in our discussion of the psychology of pain is the contribution to pain perception by the limbic system and anterior cingulate cortex. The limbic system is actually a collection of components rather than a specific anatomical area of the brain. It is often called the "emotional brain," because it is responsible for emotional aspects and responses to pain (e.g., anxiety, fear, sadness) and also for emotional memory. The anterior cingulate cortex is responsible for integrating information about pain perception. In addition to alerting the individual to potential tissue damage and evaluating how serious the danger might be, the cortex helps learning to occur (remember and avoid pain in the future) and associates memories to pain. This association may explain why athletes will cringe when they see another athlete become injured in the same manner in which they were injured. The anterior cingulate cortex is also responsible for gauging the intensity of pain. Functional magnetic resonance imaging studies have demonstrated that a signal in the anterior cingulate cortex was correlated with pain intensity. Interestingly, when this pain-related activation was accompanied by attention-demanding cognitive tasks (verbal fluency), the attention-demanding tasks increased the anterior cortex signal greater than pain activation (Davis et al, 1997). The contribution of the limbic system and anterior cingulate cortex to pain perception may also explain the reduction in pain sensitivity during stress conditions (***stress-induced analgesia***).

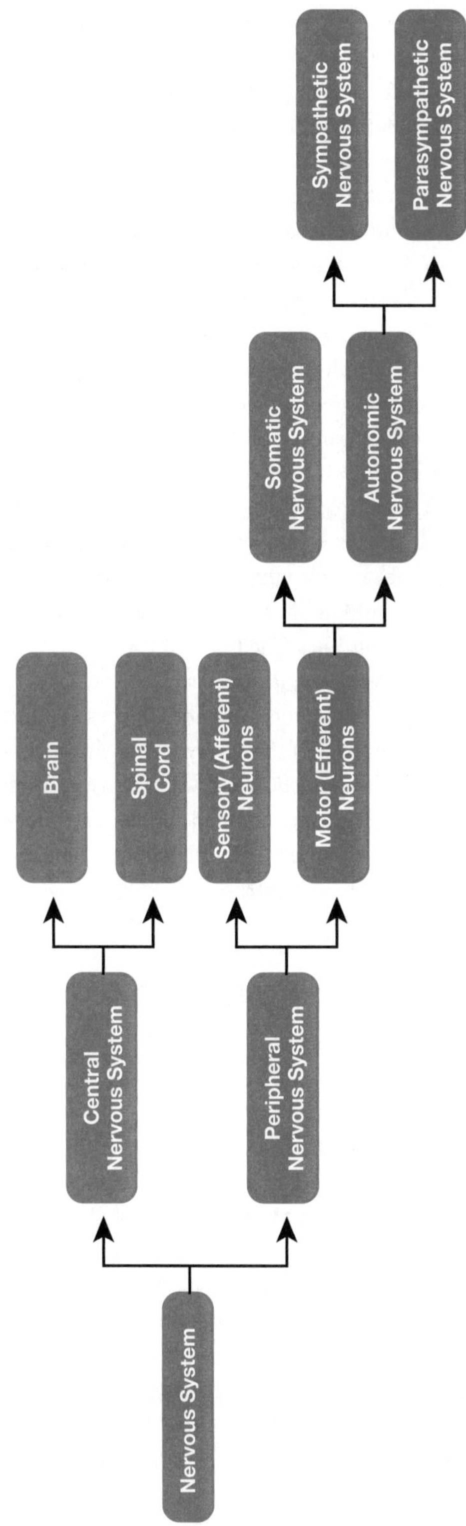

Figure 7-5 | Nervous system chart.

Stress's Influence on Pain

During acutely stressful situations, such as during exercise or sports participation, the fight-or-flight response mechanisms may cause a decrease in the physiological ***sensation*** of pain (through a stress-induced analgesia mechanism; Sternberg, 2007). In addition, the psychological perception of pain may be decreased because of the athlete's focus on factors other than pain (such as training or game components). The magnitude of the stressful situation may be linked to the decrease of the sensation and perception of pain. For example, a championship game may be more stressful for athletes; therefore, they may be able to "play through pain" better than they may otherwise be able to (such as during a routine match). This ability to perform with pain is likely linked to a combination of physiological responses related to stress-induced analgesia, as well as the psychological factors of the importance of the game and other sporting factors including the culture of risk associated with athletics.

Pain-Spasm Cycle

Athletic trainers are generally familiar with the ***pain-spasm cycle*** in which pain causes vasoconstriction and muscle spasm, which, in turn, causes more pain, which, in turn, causes more spasm; the process continues in this feedback cycle until either the pain is relieved or the spasm is decreased. Tissue damage may not necessarily begin this cycle. Stress, for example, may cause muscle tension, which may lead to the pain, which can then trigger the cycle.

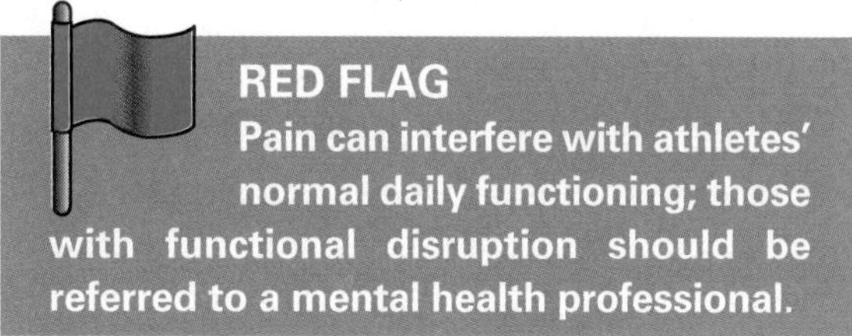

RED FLAG
Pain can interfere with athletes' normal daily functioning; those with functional disruption should be referred to a mental health professional.

Pain Threshold versus Pain Tolerance

When discussing pain perception, it is important to differentiate between ***pain sensation*** and ***pain perception***. Pain sensation occurs when nociceptors transmit a stimulus through the nervous system, whereas perception refers to the conscious interpretation of nociceptive stimulus as pain. The perception of pain can then be broken down into ***pain threshold*** or ***pain tolerance***. Pain threshold can be defined as the level of ***noxious*** stimuli required for pain to be felt. Consider what level of stimulus is required to generate a response. Pain tolerance, in contrast, is a measure of the maximum amount of pain a person can or will tolerate. Pain tolerance is often associated with the limbic system and the cerebral cortex. Both pain threshold and pain tolerance are completely subjective, extremely individualized, and can be influenced by the individual's history of pain. However, there is disagreement in the literature regarding *how* history of pain will impact subsequent pain perception. The predominant belief is that regular exposure to painful stimuli will increase pain tolerance as individuals become more conditioned to pain. However, other research has suggested that repeated or prolonged exposure to painful stimuli will result in greater perception of future pain. In this theory, repeated exposure to noxious stimuli bombards pain synapses with repetitive input, increasing their responsiveness to subsequent stimuli (this becomes a learned response).

As described by Flint (1998, p. 54), a variety of factors may influence how an athlete experiences pain:

- Personal factors include the gender and age of the athlete, the athlete's previous experience with pain and injury, the athlete's coping skills, and the athlete's personality.
- Medical factors include the amount and type of tissue that is damaged in the injury, the medical treatment that was and is provided, and the medication that the athlete may be taking.
- Social or cultural factors include cultural and ethnic norms for pain expression and social support.
- Sport context factors include sport norms for pain expression, sport situation such as score of the game and time of the season, and the importance that the athletes place on their sport.

Emotions, behaviors, and cultural/gender factors can all influence perception of pain (pain threshold) and pain tolerance. For example, multiple studies have found that males will tolerate higher levels of pain than females. Various intrinsic factors may also affect pain tolerance. For example, ***extroverts*** may express pain more freely, whereas ***introverts*** may be more sensitive to pain. The presence of peers (regardless of friend or stranger) has been shown to reduce reported perception of pain. In addition, particularly in youth athletes, individuals will tolerate more pain when they are observed by a peer than when they are alone.

If we begin to make comparisons between athletes and nonathletes, studies have found that athletes will tolerate more pain than nonathletes, and that highly competitive athletes and/or those who participate in contact sports will tolerate even more pain. The influence of overriding events can also influence pain tolerance, meaning that, when the brain is preoccupied, there may be a delay in the processing of pain stimuli or the stimuli perceived may be to a lesser extent (as was demonstrated in the functional magnetic resonance imaging study cited previously). For example, if athletes are involved in a high-stakes athletic event, they may not recognize or acknowledge significant levels of pain until hours after the event has ended, once the adrenaline rush has faded.

Cognitive-evaluative factors also influence pain tolerance. Here, past experiences and the athlete's appraisal of the perceived impact of the injury (threatening vs. nonthreatening to their athletic goals) will have a major impact on his or her pain perception and subsequent emotional and behavioral responses. Cognitive appraisal models are discussed in depth in Chapter 4.

EVIDENCE-BASED PRACTICE

Deroche, T., Woodman, T., Stephan, Y., Brewer, B. W., & Le Scanff, C. (2011). Athletes' inclination to play through pain: A coping perspective. *Anxiety, Stress & Coping, 24*(5), 579–587.

Description of the Study

The study explored athletes' pain-coping strategies related to their inclination to play through pain. Participants were 205 athletes (158 men, 47 women) from combat sports (judo, taekwondo, karate, wrestling) with a mean age of 22.73 (range 15–41) years. Demographic variables (e.g., sex, age, sport experience, number of injuries in the past year), pain intensity, pain behavior (i.e., athletes' inclination to play through pain), and pain coping strategies were reported for each participant.

Results of the Study

Pain behavior was significantly negatively related to sport experience, to previous injuries, to pain intensity, and to pain catastrophizing. Pain behavior was significantly positively related to ignoring pain. Pain catastrophizing predicted pain behavior beyond the intensity of pain experienced during sport, such that more catastrophizing was related to less inclination to play through pain. Athletes who were able to ignore pain were more inclined to play through pain at both low and high pain intensities than athletes who were less able to ignore pain.

Implications for Athletic Training Practice

Athletic trainers should be aware that an athlete's pain behavior is based on a variety of factors, including sport experience, previous injury, intensity of pain, catastrophizing about pain, and ability to ignore pain. Therefore, athletic trainers should approach athletes and their pain on an individualized basis. Although athletes may be able to alter behaviors based on personal and situational factors, care should be taken to recognize that the inclination and ability to play through pain may or may not be a desirable characteristic. For example, the inclination to play through higher pain may contribute to increased risk for injury.

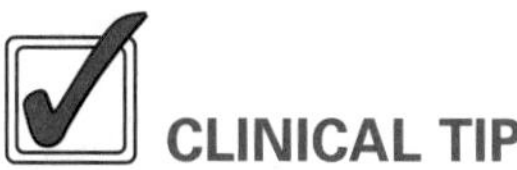

CLINICAL TIP

Because of the level of physical contact that is standard in sports such as football, ice hockey, and men's lacrosse, a certain level of post-game soreness is expected. It is common for these athletes to be unaware they have been injured until they wake up the following morning. For this reason, many athletic trainers working with these athletes schedule mandatory "check-ins" the day following a game. All athletes who participated in the game are required to report to the athletic training facility to discuss any injuries they may have sustained the previous day. This gives post-event soreness time to fade and helps athletes evaluate whether an injury may be present. It also provides an opportunity for early injury intervention by the athletic trainer.

Pain-Control Theories

The level I gate control theory (Melzack & Wall, 1965) explains how pain transmission to the brain can be blocked on ascending pathways, whereas the level II central biasing/central control theory posits that prolonged nociceptor transmission to the brain results in pain being modulated on descending pathways (consult a therapeutic modalities textbook for a thorough overview of pain-control theories). This descending pain-control theory also proposes that cognitive processes (anxiety, depression, previous experiences) can exaggerate pain perception or facilitate pain control. Consider the following examples:

- A basketball player dives for a loose ball, jamming her finger into the ball. She feels little pain initially, until she looks at her hand and sees an obvious fifth proximal interphalangeal joint dislocation. Upon sight of the deformity, her pain level increases, she goes into shock, and she is removed from the court on a stretcher (true story).
- A freshman track athlete complains of new lower extremity pain once a week. The summer between his freshman and sophomore years, he is in a car accident and sustains several serious injuries. He returns to track the following spring. By his junior year, he is an All-American and rarely reports any injuries (true story).

In the basketball example, there was no change in physical state of the tissue; however, the anxiety associated with seeing a gross deformity on her own hand increased the athlete's perception of pain, as well as her somatic symptoms. In the scenario with the track athlete, should we assume that he stopped being injured after his freshman year? More likely, his experiences with a more severe injury influenced his pain perception and ability to cope with noxious stimuli.

Pain Measurement

Being aware of the athlete's pain level and pain coping strategies can place the athletic trainer in a position to assist the athlete with pain management. Several inventories have been developed to measure and monitor pain levels and coping. Two are highlighted here: the Brief Pain Inventory (BPI) is a general measure of pain severity and interference, and the Sports Inventory for Pain (SIP) is a measure specific to athletes who are injured.

Brief Pain Inventory

The BPI was copyrighted by Cleeland in 1991 and is available in a long form and a short form (Cleeland, 2009). The BPI has two scales that ask the respondent to rate severity of pain as worst, least, average, and now (i.e., current pain), as well as interference of pain, such as how much the pain has interfered with daily activities (general activity, walking, work, mood, enjoyment of life, relations with others, sleep). The BPI also contains body diagrams and a question regarding the amount of pain relief experienced with analgesics.

Sports Inventory for Pain

The SIP (Meyers, Bourgeois, Stewart, & LeUnes, 1992) contains 25 items across 5 subscales (coping, cognitive, avoidance, catastrophizing, and body awareness) and a composite score. A shorter form of the measure (SIP15; Bourgeois, Meyers, & LeUnes, 2009) contains only 15 items across 3 subscales (coping by direct action, catastrophizing, and somatic awareness). Specific to the athletic training setting, the authors of the SIP15 suggest the measure may be used to identify athletes who are not effectively coping with pain and who may benefit from additional attention focused on pain management. In addition, as highlighted by the authors, when the SIP15 is used as a repeated measure throughout the rehabilitation process, it can help identify athletes who have a change in pain management, and thus may benefit from implementation of psychosocial strategies.

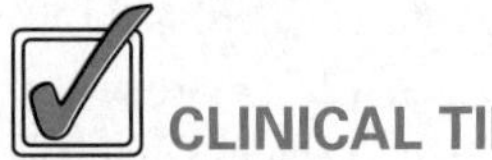

CLINICAL TIP

The SIP (Meyers et al, 1992) and revised 15-item measure (SIP15; Bourgeois et al, 2009) can be used to help identify athletes who may not be coping effectively with pain, and thus may benefit from a mental health referral.

INTERPRETING PAIN SENSATIONS

Although pain is unavoidable, athletic trainers recognize that pain can be one of the most challenging obstacles to effective rehabilitation. As has been discussed in this chapter, pain has significant negative physical and emotional implications. For these reasons, it is essential that athletes be educated about their pain, including differentiating between benign and harmful pain, and gaining an understanding of acute versus chronic pain.

Benign versus Injury Pain

For athletes, pain can become a normal, persistent part of athletic participation. However, learning to interpret this pain can provide important information about what is occurring in the body (Table 7-1 includes common descriptors of pain). Different types of pain result in different physical, psychological, and emotional responses. For example, pain in uninjured athletes is often viewed as positive. This type of benign "performance" pain indicates athletes are putting forth a strong effort and pushing their limits in the pursuit of improved performance (Taylor & Taylor, 1997). Many athletes say that this type of pain motivates them to work harder ("I don't feel like I worked hard in a workout unless I'm sore the next day."). Conversely, pain in injured athletes is often viewed as negative. This type of harmful "injury pain" is commonly associated with further damage and signals a need to protect the area. If athletes can differentiate between performance and injury pain, then pain can be used as a source of information

TABLE 7-1 Common Descriptors of Pain

Burning	Shooting
Stabbing	Sharp
Shocklike	Cramping
Dull	Hot
Aching	Tingling
Tender	Stinging
Stiff	Sore
Throbbing	Piercing
Radiating	Cold
Annoying	Crushing

to adjust and monitor their recovery (Table 7-2). For example, an understanding of benign pain will prevent an athlete from backing off from rehabilitation if this pain can be viewed as a normal, healthy part of healing. Conversely, athletes who can recognize harmful pain may actually speed their own rehabilitation program if they recognize when rest periods are warranted.

College athletes have reported knowing when to report an injury to medical staff based on their pain associated with the injury (Granquist & Liang, 2012). Specifically, they said they know when to report the pain:

- "When the pain gets to the point where I need to"
- "When I notice the pain, and it is not going away"
- "When it is really severe, and I cannot deal with the pain"

This same group of athletes described pain as one of the criteria by which they judge the severity of their injury:

- "Depending on the pain I'm in"
- "Level of discomfort"
- "How bad it hurts"

They based their reporting of injury on previous injury experiences:

- "Based on past experiences. Knowing if I'm hurt or injured. There is a big difference between those two."
- "Comparing it to previous injuries."
- "I've been through injuries. In football, you get bruises and scrapes around your body. I wouldn't report unless there is a sharp pain, blood, or deformity."

Acute versus Chronic Pain

Acute pain is pain of recent and sudden onset, typically high-intensity pain localized at or near the site of injury. Acute pain is generally easily diagnosed and managed. Conversely, ***chronic pain*** is defined as pain that persists beyond the normal time expected for healing (typically a minimum of 3–6 months, depending on various sources). For example, pain as the result of a medial collateral ligament sprain could be defined as chronic if it was expected to heal within 6 weeks but pain has persisted for 3 to 6 months. Chronic pain is often no longer located in the area of the original tissue trauma and is nonresponsive to treatment attempts. The

TABLE 7-2 Benign versus Injury Pain

	Pain Characteristics	Injury Characteristics	Patient Perceptions	Patient Responses
Benign pain	• Dull • Generalized • Short-lasting	Not associated with swelling, tenderness, lasting soreness	• Viewed as positive • Acute • Short in duration • Produced voluntarily • Under control of the athlete • Can be reduced at will	• Satisfaction and inspiration • Creates positive emotions • Facilitates performance • Enhances well-being
Injury pain	• Sharp • Localized • Occurs during and persists after exertion	Associated with swelling, tenderness, lasting soreness	• Viewed as negative • Chronic • Uncontrollable • Signals danger to physical well-being • Motivates to protect injured area	• Increased anxiety • Feelings of fear and dread • Loss of confidence and motivation

Adapted from Heil, J. (1993). Psychology of Sport Injury. *Champaign, IL: Human Kinetics; and Rians, C. B. (1990). Principles and practices of sports medicine. In: J. Taylor & S. Taylor (1997).* Psychological Approaches to Sports Injury Rehabilitation *(p. 223). Philadelphia, PA: Lippincott Williams & Wilkins.*

term ***persistent pain*** has been used recently to differentiate pain that meets the time frame defined as chronic but is actually a symptom of a treatable condition (e.g., a baseball player diagnosed with rotator cuff tendonitis at the start of the season who continues to play throughout the full season). Persistent pain is common in athletics, because many athletes are unwilling to rest for the amount of time needed for symptoms to resolve. It is important for athletic trainers to differentiate true chronic pain from persistent pain. True chronic pain is much more difficult to treat because it often involves more social, emotional, and psychological input than acute pain. As a result of these additional factors, chronic pain can be perpetuated with much less tissue damage. Even therapeutic modalities textbooks are beginning to recognize the psychosocial impact of chronic pain.

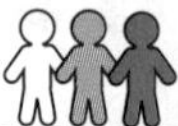

SPECIAL CONSIDERATIONS

Athletes with chronic pain are likely to experience more psychological impacts of their pain (Knight & Draper, 2013). For example, the following may be demonstrated:

- Prescription drugs are more likely to be misused or abused
- Physical activity is diminished or absent
- Social activity is diminished or absent
- There is increased risk for suicide attempt or ideation

Complex regional pain syndrome (CRPS) type I, also known as reflex sympathetic dystrophy syndrome (RSDS), may follow a minor nerve injury (e.g., sprain, strain, surgery), and CRPS type II, also known as causalgia, may follow a major nerve injury. In CRPS, the sympathetic nervous system seems to assume an abnormal function after an injury. For additional information, as well as photos, review the comprehensive article by Marinus et al (2011). Also available is a guide for medical practitioners by Turner-Stokes and Goebel (2011).

This condition often does not receive much attention, but athletic trainers who work with athletes who are reporting ongoing pain should be aware of the signs, symptoms, and treatment of CRPS. It is commonly accepted that athletes with CRPS should not be treated with ice because it can cause additional nerve damage and may lead to the condition worsening and spreading to other areas of the body. Signs and symptoms include, but are not limited to:

- Constant burning pain, including ***allodynia*** and/or hyperalgesia
- Pain that is disproportionate in intensity to the inciting (original) event
- Inflammation that may affect the appearance of the skin (e.g., bruising)
- Swelling of the distal extremity, especially in the acute phase
- Excessive sweating
- Changes in skin temperature
- Muscle spasms of the extremities
- Abnormal hair and nail growth
- Insomnia
- Cognitive problems (e.g., memory and concentration issues) and emotional disturbance

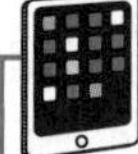

VIRTUAL FIELD TRIP

Go to http://davisplus.fadavis.com for links to resources related to CRPS.

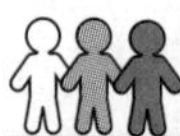

SPECIAL CONSIDERATIONS

The American Chronic Pain Association estimates that one in three Americans suffers from some type of chronic pain, resulting in an annual economic burden of $70 billion. One of the most common classes of medications used in treating pain is the opioids. An opioid is a chemical substance that has a morphine-like action in the body (Fig. 7-6). These narcotic drugs are the most powerful analgesics agents available today to manage pain. Although these medications are ideal for short-term pain reduction, there is potential for physical dependence and addiction among long-term chronic pain sufferers. Prescription opioid misuse in the

United States has increased more than threefold since 1990 to epidemic proportions (Hall et al, 2008). Physiological dependence involving withdrawal symptoms may occur even at prescribed doses in nonaddicted individuals (Ling, Mooney, & Hillhouse, 2011). Addiction, including psychological craving for medication that can lead to self-destructive behavior, can occur with prolonged use. The most commonly abused opioid medications are codeine, hydrocodone, oxycodone, morphine, meperidine, hydromorphone, fentanyl, and methadone. The Diagnosis, Intractability, Risk, Efficacy (DIRE) instrument (Belgrade, Schamber, & Lindgren, 2006) has been developed to predict risk for dependence or addiction to prescribed opioids.

VIRTUAL FIELD TRIP

Visit http://davisplus.fadavis.com for information from the FDA about safe use of pain medicine, including analgesics such as acetaminophen and NSAIDs.

ROLE OF PAIN THROUGHOUT THE REHABILITATION PROCESS

As injured athletes progress through their rehabilitation program, they are likely to experience different pain sensations during various phases of rehabilitation. Injured athletes place more importance on knowledge of the rehabilitation process than on details of injury, meaning that, once the initial injury has been explained, athletic trainers should focus on educating athletes on what will happen (rather than what has happened). An understanding of the role of pain during each rehabilitation phase can aid athletes in coping with these pains and discomforts, and can assist them in using pain as information about physiological processes that are happening. Athletes need to understand how their injury will progress, and what levels of pain and disability are to be expected following surgery (if necessary) and at each phase of recovery. Our research has found that, when athletes are educated about the source of pain, they are more at ease when pain occurs because they understand why they are experiencing it and are able to view it as a normal part of recovery. Many therapeutic exercise textbooks will break the rehabilitation process into three basic stages: (1) flexibility and range of motion (ROM),

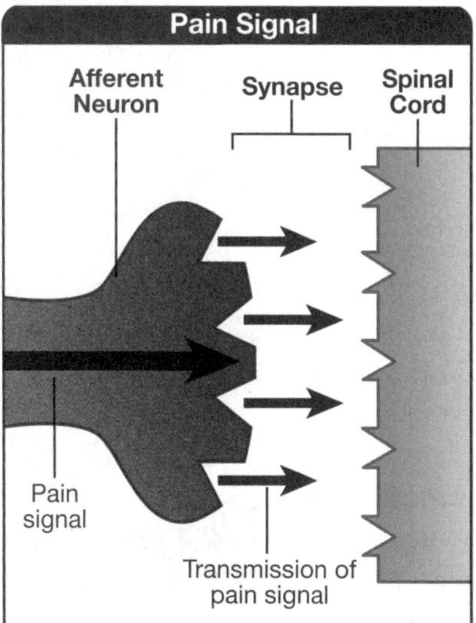

The pain signal is transmitted from the afferent nerve to the spinal cord.

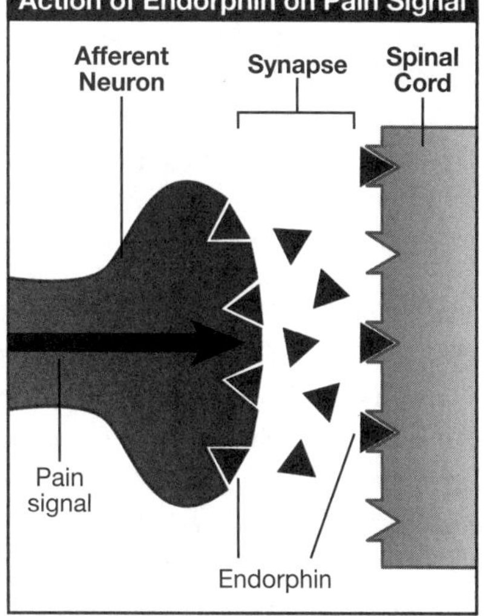

Endorphins block transmission of pain signals on the afferent neuron and block reception of pain signals by the spinal cord.

Figure 7-6 | How opioids work to decrease pain.

(2) strength and muscular endurance, and (3) coordination and agility. Typical pain sensations will be discussed within the scope of these three stages.

Flexibility and Range of Motion

Pain is typically the most severe during this first stage of rehabilitation. In addition, the fact that pain is new and unknown contributes to and heightens the emotional and mental implications of the pain. For these reasons, education is extremely important during this phase. The fear of the unknown is one of the greatest fears; however, if athletes are educated about the cause and source of pain, and understand what causes it and when it is likely to occur, that can aid in decreasing anxiety surrounding the physical sensations and decreasing their perception of pain. Understanding when pain is likely to occur can also aid in athletes' use of pain-management strategies (discussed later in this chapter), thereby increasing their sense of control over their own pain and the rehabilitation process.

Strength and Muscular Endurance

By the strength and muscular endurance stage, the athlete typically has seen some progress during rehabilitation, and initial injury pain has decreased. However, this phase is often more psychologically intimidating than the last because the injured part is likely being tested for the first time. Here, athletes are performing less "rehabilitation" exercises (e.g., ROM, Thera-Band) and beginning to move back into exercises they did before injury (e.g., Nautilus weight-lifting machines). Soreness is to be expected; therefore, it is extremely important to help athletes learn to differentiate between benign pain (e.g., scar tissue being broken up) and harmful injury pain (e.g., healing tissue being torn or reinjured).

Coordination and Agility

During the coordination and agility stage, the pain sensations may be replaced more by fatigue. As the injured athlete shifts the rehabilitation focus to proprioception, coordination, and agility tasks, it is especially important to pay attention to fatigue. Continuing to exercise after the injured area has become fatigued may result in further or repeated injury. It is important to educate athletes about the importance of rest during this sport-specific phase of rehabilitation.

Nonadaptive Behaviors Following Injury

Pain may influence behaviors following injury and during rehabilitation. The athletic trainer should be aware of nonadaptive behaviors, such as those that disrupt the athlete's daily functioning (e.g., eating, sleeping, school, work, sport, relationships) and the rehabilitation process. As discussed in Chapter 6, athletes who exhibit behaviors that are a disruption to their daily functioning should be referred to a mental health professional.

These nonadaptive behaviors following injury and during rehabilitation may be related to one or more factors. Using a biopsychosocial approach to rehabilitation (this approach is discussed in detail in Chapter 8), the athletic trainer should consider the characteristics of the injury (e.g., type, severity) and the sociodemographic factors (e.g., age, gender) related to the athlete's behavior. Also, based on a biopsychosocial perspective, biological factors (e.g., sleep, tissue repair), psychological factors (e.g., personality, cognition, emotions), and social/contextual factors (e.g., social support, life stress, rehabilitation environment) influence behavior.

RED FLAG

Injured athletes who suffer from chronic pain may be at increased risk for suicide. Although athletes may consider suicide at lower rates than nonathletes, experts have found that athletes are more likely to either kill themselves or be seriously injured if they do attempt suicide. According to Swift (2006), "An emotionally troubled athlete is more dangerous to himself than an emotionally troubled nonathlete" (p. 60). Although few statistics are available on the incidence of suicide among athletes (current, cut from team, dropped out), we do know that the prevalence of suicidal thoughts, suicide planning, and suicide attempts is significantly higher among high-school and college-aged individuals (young adults aged 18–29 years) than among those older than

30 years. Suicide is the third leading cause of death among persons aged 15 to 24 years, accounting for 20% of all deaths annually (Centers for Disease Control and Prevention, 2010). In 2011, students in grades 9 to 12 were surveyed regarding suicidal thoughts and behaviors within the previous 12 months. Almost 16% (15.8%) reported that they had seriously considered attempting suicide, 12.8% reported that they made a plan about how they would attempt suicide, 7.8% reported having attempted suicide one or more times, and 2.4% reported that a suicidal attempt resulted in injury, poisoning, or an overdose that required medical attention (Centers for Disease Control and Prevention, 2012). With any number of high-profile athlete suicides populating news stories (recently, the December 2012 murder-suicide involving Jovan Belcher, the 25-year-old linebacker for the Kansas City Chiefs), athletic trainers must be aware of the psychological impact of pain and forced inactivity (learn more about psychosocial intervention and referral in Chapter 6).

Nonpharmacological Pain Management

Nonpharmacological pain-management strategies include psychosocial strategies that are discussed later in this chapter. In addition, the athletic trainer can use such methods as visual distraction (providing something interesting on which the athlete can focus), auditory distraction (can be as easy as talking to the athlete throughout painful ROM exercises), music (can serve as a distraction technique), massage, and transcutaneous electrical nerve stimulation (or other pain-control therapeutic modalities). The athletic trainer may also consider referring the athlete to a professional for methods such as hypnosis, acupressure, acupuncture, or biofeedback.

The Placebo Effect

The placebo effect is suspected to have occurred when pain reduction is obtained through mechanisms *other than* physiological effects of treatment. It has been said that the best research on pain should come from veterinary medicine—if you treat a horse and he walks, you know it's not the placebo effect. The placebo effect is linked to a psychological mechanism whereby if the athlete believes the treatment is beneficial, then pain can be reduced. Research on pain-control theories supports the existence of the placebo effect. Consider the level II descending pain-control theory (central biasing/central control). This is a change in the perception of pain *without* any physiological (healing) change in the tissue. This method of pain control can be facilitated by cognitive processes. All modalities (and other therapeutic strategies used by athletic trainers) have some degree of placebo effect, and this effect can be increased if the modality is applied with enthusiasm and faith on the part of the athletic trainer.

PSYCHOSOCIAL STRATEGIES

The aim with psychosocial strategies in pain management is to diminish both autonomic changes associated with pain (e.g., vasoconstriction, muscle spasm) and psychological distress. As is discussed throughout this textbook, education of the athlete is a key to the implementation of psychosocial strategies. Specifically with pain management, the athlete should be educated on the pain-spasm cycle (refer to Figure 8-4 in Chapter 8) and how stress influences this cycle. Athletes should also be educated on the process of pain sensation and perception. Specific to pain management, a focus should be placed on the management of stress and pain-related thoughts. To do this, athletic trainers can help athletes identify stress that they may be experiencing and then help them normalize that stress is a part of life. They can then introduce stress-management techniques such as deep breathing and progressive muscle relaxation. Imagery can be implemented both for relaxation to reduce stress to decrease pain and for pain management directly.

Athletic trainers may also work with athletes who have pain during rehabilitation or have chronic or persistent pain to create a "pain plan." This plan may include both dissociative and associate strategies for pain management (Fig. 7-7). Dissociative strategies are techniques that

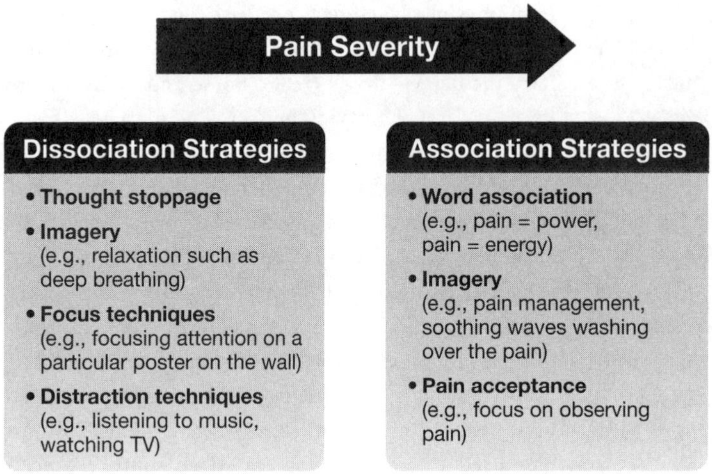

Pain Severity →

Dissociation Strategies

- **Thought stoppage**
- **Imagery**
  (e.g., relaxation such as deep breathing)
- **Focus techniques**
  (e.g., focusing attention on a particular poster on the wall)
- **Distraction techniques**
  (e.g., listening to music, watching TV)

Association Strategies

- **Word association**
  (e.g., pain = power, pain = energy)
- **Imagery**
  (e.g., pain management, soothing waves washing over the pain)
- **Pain acceptance**
  (e.g., focus on observing pain)

Figure 7-7 | Dissociation and association strategies for pain management.

distract athletes from the pain and focus their attention in a different direction, such as imagery scripts. Associative strategies are techniques to help athletes reinterpret the pain. An example of an associative strategy is to use the word association "pain = power!"

Deep Breathing

Deep breathing is the focus on the breath and breathing patterns. Deep-breathing techniques are useful because they are readily available (everyone breathes!) and can have physiological effects on the body that may decrease pain (e.g., increased relaxation of muscles), as well as psychological effects that may focus attention away from the pain. Counting breaths or breathing to an inhalation-exhalation ratio may serve as distraction from the pain.

Progressive Muscle Relaxation

Progressive muscle relaxation, systematic tensing and relaxing of muscle groups, should only be used if it does not cause additional pain or tissue damage. Similar to deep breathing, it can have both physiological and psychological effects.

Imagery

Imagery can be used as a relaxation strategy to distract the athlete from focusing on injury-related pain. Relaxation imagery and pain-management imagery can be introduced by the athletic trainer to the athlete as part of the pain plan. Imagery is discussed in detail in Chapter 10.

Relaxation

Many imagery scripts are available for relaxation. Sample scripts may ask athletes to imagine they are in a relaxing setting, such as at the beach or in a peaceful forest. These relaxation scripts can be used during stationary times in rehabilitation (such as during heating or icing) and may be useful to athletes to listen to if they have trouble sleeping.

Pain Management

Pain-management imagery focuses attention on a visual stimulus to produce specific images to promote pain management. Imagery for pain management may use a variety of strategies such as seeing the pain float away or seeing the pain decrease in size (Table 7-3). Athletes should be encouraged to try these different strategies to find the one that works best for them and their pain. An example of a pain-management imagery script is in Table 7-4.

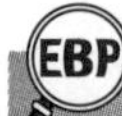

EVIDENCE-BASED PRACTICE

Cupal, D. D., & Brewer, B. W. (2001). Effects of relaxation and guided imagery on knee strength, reinjury anxiety, and pain following anterior cruciate ligament reconstruction. *Rehabilitation Psychology, 46*(1), 28–43. doi:10.1037/0090-5550.46.1.28

Description of the Study

The purpose of the study was to examine the effects of a relaxation and guided imagery intervention on knee strength, reinjury anxiety, and pain. Thirty patients (16 men, 14 women; age range 18–50 years) who were participating in rehabilitation following anterior cruciate ligament (ACL) reconstructive surgery participated in this study. Participants were randomly assigned to either a treatment group that received 10 identical individual relaxation and guided imagery sessions; a placebo group that received attention, encouragement, and support during sessions; or a control group that received no intervention. All participants received a normal course of rehabilitation. At 2 weeks after surgery, participants completed a reinjury anxiety scale and a pain scale. Data on the reinjury anxiety scale, pain scale, and knee strength were collected at 24 weeks after surgery.

Results of the Study

One-way analysis of variance indicated that participants in the treatment group demonstrated significantly greater knee strength than participants in the placebo or the control group. One-way analyses of covariance indicated that participants in the treatment group reported significantly less reinjury anxiety and pain than participants in the placebo or control groups.

Implications for Athletic Training Practice

Based on the findings of this study, athletic trainers should integrate psychosocial strategies, specifically relaxation and imagery, into athletes' rehabilitation protocols to enhance outcomes, specifically strength, reinjury anxiety, and pain. The reduction of pain may lead to a more pleasant rehabilitation process and assist in rehabilitation adherence.

TABLE 7-3 **Imagery Techniques for Pain Management**

Managing pain associated with participation (10–15 minutes of guided imagery)

There are a few easy ways to use scripts to create a *pain-controlled* environment for the athlete. The athlete can either associate with the pain or disassociate; both techniques will be shared. Remember that the brain *perceives pain*; thus, we have control of "how" pain is perceived.

Technique	Description
1. Imagine the painful area as a red object.	Take a deep breath in and imagine a cool sensation, almost icy, a flow of air going right to that spot and cooling it down, so it changes color, a lighter shade, like red, then to pink. With each exhalation, draw all the pain out of that area. With each deep breath in, see the color changes as your pain lessens. Breathing in, cooling it more, changing it to a paler shade of pink, then even cooler, to almost white, then to light blue. Breathing out, drawing the pain out with your breath. All the while, you are exhaling any discomfort right out of your body. *This associative technique can also be used by using a red balloon lifting off and floating away into the distant cool blue sky.*

Continued

TABLE 7-3 **Imagery Techniques for Pain Management—cont'd**

Technique	Description
2. Change your pain into a sound.	No matter how loud or bothersome the sound, you can always make it softer, less distracting, by turning the volume down. See the pain being controlled by a dial on a stereo system for which you have the remote control. You have complete control of the sound. You can turn the volume down to a level that won't bother you anymore. You may want to turn the sound off completely. You are in control of the sound. You are in control of your pain. *This is an additional associative technique.*
3. Find a special relaxing place.	Sometimes you might find it easier to take your mind to an amazing place. A place of comfort, like a vacation, somewhere where you can go to get away and really relax. Maybe it is somewhere you have been, somewhere full of happy, pleasant feelings, soothing sounds, fresh scents, that bring you back to a time, a place, where you felt so good, so free, no worries, no stress, just relaxation and comfort. Maybe you can go somewhere you have never been, imagining how good you can feel, how wonderful it is to be free, to feel totally relaxed in this new place of comfort. I don't know where your mind can take you, but I know there has been a time when you felt really good. *This is a dissociation technique, or ignoring the pain signal, instead of attending to the pain and attempting to manage it (associative). Many types of distraction techniques can be used with athletes throughout the rehabilitation process (e.g., watching TV while in a prone-hang, listening to music in the cold whirlpool).*
4. Count.	All you have to do to feel this relaxation is count, nice and slow, in your mind, from 10 down to 1, like this: 10, allowing my body to relax; 9, getting even more relaxed; 8, deeper relaxed with each number; 7, every muscle feeling better; 6, more and more relaxed; 5, so nice, so comfortable; 4, deeper and deeper relaxed; 3, feeling good; 2, feeling better, and 1. It doesn't matter what you say to yourself as you count, just that you know you will feel more and more relaxed with each and every count; every breath will bring more and more comfort. *Most useful for pain that is due to muscle spasm alone.*

Adapted from Hamson-Utley, J. Pain Management Strategies, *presented at the National Athletic Trainers' Association Clinical Symposium, 2011, used by permission.*

TABLE 7-4 **Sample Imagery Script for Pain Management**

Description

This pain-management relaxation script will guide you to focus on observing and accepting your pain. Then, you will be guided to transform your pain into something that you can manage, that you can change, that you can control.

Script

- Find a comfortable position, making sure that your back is supported, lying down or sitting in a reclined chair with head support. (pause 10 seconds+)
- Pain management begins with observation. As you nest into a comfortable position, notice how you are feeling at this moment. Without trying to change anything, just observe your body and mind right now. (pause 15 seconds+)
- Now, start attending to your breathing. Using a 4 count, take a deep breath in and hold the air in your lungs, now exhale over a 4 count. Do this again, establishing a breathing rhythm that leads your body to relax. Continue with this 4 count inhale and exhale throughout this session.
- Now, pay attention to your pain. Where is your pain located? Do not try to make anything happen. Notice how your whole body feels. Passively observe, not trying to change anything. Simply take note of how your body feels. (pause 15 seconds+)
- Take another deep breath in 1, 2, 3, 4 ... now exhale 1, 2, 3, 4.
- Continue to breathe slowly, smoothly.
- Take a few moments now and think about your pain. (pause) You may not be in pain right now. Just observe the state of your pain at this moment. (pause 15 seconds+) The way your body feels is always changing. The way you feel is different from moment to moment. Just observe as each moment passes. (pause 30 seconds+)
- Although pain is unwanted and difficult to tolerate, try for the next few moments to regard your pain with acceptance. Accept the way you are feeling right now physically and emotionally, whether positive or negative; allow your body and mind to just be in the moment. Accepting and observing.
- Now, repeat a few pain-management affirmations:
  - I accept this pain I experience, the whole of it; I accept it, letting go of the need to control or to change in this moment.
  - I accept the pain, and I accept myself.
  - I release myself from the need to do anything right now, except just be.
- Now just relax for a few moments and let go. Just be. There is nothing you need to be doing in this moment, besides accepting this moment just as it is. (pause 30 seconds+)
- Observe again your pain and notice that you can alter the pain slightly. See if you are able to transform the feeling, just a little.
- Picture the pain as (*insert one technique from above*). (pause after 15 seconds+; skip next section or go through it)
- Now focus in on this area again and imagine a slightly different feeling of your choice. You may wish to imagine the sensation of pleasant tingling ... warmth ... or soft but firm, comfortable pressure.
- Imagine this sensation now. Imagine the sensation of replacing just a slice of the pain with this new pleasant sensation. Now, replace another slice, and another. Feel this new sensation growing, pleasantly, providing some relief and allowing you to relax. (pause 15 seconds+)

Continued

TABLE 7-4 **Sample Imagery Script for Pain Management—cont'd**

• Take a deep breath in, 1, 2, 3, 4, and exhale, 1, 2, 3, 4. Continue to breathe slowly and rhythmically as you now meditate in this calm, pain-free space in your mind.
• You *can choose any phrase you want* to focus on for the meditation portion of this pain-management relaxation. This will be your focus word. Focus your attention on this word with each breath. Every time your thoughts drift, focus in again using this word. Don't worry about making anything happen or doing this meditation a certain way. Whatever happens is right for you at this moment.
• Keep an attitude of passive acceptance. Just accept the state you are in and continue to focus your mind on the word you will be repeating.
• Breathe in 1, 2, 3, 4 (repeat word); breathe out 1, 2, 3, 4 (repeat word).
• Continue to use this word cue as you breathe, steadily increasing your relaxed state. Take note of how your body feels now. See how relaxed your muscles are. Notice how calm your mind is. Enjoy this feeling of relaxation for a few moments more.
• Keep this feeling of relaxation with you as you return to your regular activities. Memorize this peaceful, relaxed feeling, so you can return to this state whenever you choose to. Slowly reawaken your body now. Take a deep breath in 1, 2, 3, 4 and exhale 1, 2, 3, 4. Feel your mind and body becoming more awake and alert. Begin to move your arms and legs, and stretch your muscles to let them reawaken.
• Sit relaxed for a moment with your eyes open, observing the room and things around you. When you are ready, return to your usual activities, keeping with you a sense of calm and relief.

Adapted from Hamson-Utley, J. Pain Management Strategies, *presented at the National Athletic Trainers' Association Clinical Symposium, 2011, used by permission.*

ATHLETE INSIDER CONCLUSION

Jayda is experiencing ongoing pain following a series of surgeries to her lower leg. During one of the team meetings, Jayda's coach tells the athletic trainer that she "doesn't really know what to do with Jayda, doesn't really know if she wants to play, and doesn't know what's going on...." Jayda has fear over her return to participation—especially at the field where she sustained the tibia-fibula fracture. Trusting the medical staff that she is cleared to play, she expresses interest in pain-management strategies. Jayda also agrees to work on her feelings of "personal exhaustion" with a mental health professional in the university counseling center.

Effective Psychosocial Strategies for the Athletic Trainer to Use With Jayda

The following psychosocial strategies can be used with Jayda as she returns to participation:

1. Help Jayda learn to differentiate between benign pain and injury pain. This understanding will decrease the anxiety she feels over every pain sensation.
2. Educate Jayda and her coach about the pain sensation and perception process, and about effective psychosocial strategies that she can use to assist with pain management.
3. Implement stress-management strategies. As discussed in this chapter, stress contributes to pain; therefore, stress management may be an effective strategy for decreasing or managing pain, or both. Specifically, relaxation strategies can be used.
4. Help Jayda identify and implement dissociative and associative pain-management strategies.
5. Create a comprehensive "pain plan" that includes preventive strategies, management strategies, and a refocus plan.

CONCLUSION

This chapter introduced the concept of pain and provided an overview of basic concepts related to it, including the physiology of pain. While emphasizing that pain is a complex physiological, cognitive, and emotional process, this chapter provided guidance for the athletic trainer in educating the athlete about pain, as well as the role of pain throughout the rehabilitation process. Benign (performance) pain was differentiated from injury pain, and acute pain was differentiated from chronic pain. Finally, this chapter provided psychological strategies that the athletic trainer can apply to the rehabilitation process and aid in pain management for the athlete.

REFERENCES

Belgrade, M. J., Schamber, C. D., & Lindgren, B. R. (2006). The DIRE score: Predicting outcomes of opioid prescribing for chronic pain. *Journal of Pain, 7*(9), 671–681.

Bourgeois, A. E., Meyers, M. C., & LeUnes, A. (2009). The Sports Inventory for Pain: Empirical and confirmatory factorial validity. *Journal of Sport Behavior, 32*(1), 19–35.

Centers for Disease Control and Prevention, National Center for Injury Prevention and Control. (2010). Web-based Injury Statistics Query and Reporting System (WISQARS). Retrieved February 26, 2013, from http://www.cdc.gov/injury/wisqars/index.html.

Centers for Disease Control and Prevention. (2012). Youth risk behavior surveillance—United States, 2011. *MMWR, Surveillance Summaries*, 61(SS-4), 1–162. Retrieved February 26, 2013, from www.cdc.gov/mmwr/pdf/ss/ss6104.pdf.

Cleeland, C. S. (2009). *The Brief Pain Inventory user guide*. Retrieved February 26, 2013, from www.mdanderson.org/education-and-research/departments-programs-and-labs/departments-and-divisions/symptom-research/symptom-assessment-tools/BPI_UserGuide.pdf

Cupal, D. D., & Brewer, B. W. (2001). Effects of relaxation and guided imagery on knee strength, reinjury anxiety, and pain following anterior cruciate ligament reconstruction. *Rehabilitation Psychology, 46*(1), 28–43. doi:10.1037/0090-5550.46.1.28

Davis, K. D., Taylor, S. J., Crawley, A. P., Wood, M. L., & Mikulis, D. J. (1997). Functional MRI of pain- and attention-related activations in the human cingulate cortex. *Journal of Neurophysiology, 77*(6), 3370–3380.

Deroche, T., Woodman, T., Stephan, Y., Brewer, B. W., & Le Scanff, C. (2011). Athletes' inclination to play through pain: A coping perspective. *Anxiety, Stress & Coping, 24*(5), 579–587.

Flint, F. (1998). *Psychology of sport injury: A professional achievement self-study program course*. Champaign, IL: Human Kinetics.

Granquist, M. D., & Liang, C. T. H. (2012). *Athletes' perspectives on reporting, treatment seeking, and severity of sport injuries*. Presentation at the Association of Applied Sport Psychology Annual Conference, Atlanta, GA.

Hall, A. J., Logan, J. E., Toblin, R. L., et al. (2008). Patterns of abuse among unintentional pharmaceutical overdose fatalities. *Journal of the American Medical Association, 300*(22), 2613–2620.

Heil, J. (1993). *Psychology of Sport Injury*. Champaign, IL: Human Kinetics.

Knight, K. L., & Draper, D. O. (2013). *Therapeutic Modalities: The Art and Science*. Philadelphia, PA: Lippincott Williams & Wilkins.

Ling, W., Mooney, L., & Hillhouse, M. (2011). Prescription opioid abuse, pain and addiction: Clinical issues and implications. *Drug and Alcohol Review, 30*(3), 300–305.

Marinus, J., Moseley, G. L., Birklein, F., et al. (2011). Clinical features and pathophysiology of complex regional pain syndrome. *The Lancet Neurology, 10*(7), 637–648.

Melzack, R., & Wall, P. D. (1965). Pain mechanisms: A new theory. *Science, 150*(3699), 971–979.

Merskey, H., Albe-Fessard, D. G., Bonica, J. J., et al. (1979). Pain terms: A list with definitions and notes on usage: Recommended by the IASP Subcommittee on Taxonomy. *Pain, 6*(3), 249–252.

Meyers, M. C., Bourgeois, A. E., Stewart, S. S., & LeUnes, A. A. (1992). Predicting pain response in athletes: Development and assessment of the Sports Inventory for Pain. *Journal of Sport & Exercise Psychology, 14*(3), 249–261.

Rians, C. B. (1990). Principles and practices of sports medicine. In: J. Taylor & S. Taylor (1997). *Psychological Approaches to Sports Injury Rehabilitation* (p. 223). Philadelphia, PA: Lippincott Williams & Wilkins.

Sternberg, W. F. (2007). Pain: Basic concepts. In: D. Pargman (Ed.), *Psychological Bases of Sport Injuries* (3rd ed., pp. 305–317). Morgantown, WV: Fitness Information Technology.

Swift, E. M. (2006). What went wrong in Winthrop? One high school football team, five suicides in three years. Can we learn anything? *Sports Illustrated, 104*(1), 60.

Taylor, J., & Taylor, S. (1997). *Psychological Approaches to Sports Injury* (pp. 221–223). Philadelphia, PA: Lippincott Williams & Wilkins.

Turner-Stokes, L., & Goebel, A. (2011). Complex regional pain syndrome in adults: Concise guidance. *Clinical Medicine, 11*(6), 596–600.

BOARD OF CERTIFICATION STRATEGIES AND COMPETENCIES

As the Sixth Edition of the Board of Certification's Role Delineation Study outlines, athletic trainers are involved in the prevention and care of athletic injury (Domain 1), as well as reconditioning participants for optimal performance and function (Domain 4). The Fifth Edition Athletic Training Education Competencies include knowledge and skills in the content area of Psychosocial Strategies and Referral (PS), and concepts related to pain are included within this content area. Specifically, describing psychosocial factors that influence pain sensation and perception, identifying multidisciplinary approaches for managing persistent pain (PS-9), and selecting and integrating psychosocial techniques into the rehabilitation program to address pain management (CIP-7) are included in the Psychosocial Strategies and Referral content area.

Board of Certification Style Questions

1. Which of the following are types of nociceptors? (Select all that apply.)
   a. Electrical
   b. Mechanical
   c. Thermal
   d. Chemical

2. Pain sensation may be influenced by (select all that apply):
   a. stress.
   b. repetition of stimuli.
   c. situational factors.
   d. environmental factors.

3. An athlete's pain perception is (select all that apply):
   a. directly related to amount of tissue damage.
   b. the same as pain sensation.
   c. physiological.
   d. influenced by personal and situational factors.

4. Which of the following are components of pain perception? (Select all that apply.)
   a. Pain threshold
   b. Pain tolerance
   c. Nociceptor stimulation
   d. Reduction in pain sensitivity during stress conditions

5. Which of the following would be considered performance (benign) pain?
   a. Lateral ankle pain during therapeutic rehabilitation following sprain
   b. Anterior shin pain that occurs midway through a 5K race
   c. Bilateral quadriceps pain the day after a strength training session
   d. Anterior shoulder pain after throwing 75 pitches

END-OF-CHAPTER EXERCISES

1. Differentiate between pain sensation and pain perception.

2. Describe stress-induced analgesia.

3. Reflect on examples from your clinical experiences of athletes who have had the following types of pain: acute, chronic, persistent, benign pain, or injury pain. Identify characteristics of pain/pain descriptions that led you to determine the type of pain.

4. Consider an injury that you have personally experienced several times. What personal and/or situational factors played into your interpretation of pain at the different time points?

5. How do you ask your athletes to quantify their pain? Based on what you learned in this chapter, how could you make this scale more objective?

6. Consider a time when you experienced pain without any physical damage. How can you explain this pain sensation in light of what you read in the chapter?

7. Discuss personal, cultural, and gender factors that you have witnessed that influence pain perception and pain tolerance in your athletes.

8. Discuss pain sensations that you have found to be common during each phase of rehabilitation: flexibility and ROM, strength and muscular endurance, coordination and agility.

Chapter 8

Psychosocial Aspects of Rehabilitation

Megan D. Granquist with Britton W. Brewer

CHAPTER OUTLINE

KEY TERMS

Athletic identity The degree to which a person identifies the self as an athlete.

Autonomy A sense of choice or control over one's actions and behaviors.

Biopsychosocial perspective The view that biological, psychological (e.g., thoughts, emotions, behaviors), and social factors all play a significant role in human functioning in the context of disease or illness.

Cognitive appraisal Interpretation of a situation.

Compliance An individual completing a required behavior.

Macrotrauma Injury resulting from a single impact or force that creates tissue damage (e.g., fracture, sprain, or dislocation).

Microtrauma Injury resulting from repeated smaller forces that gradually result in tissue damage over time (e.g., stress fracture, tendinitis).

Pain-spasm cycle Pain that causes vasoconstriction and muscle spasm, which, in turn, causes more pain, which, in turn, exacerbates the cycle; sometimes referred to as the pain-spasm-pain cycle.

Rapport The harmonious or synchronous relationship of two or more people who relate well to each other.

Rehabilitation adherence Behaviors an athlete demonstrates by pursuing a course of action that coincides with the recommendations of the athletic trainer and is aimed at recovery from injury.

Rehabilitation antecedents Biopsychosocial factors (injury characteristics, biological factors, psychological factors, sociodemographic factors, social/contextual factors) that influence rehabilitation adherence and outcomes.

Rehabilitation nonadherence The athlete working either too little (i.e., underadherence) or too much (i.e., overadherence) based on recommendations of the athletic trainer.

Rehabilitation outcomes Results of rehabilitation; examples include, but are not limited to, functional ability, strength, range of motion, readiness to return to sport, treatment satisfaction, quality of life.

Rehabilitation overadherence The athlete doing more than the rehabilitation program calls for.

Rehabilitation underadherence The athlete doing less than the rehabilitation program calls for.

Self-efficacy Confidence in one's ability to perform a particular task in a specific situation.

CHAPTER OBJECTIVES

After reading this chapter, you will be able to:

1. Identify and describe factors that influence sport injury rehabilitation from a biopsychosocial perspective.
2. Discuss detection and consequences of underadherence and overadherence.
3. Describe the concept of sport injury rehabilitation as performance.
4. Describe the psychosocial strategies that the athletic trainer can use to motivate the athlete during injury rehabilitation.
5. Select and integrate appropriate psychosocial strategies into an athlete's rehabilitation program to enhance rehabilitation adherence, return to participation, and overall outcomes.

ATHLETE INSIDER

José had been looking forward to joining the high-school cross-country team, affectionately called the "Cross-Country People," since he was in elementary school and watched his older sister win her first race. With both his mother and father as amateur runners, running was part of José's family. During his freshman year on the team, he was training particularly hard and taking extra hill runs along the road on the weekends to try and better his times. Partway through the season, he started to notice pain on the lateral side of his right knee. He tried to run through and ignore the pain, but he eventually mentioned it to his father. His father recommended that he speak with the athletic trainer at the high school before it got worse. José was reluctant to talk to the athletic trainer because he did not want to stop running; however, he followed his father's recommendation. The athletic trainer took José's injury history from a biopsychosocial perspective. José found that the athletic trainer was very helpful by listening to him, assessing his pain as coming from the iliotibial (IT) band, and providing him with treatment advice. The athletic trainer also wanted to set up José on a rehabilitation program, but José declined because he did not want to be late for practice. As per the athletic trainer's recommendations, José agreed to begin icing and stretching, and planned to return to the athletic training room for instruction on foam-roller exercises. Although not consistent with the athletic trainer's recommendations, José also planned to continue his weekend runs so that he would not give up a spot on the team.

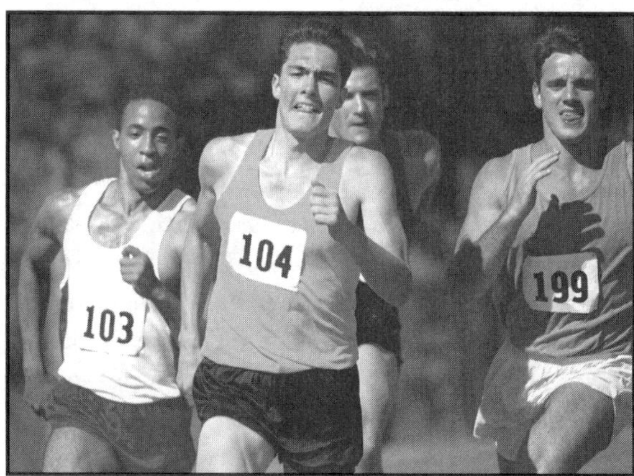

Figure 8-1 | Athlete Insider

INTRODUCTION

The terms ***rehabilitation adherence*** and ***compliance*** are often used interchangeably (Bassett & Prapavessis, 2007; Taylor & May, 1996). However, the term *adherence* is typically associated with a description of behaviors that are aimed at a particular outcome, whereas *compliance* can be defined as an individual completing a required behavior; alternately stated, adherence can be seen as a range of behaviors, whereas compliance is seen as a specific behavior either being completed or not completed. For example, an athlete may be compliant with wearing the prescribed brace but may not be adherent to the overall rehabilitation protocol. Thus, in this chapter, the term *rehabilitation adherence* is used to describe a set of behaviors that are aimed at recovery from injury.

Rehabilitation nonadherence (e.g., athlete working either too little or too much) may decrease overall ***rehabilitation outcomes*** (e.g., functional ability, strength, range of motion [ROM], readiness to return to sport, treatment satisfaction, quality of life) and may increase the chance of reinjury. Despite the ease of access for athletes to receive rehabilitation services, issues with rehabilitation adherence commonly occur and are recognized by athletic trainers as a problem that affects rehabilitation in the athletic training setting. This chapter provides an overview of the factors that influence sport injury rehabilitation adherence from a ***biopsychosocial perspective***, and discusses detection and consequences of ***rehabilitation underadherence*** and ***rehabilitation overadherence***.

Within this chapter, sport injury rehabilitation will be likened to athletic performance (i.e., athletes may not be currently performing in their sport, but they must still perform in rehabilitation); thus, psychosocial strategies athletes practice in the sport setting can be applied to rehabilitation. Within this chapter, motivational strategies are discussed, and similar to Chapter 7, psychosocial strategies for rehabilitation are overviewed, with more detail provided in Chapter 10. Although rehabilitation most often leads to return to participation, this chapter focuses on the rehabilitation process, and Chapter 11 is dedicated to that topic.

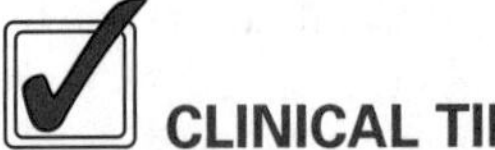

CLINICAL TIP

Consistent with a patient-centered approach, athletic trainers should refer to athletes as "athlete with injury" rather than "injured athlete."

The athletic training room provides a distinct rehabilitation environment. Typically, free services, convenient hours, and the location of the athletic training room allow athletes easy access to rehabilitation services. Athletes also often have established ***rapport*** with the athletic trainers who work and travel with their teams. The unique factors associated with rehabilitation in the athletic training room require athletic trainers to approach the rehabilitation process differently than they might in a physical therapy or hospital rehabilitation setting. Because athletes are often motivated to return to athletic performance and a high level of physical activity, it may be helpful to view rehabilitation as a performance. Viewing rehabilitation as performance starts at the beginning of rehabilitation and continues throughout the course of rehabilitation and return to participation. Particularly for those athletes with a strong ***athletic identity***, this framework sets the tone for athletes to approach rehabilitation with the same dedication and intensity with which they would approach athletic conditioning, practice, and competition. This is also where, although nuanced, the terminology of "athlete with injury" is preferred over "injured athlete"; the aim is to have athletes retain their athletic identity rather than the injury identity.

CLINICAL TIP

During the beginning of rehabilitation, athletic trainers can initiate a conversation with athletes to find out how they approach performance in their sport (i.e., the attitude they bring to training, the effort and dedication involved in their practice). Athletic trainers can say something such as "Great! That's exactly the way we are going to approach your rehabilitation." This approach achieves several goals: (a) it highlights the active rather than passive role athletes must take in rehabilitation, (b) it lets athletic trainers know what skills (e.g., imagery, positive self-talk) athletes are familiar with, and (c) it sets the stage for transfer of skills from one domain to another (e.g., sport to rehabilitation, rehabilitation to return to participation).

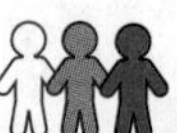

SPECIAL CONSIDERATIONS

Depending on the recovery time and rehabilitation progress, athletes' athletic identity may decrease during the course of rehabilitation (Brewer, Cornelius, Stephan, & Van Raalte, 2010). This may influence their motivation toward rehabilitation and return to participation. Therefore, psychosocial strategies aimed at motivational techniques are of particular importance for rehabilitation programs that are long in duration.

FACTORS THAT INFLUENCE ADHERENCE TO REHABILITATION PROGRAMS

It is common for athletes who sustain injuries to be prescribed rehabilitation programs. The programs are assumed to be successful to the degree that the athletes complete—or adhere to—them. In the context of sport injury rehabilitation, adherence refers to the extent to which athletes engage in behaviors as part of a treatment regimen designed to facilitate their recovery from injury. Depending on the specific injury and rehabilitation program prescribed, adherence to sport injury rehabilitation may involve a wide variety of behaviors. Some of the behaviors occur in the athletic training environment, whereas other behaviors occur away from the clinical setting. Adherence behaviors typical in athletic training settings include attending scheduled appointments, performing rehabilitation exercises, and participating in therapeutic modalities. Outside of the rehabilitation environment, athletes may be asked to engage in such behaviors as completing home rehabilitation exercises, refraining from engaging in potentially harmful activities, taking medication, and self-administering therapeutic modalities (e.g., icing).

Given the importance of adherence to achieving successful rehabilitation outcomes, many studies have been conducted to identify potential contributors to adherence to sport injury rehabilitation programs. Researchers have drawn on various theoretical models to guide their investigations of factors related to adherence. In the biopsychosocial model (Brewer, Andersen, & Van Raalte, 2002), which provides a general framework for more specific examination of the process of sport injury rehabilitation, adherence is considered a behavioral factor and is subject to the influence of injury-related, biological, social/contextual, and other psychological factors. When injuries occur, the characteristics of the injuries (e.g., type, course, severity, location, history) and sociodemographic factors (e.g., age, gender, race/ethnicity) are thought to have a direct effect not only on biological factors (particularly with respect to body parts involved with the injuries), but on psychological (including thoughts, emotions, and actions) and social/contextual factors (including life stress and characteristics of the situation and the rehabilitation environment) as well. Table 8-1 provides additional examples of biopsychosocial factors. It is easy to see, for example, how an ankle injury to a 13-year-old girl might produce inflammation in the area of the injury (biological factor), create fearful emotions (psychological factor), and inject stress into her daily life (social/contextual factor). The girl's emotions, in turn, can both affect and be affected by the amounts of inflammation and stress she is experiencing (i.e., an abundance of inflammation and stress can increase fear, and elevations in fear [and the corresponding hormonal response] can increase inflammation and create more stress in the social system). This complex set of multiple interacting influences establishes the context in which rehabilitation adherence occurs.

In addition to the proposed influences of injury characteristics, sociodemographic factors, biological factors, and social/contextual factors on rehabilitation adherence, other psychological factors are thought to affect athletes' completion of their rehabilitation program. Multiple psychologically based models have been developed to explain rehabilitation adherence. In these models, some combination of social/contextual factors, personal factors (i.e., personality), cognitive responses, emotional responses, and behavioral responses is thought to contribute to athletes' adherence behavior. Among the theoretical perspectives that have been used to help identify predictors of rehabilitation adherence are personal investment theory (Maehr & Braskamp, 1986), protection motivation theory (Maddux & Rogers, 1983), and the integrated model of psychological response to sport injury (Wiese-Bjornstal, Smith, Shaffer, & Morrey, 1998). Of particular note, cognitive factors figure prominently and are considered proximal to rehabilitation adherence in each of these three approaches. In applying personal investment theory to examine rehabilitation adherence, beliefs about personal incentives to adhere, one's sense of self (e.g., confidence, motivation), and perceived options (e.g., treatment efficacy, future sport plans) can be used as potential predictors of adherence (see Duda, Smart, & Tappe, 1989). In protection motivation theory, athletes are deemed most likely to adhere when they perceive their injuries as severe, view themselves as vulnerable to further damage if they do not complete their rehabilitation, believe that rehabilitation will be effective in treating their injuries, and

TABLE 8-1 Examples of Biopsychosocial Factors

Injury Characteristics	Sociodemographic Factors	Biological Factors	Psychological Factors	Social/Contextual Factors
• Type • Course • Severity • Location • History	• Age • Gender • Race/ethnicity • Socioeconomic status	• Tissue repair • Immune functioning • Nutrition • Sleep	• Personality • Emotional responses • Cognitive responses • Behavioral responses (adherence)	• Life stress • Social support • Situational characteristics • Rehabilitation environment

believe that they are capable of completing rehabilitation activities (see Taylor & May, 1996). In the integrated model, rehabilitation adherence is considered a behavioral factor that is reciprocally related to both cognitive and emotional factors, and is affected by the interaction between personal (e.g., personality) and situational (e.g., social support) factors.

Factors predictive of sport injury rehabilitation adherence can readily be mapped onto the framework of the biopsychosocial model. Although biological variables associated with adherence to rehabilitation have not been identified, potential contributors to adherence have been found among the characteristics of the injury, sociodemographic factors, social/contextual factors, and psychological factors categories of the biopsychosocial model.

Characteristics of the Injury

Few characteristics of sport injuries have been examined as prospective predictors of adherence to sport injury rehabilitation, but athletes with more severe injuries have been found to adhere better to their rehabilitation program than those with less severe injuries (Taylor & May, 1996). It is important to note that, for injury severity and most of the other biopsychosocial factors described in this section of the chapter, evidence of association with rehabilitation adherence is based on the self-reports of athletes with injuries. This means that each of the biopsychosocial factors is filtered through the athletes' perceptions of those factors, and that the observed relationships with adherence may have more to do with the athletes' perceptions than with the biopsychosocial factors themselves.

Sociodemographic Factors

Age is the sole sociodemographic factor that has been identified as a predictor of adherence to sport injury rehabilitation. Specifically, young athletes have displayed better adherence to their rehabilitation programs than older athletes (Levy, Polman, & Borkoles, 2008; Levy, Polman, & Clough, 2008). Age has also been shown to moderate the relationship between other variables and sport injury rehabilitation adherence. In one study (Levy, Polman, & Borkoles, 2008), for example, young athletes demonstrated high levels of adherence to clinic-based rehabilitation activities regardless of their level of perceived ***autonomy*** support, whereas older athletes were substantially less adherent to clinic-based rehabilitation activities when perceived autonomy support was low than when it was high.

Social/Contextual Factors

Several social/contextual factors have been found to be predictive of sport injury rehabilitation adherence. Athletes tend to adhere better to their injury rehabilitation programs when they perceive: (a) the clinical environment as comfortable (Fields, Murphey, Horodyski, & Stopka, 1995; Fisher, Domm, & Wuest, 1988), (b) scheduling of rehabilitation appointments as convenient (Fields et al, 1995; Fisher et al, 1988), (c) rehabilitation practitioners as expecting them to adhere (Taylor & May, 1995), and (d) others as supportive of their rehabilitation activities (Byerly, Worrell, Gahimer, & Domholdt, 1994; Duda et al, 1989; Fisher et al, 1988; Johnston & Carroll, 2000; Levy, Polman, & Borkoles, 2008; Levy, Polman, & Clough, 2008). Also, in a study of athletes undergoing rehabilitation after anterior cruciate ligament (ACL) reconstruction surgery (Chan, Lonsdale, Ho, Yung, & Chan, 2009), autonomy-supportive behaviors of physiotherapists were positively associated with the athletes' autonomous treatment motivation, which, in turn, was positively associated with the athletes' adherence to the rehabilitation program. Thus, social/contextual factors may contribute to other factors that are facilitative of sport injury rehabilitation adherence.

Psychological Factors

Numerous psychological factors have been identified as potential contributors to sport injury rehabilitation adherence. As would be expected from a biopsychosocial perspective, predictors of adherence have been documented from among the personal, cognitive, emotional, and behavioral aspects of psychological functioning.

Personal Factors

Associations between several personality characteristics and adherence to sport injury rehabilitation programs have been reported. Athletes who adhere well to rehabilitation tend to be tolerant of pain (Byerly et al, 1994; Fields et al, 1995; Fisher et al, 1988), motivated by the desire to improve rather than to beat others (Duda et al, 1989), self-motivated (Brewer, Daly, Van Raalte, Petitpas, & Sklar, 1999; Brewer, Van Raalte, Cornelius et al, 2000; Duda et al, 1989; Fields et al, 1995; Fisher et al, 1988; Levy, Polman, & Clough, 2008; Noyes, Matthews, Mooar, & Grood, 1983), task involved (Duda et al, 1989), and tough minded (Wittig & Schurr, 1994). Adherent athletes also tend to be consistent across situations in their belief that their behavior can affect their health status (Murphy, Foreman, Simpson, Molloy, & Molloy, 1999). Depending on the type of adherence under consideration, mental toughness may be helpful or harmful with respect to athletes' involvement in rehabilitation activities (Levy, Polman, Clough, Marchant, & Earle, 2006). Similarly, for young athletes, but not for older athletes, those who strongly identify with the athlete role have been found to adhere better to home exercise activities than people who are less strongly identified (Brewer et al, 2003b).

Cognitive Factors

Among the many cognitive factors for which associations with adherence to sport injury rehabilitation have been reported, many of the cognitions pertain directly to sport injury, rehabilitation, and recovery. Reflecting the proposed direct link between cognition and behavior in the biopsychosocial model, athletes are more likely to adhere to injury rehabilitation activities when they believe that their treatment is effective (Brewer et al, 2003a; Duda et al, 1989; Noyes et al, 1983; Taylor & May, 1996), value their rehabilitation highly (Taylor & May, 1996), perceive their level of exertion as high during rehabilitation activities (Fisher et al, 1988), report experiencing few threats to their self-esteem (Lampton, Lambert, & Yost, 1993), consider themselves as motivated largely by self-determination (Chan et al, 2009), identify stable and personally controllable factors as responsible for their recovery (Laubach et al, 1996), express confidence in their ability to cope with their injuries (Daly, Brewer, Van Raalte, Petitpas, & Sklar, 1995; Levy, Polman, & Clough, 2008), and complete their rehabilitation program (Brewer et al, 2003a; Levy, Polman, & Clough, 2008; Milne, Hall, & Forwell, 2005; Taylor & May, 1996). Athletes who indicate that they use the cognitive strategies of goal setting, positive self-talk (Scherzer et al, 2001), and imagery (Milne et al, 2005; Scherzer et al, 2001) tend to achieve higher levels of sport injury rehabilitation adherence than those who report not using those strategies. Experimental evidence that goal setting produces favorable effects on adherence has been found in two studies (Evans & Hardy, 2002; Penpraze & Mutrie, 1999).

Emotional and Behavioral Factors

Compared with personal and cognitive factors, few emotional and behavioral factors have been identified that are predictive of adherence to sport injury rehabilitation. Athletes with mood disturbance tend to adhere less well to their rehabilitation programs than athletes without mood disturbance (Alzate Saez de Heredia, Muñoz, & Artaza, 2004; Daly et al, 1995). With regard to behavior, athletes who adhere well to their rehabilitation program tend to report seeking information about their injuries and engaging in other similar instrumental coping behaviors to a greater extent than less adherent athletes (Udry, 1997).

CONSEQUENCES OF NONADHERENCE

Whether athletes adhere to their rehabilitation programs can have important implications for the outcomes they experience. When athletes depart from the program recommended by their athletic trainer, they are said to be *nonadherent*. There are two main types of nonadherence: underadherence and overadherence. Doing less than the rehabilitation program calls for is considered underadherence, whereas doing more than the program requires is overadherence. Both underadherence and overadherence have the potential to hamper the rehabilitation of athletes with injuries. In the context of sport injury rehabilitation, underadherence typically involves failing to attend rehabilitation sessions, complete agreed-on clinic- and/or home-based exercises, self-administer therapeutic modalities, restrict potentially harmful physical activity appropriately, or take prescribed medication. Underadherence to medical regimens in general (for a review, see Christensen, 2004) and sport injury rehabilitation programs in particular has been well documented. Estimates of the prevalence rates of adherence to sport injury rehabilitation have ranged from 40% to 91% (Brewer, 1999), suggesting that, on average, groups of athletes tend to underadhere to certain aspects of rehabilitation regimens. Underadherence can slow the progress of athletes in rehabilitation and leave them inadequately prepared for a return to sport, thereby placing them at increased risk for injury or reinjury. If athletic trainers are not aware of athletes' underadherence, they may advance the athletes too quickly through the rehabilitation program, which can further increase athletes' risk for injury.

Overadherence includes such behaviors as self-administering more of a therapeutic modality than prescribed or doing home exercises at greater frequency or intensity than indicated by the rehabilitation protocol. Less is known about overadherence than underadherence, in part because the most common methods of assessing adherence to sport injury rehabilitation (e.g., attendance at rehabilitation sessions, athletic trainer ratings of athlete adherence) generally do not allow for values greater than 100%. Nevertheless, Frey (2008) suggested that overadherence can prolong recovery, increase injury risk, decrease motivation, elevate fatigue, and lead to burnout.

CLINICAL TIP

The athletic trainer should tell athletes that during rehabilitation, "more is not necessarily better," and should make athletes aware that overadherence can sometimes lead to further injury and potentially set the athlete back even further in recovery. During this conversation, athletic trainers should educate athletes about the injury-healing process and how this relates to the phases of their rehabilitation program and the exercises and activity restrictions during each phase.

Understanding the potential impact of nonadherence on rehabilitation outcomes requires evidence of a dose–response relationship between the rehabilitation activities that athletes are being asked to adhere to and the outcomes that rehabilitation protocols are designed to achieve. In particular, it is necessary to know not only the amount (or "dose") of a given rehabilitation activity required to achieve optimal treatment outcomes, but also the minimum amount needed to produce acceptable treatment outcomes and the amount past which further activity compromises treatment outcomes (Brewer, 1999). Unfortunately, such information is known for few rehabilitation activities. Without knowledge of dose–response relationships, it is premature to devote extensive resources to enhancing adherence, especially when considering that, for many injuries, factors other than whether athletes complete the rehabilitation protocol (e.g., heredity, previous injuries, state of health) contribute to healing. In these sorts of situations, some athletes recover rapidly despite adhering poorly to the rehabilitation program, whereas other athletes recover slowly despite diligently following the rehabilitation program to the letter. Knowing dose–response relationships can help guide the formulation of rehabilitation protocols and provide concrete, evidence-based targets for adherence.

EVIDENCE-BASED PRACTICE

Boyce, D., & Brosky, J. A. (2008). Determining the minimal number of cyclic passive stretch repetitions recommended for an acute increase in an indirect measure of hamstring length. *Physiotherapy Theory and Practice, 24*(2), 113–120. doi: 10.1080/09593980701378298

Description of the Study

The study examined the dose–response relationship between cyclic passive hamstring stretches and hamstring length. Healthy male participants (n = 18, age range 19–37 years) performed a series of ten 15-second passive stretches. Hamstring length was assessed indirectly after each stretch through measurement of knee extension ROM.

Results of the Study

The results of the study indicated that knee extension ROM increased the most between the first and second stretches, and increased significantly through each of the first five stretches, after which no significant gains were observed.

Implications for Athletic Training Practice

The study provides evidence of a dose–response relationship between passive hamstring stretches and hamstring length, and establishes an empirical basis for determining the specifications of a hamstring stretching program. Athletic trainers can use this information to estimate the effects of underadherence and overadherence on the hamstring stretching protocol.

CLINICAL TIP

Based on a review of the literature related to rehabilitation adherence, Brewer (2004) concluded that athletes and other clients undergoing rehabilitation are most likely to adhere when they:

- have personal characteristics that enable adherence to rehabilitation programs that may be challenging.
- are part of a rehabilitation environment that is conducive to adherence.
- recognize their injury as serious enough to warrant care.
- are not overwhelmed by pain or emotions.
- attribute their recovery to behaviors within their control.
- trust in the value of their rehabilitation program.
- are confident in their ability to successfully complete the rehabilitation program.

MEASURING AND MONITORING ADHERENCE

Given the importance of adherence in sport injury rehabilitation in general and in establishing dose–response relationships in particular, it is imperative to be able to measure adherence accurately and monitor the adherence of athletes efficiently. To be useful, measures of adherence must take into account the multiple contexts in which sport injury rehabilitation occurs. The primary contexts for sport injury rehabilitation are in the clinic (or athletic training room) and at home.

Measures of Adherence to Clinic-Based Activities

Because athletic trainers are present for most of the clinic-based rehabilitation activities in which athletes with injuries are engaged, it is easier to monitor adherence in the clinic than at home. As noted earlier, in clinical settings, athletes are asked to attend rehabilitation appointments, perform rehabilitation exercises, and participate in therapeutic modalities. Athletic trainers can easily monitor attendance at rehabilitation appointments by recording the presence (or absence) of athletes and creating an attendance index by dividing the number of appointments attended by the number of appointments scheduled. Such an index is surely objective and is ideal for identifying athletes who fail to show up for rehabilitation appointments, but it contains no information about what athletes actually do when they are at the rehabilitation appointments. An athlete could, for example, attend every rehabilitation appointment but fail to exert much effort when there. The athlete would be judged fully adherent in terms of attendance, but the quality of the athlete's performance of rehabilitation exercises would suggest less than full adherence to clinic-based activities.

To determine how adherent athletes are during rehabilitation sessions, it is necessary to observe their behavior and record the results of such observations. The Sports Medicine Observation Code (SMOC; Crossman & Roch, 1991) was developed to facilitate direct, systematic observation of athletes during rehabilitation sessions. Observers record the duration and frequency of 13 behaviors (e.g., active rehabilitation, waiting, initial diagnosis, preventive treatment) occurring at selected points in time over the course of rehabilitation sessions. The SMOC yields a detailed account of how athletes spend their time during rehabilitation sessions, but it only provides information about adherence to the extent that the observed frequency and duration of on- and off-task behaviors is compared with those specified in the rehabilitation protocol. Moreover, the SMOC is time consuming and labor intensive to use and, consequently, is impractical for application in most clinical settings.

An approach for gauging athlete behavior during rehabilitation sessions that is more realistic than direct observation is to have athletic trainers record their perceptions of athletes' adherence to the rehabilitation protocol during their clinic appointments. Such information can be recorded informally, but it is difficult to compare informal observations over time and across athletes. Standardized instruments are available for recording perceptions of athletes' adherence to clinic-based rehabilitation activities.

Tailored specifically for assessing adherence to rehabilitation that occurs in the athletic training environment, the Rehabilitation Adherence Measure for Athletic Training (RAdMAT; Granquist, Gill, & Appaneal, 2010) is a 16-item questionnaire on which athletic trainers rate the behavior of athletes with respect to communication, attitude/effort, and attendance at and participation in rehabilitation sessions. The RAdMAT has been shown to discriminate among high, moderate, and low levels of adherence, and can be useful for identifying athletes who fail to participate adequately in rehabilitation activities, who do not communicate effectively with their athletic trainers, or who just "go through the motions" in rehabilitation. Because the RAdMAT measures multiple aspects of adherence, it is possible for athletic trainers to determine which behaviors to target for intervention (e.g., attendance, communication, effort). Tailoring interventions to the specific needs of athletes may have desirable effects on both adherence and rehabilitation outcomes.

Another tool that athletic trainers can use to measure the adherence of athletes to clinic-based rehabilitation activities is the Sport Injury Rehabilitation Adherence Scale (SIRAS; Brewer, Van Raalte, Petitpas, et al, 2000). The SIRAS, which can be used to refer to a single rehabilitation session or to multiple rehabilitation sessions, consists of items that assess the intensity of athletes' efforts in completing rehabilitation activities, the degree to which athletes followed their athletic trainer's instructions and advice during rehabilitation, and athletes' receptivity to changes in the rehabilitation protocol. Like the RAdMAT, the SIRAS can discriminate among high, moderate, and low levels of adherence (Brewer, Avondoglio, Cornelius, et al, 2002; Kolt, Brewer, Pizzari, Schoo, & Garrett, 2007). With only three items, however, the SIRAS is briefer but far less comprehensive than the RAdMAT. Consequently, the RAdMAT would be the instrument of choice if the purpose is to identify areas of clinic-based rehabilitation adherence in need of enhancement, whereas the SIRAS may be the more suitable instrument for repeated administrations over the course of rehabilitation.

Overall, although rating scales such as the RAdMAT and the SIRAS may provide less detailed information about athletes' clinic-based rehabilitation behavior than direct observation systems such as the SMOC, they are substantially more practical and user friendly. Moreover, they likely are less susceptible to social desirability bias than athlete self-reports of adherence and more nuanced than mere tallies of rehabilitation activities completed in that they measure both the volume of activities completed and the intensity of effort expended in completing the activities. Table 8-2 provides a summary of these measures.

TABLE 8-2 **Clinic-Based Measures of Rehabilitation Adherence**

Sports Medicine Observation Code (SMOC; Crossman & Roch, 1991)	Rehabilitation Adherence Measure for Athletic Training (RAdMAT; Granquist, Gill, & Appaneal, 2010)	Sport Injury Rehabilitation Adherence Scale (SIRAS; Brewer, Van Raalte, Petitpas, et al, 2000)
Consists of 13 behaviors that observers record the duration and frequency of during rehabilitation.	Consists of 16 items with ratings on a 4-point Likert-type scale (range 16–64, with higher scores indicating greater adherence).	Consists of three items with ratings on a five-point Likert-type scale (range 3–15, with higher scores indicating greater adherence).
Behaviors:	Contains three subscales:	Asks the sport medicine professional to rate the patient's:
• Active rehabilitation (e.g., icing, ultrasound) • Initial treatment (e.g., first aid)	• Attendance/participation (e.g., "arrives at rehabilitation on time," "follows the prescribed rehabilitation plan"; subscale range 5–20)	• Intensity of rehabilitation completion • Frequency of following instructions and advice

TABLE 8-2 Clinic-Based Measures of Rehabilitation Adherence—cont'd

Sports Medicine Observation Code (SMOC; Crossman & Roch, 1991)	Rehabilitation Adherence Measure for Athletic Training (RAdMAT; Granquist, Gill, & Appaneal, 2010)	Sport Injury Rehabilitation Adherence Scale (SIRAS; Brewer, Van Raalte, Petitpas, et al, 2000)
• Attending related (e.g., athlete listens to clinic personnel, related to injury) • Attending unrelated (e.g., athlete listens to clinic personnel, unrelated to injury) • Interaction related (e.g., athlete interacts verbally with clinic personnel, related to injury) • Interaction unrelated (e.g., athlete interacts verbally with clinic personnel, unrelated to injury) • Waiting • Initial diagnosis • Preventative treatment (e.g., taping) • Maintenance (e.g., scheduling next appointment) • Nonactivity • Unrelated activity (e.g., reading a book) • Exclusion (e.g., athlete visits rest room)	• Communication (e.g., "communicates with the athletic trainer if there is a problem with the exercises," "provides the athletic trainer feedback about the rehabilitation program"; subscale range 3–12) • Attitude/effort (e.g., "gives 100% effort in rehabilitation sessions," "is self-motivated in rehabilitation sessions"; subscale range 8–32)	• Receptivity to changes in rehabilitation **NOTE:** The instructions of the SIRAS can be modified to refer to a single rehabilitation session or to multiple rehabilitation sessions over a period of time.

Measures of Adherence to Home-Based Activities

Measuring adherence to home-based activities can be even more challenging than measuring clinic-based activities in sport injury rehabilitation because the behaviors being assessed occur outside of the view of athletic trainers. It may be tempting to infer how well athletes are adhering to their home rehabilitation protocols on the basis of their recovery progress—with athletes recovering quickly presumed to be adhering and athletes recovering slowly presumed not to be adhering—but such inferences are inappropriate. Some athletes may recover quickly in spite of not adhering to home rehabilitation activities, whereas other athletes may recover slowly even though they follow through religiously on their home rehabilitation program. Factors other than adherence to home-based rehabilitation activities contribute to recovery from sport injuries (e.g., heredity, clinic-based treatment).

A frequently used method of measuring adherence to home-based activities in sport injury rehabilitation is simply to ask athletes about the extent to which they are adhering to the home program. The desirable aspect of this method is that it involves obtaining information directly from the source of the behavior. Unfortunately, athlete self-report measures are subject to the effects of forgetting and responding in a socially desirable manner. Inaccuracy because of memory loss can be reduced by taking measurements frequently (e.g., daily), but inaccuracy caused by biased responding is more difficult to eliminate. Suspicions of nonadherence can be investigated by having athletes recall or replicate their prescribed home rehabilitation program. If athletes are unable to remember what they were supposed to do or do what they were supposed to do incorrectly, it is reasonable to infer that they may not be completing their rehabilitation program as recommended (for an overview, see Brewer, 2004).

For some home-based rehabilitation activities, objective measures of adherence can be used to avoid the limitations of athlete self-report. With regard to adherence to prescribed medication regimens, for example, multiple well-established objective indices have been developed, including medication measurement (e.g., pill counts), review of pharmacy data (e.g., regimen prescribed, amount of medication dispensed, timing of refills), electronic medication monitors, biochemical analysis (e.g., blood, urine), and direct observation (Rand & Weeks, 1998). There are limitations to each of these methods, but they can nevertheless be used to validate self-reports and identify potential inaccuracies or discrepancies with athlete self-reports.

Assessing appropriate restriction of physical activity can be especially challenging because the target of assessment is not a behavior but is instead a lack of behavior, and it is more difficult to measure a lack of behavior than it is to measure a behavior. Measuring self-administration of therapeutic modalities presents similar obstacles. Electronic monitoring has, however, made objective assessment of adherence possible for some home rehabilitation exercise regimens. Electronic monitoring devices have been embedded in accelerometers, ankle exercisers, biofeedback units, splints, and videocassettes used during home exercises (for an overview, see Brewer, 2004). In general, although objective assessment of adherence to home rehabilitation activities is desirable, there are many instances where it is impractical, cost prohibitive, or simply not possible. In such situations, it is necessary for athletic trainers seeking to measure how well the athletes in their care are adhering to their home rehabilitation programs to be creative in using the means at their disposal.

ENHANCING REHABILITATION ADHERENCE AND OUTCOMES

To achieve optimal outcomes following sport injury rehabilitation, athletic trainers must identify and address multiple biological, psychological, and social factors that influence rehabilitation adherence. This section describes a step-by-step process for obtaining an athlete's background based on a biopsychosocial perspective, identifying potential barriers to rehabilitation, and identifying and implementing strategies to reduce these barriers. Ideally, this process would be a collaborative effort between the athletic trainer and the athlete at the beginning of the rehabilitation program. The process of identifying potential barriers and implementing strategies to avoid or reduce these barriers may serve to build rapport between the athletic trainer and athlete. In addition, the awareness of the steps and the integration of these into the rehabilitation process may be helpful to enhance rehabilitation adherence and overall rehabilitation outcomes.

Obtaining Athlete Background Based on a Biopsychosocial Perspective

The first step of this process is a modification of a routine injury history and intake at the beginning of the rehabilitation process. In this manner, the athletic trainer compiles an athlete's background from a biopsychosocial perspective. Athletic trainers may tend to focus on the injury characteristics and biological factors related to injury (the physical aspects), and the sociodemographic factors, social/contextual factors, and psychological factors may receive less attention. Therefore, completing a history using a biopsychosocial approach allows a more comprehensive background to be compiled. Figure 8-2 provides an example of how the athletic trainer may complete the framework.

CLINICAL TIP

Information gathered from a biopsychosocial perspective would fit nicely in the History section of a HOPS (History, Observation, Palpation, Special Tests) medical note.

Characteristics of the Injury	• Grade III ACL sprain • Left knee • Allograft reconstruction • Brace with play • First severe injury
Sociodemographic Factors	• 19 years old • Male • Nonscholarship • Loss of summer employment
Biological Factors	• Good health • Moderate nutrition • Reports sleep difficulty
Psychological Factors	• Shows frustration • Reports stress • First severe injury
Social/Contextual Factors	• Good team and family support • Coach wants a quick return • Rehabilitation done in the athletic training room

Figure 8-2 | Example of athlete's background based on a biopsychosocial perspective.

As can be seen in Figure 8-2, Taylor is a 19-year-old male athlete who plays soccer at the NCAA Division III level. He tore his ACL at the end of spring soccer, and he aims to return in the fall. This is his first significant injury. Although his coach is pushing him for a quick return to participation, Taylor reports that he has good family and team support.

A blank form similar to Figure 8-2 could be kept in the athletic training room for use during intakes with the athlete. In addition to a comprehensive history, this framework can also serve as an opening for the athletic trainer to educate the athlete on the biopsychosocial aspects related to rehabilitation adherence and outcomes. This, in turn, may facilitate an opportunity for the athletic trainer to discuss the aspects related to stress management and other coping skills that may serve to enhance the rehabilitation process. This form could be filed with the athlete's medical records and may function as a tool for athletic trainers to reflect on the biopsychosocial aspects related to the athlete with whom they are working in rehabilitation and guide questions that may assist in the rehabilitation process.

Identifying Potential Biopsychosocial Barriers

The next step of this process is to identify potential barriers that may interfere with rehabilitation or return to participation; this is also based on a biopsychosocial perspective. As listed in Table 8-3, for example, potential barriers can be identified in each of the following areas: injury characteristics, biological factors, sociodemographic factors, social/contextual factors, and psychological factors. With their knowledge of the athlete's background and their experience working with athletes in rehabilitation, athletic trainers can come up with areas that may be a hindrance during rehabilitation.

As shown in the example in Table 8-3, potential barriers to rehabilitation and return to participation can include, but certainly may not be limited to, wearing a brace, sleep concerns, loss of employment, pressure from the coach, and stress. Again, a blank form similar to Table 8-3 could be completed by the athletic trainer as part of the intake and rehabilitation program planning. As discussed previously, this process of identifying potential barriers and subsequently identifying and implementing strategies to avoid or reduce the potential barriers should be a collaborative process between the athletic trainer and athlete. As such, the athlete should play a joint role in brainstorming barriers and strategies.

Identifying Strategies to Avoid or Reduce Barriers

As listed in Table 8-3, once potential barriers are identified, strategies for avoiding or reducing barriers can be identified. This identification of barriers may be the athletic trainer's and athlete's best guess at what may arise during the rehabilitation and return-to-participation process, and so, too, is the identification of possible strategies. However, the identification and subsequent implementation of strategies can serve as "an ounce of prevention." With practice and experience, athletic trainers can build a psychosocial

TABLE 8-3 **Potential Barriers and Possible Strategies**

Potential Barriers	Guide	Possible Strategies
Injury Characteristics		
• Athlete must wear brace for physical activity and on return to participation.	→	• Athletic trainer educates athlete on purpose of the brace. • Athlete does performance imagery.
Biological Factors		
• Athlete experiences sleep disruptions.	→	• Athletic trainer educates athlete on stress related to sleep. • Athlete engages in stress-management and relaxation techniques.
Sociodemographic Factors		
• Athlete has limited summer employment because of activity restrictions.	→	• Athlete engages in reframing of importance of rehabilitation for a full recovery.
Social/Contextual Factors		
• Coach is pushing for a quick return to participation of the athlete.	→	• Athletic trainer discusses rehabilitation and return-to-participation process with coach. • Athletic trainer encourages coach to be supportive of the athlete during rehabilitation.
Psychological Factors		
• Athlete is frustrated at limited activities and is experiencing stress over trying to quickly return to play.	→	• Athletic trainer engages in collaborative goal setting with the athlete. • Athlete engages in stress-management and relaxation techniques.

strategies toolbox and may be better able to assist athletes with identifying strategies to avoid or reduce barriers.

Implementing Strategies to Avoid or Reduce Barriers

After identifying possible strategies to avoid or reduce barriers that may be encountered in rehabilitation and return to participation, athletic trainers can implement these strategies. Many of these strategies can be seamlessly integrated into the rehabilitation program (as discussed in detail in Chapter 10), but sport psychology consultants can be of assistance if they are available.

As listed in Table 8-3, for example, the athletic trainer may educate the athlete on performance imagery or refer the athlete to a sport psychology consultant for imagery training. The athletic trainer can also educate the athlete on stress-management and relaxation techniques, discuss the rehabilitation with the coach as part of the sports medicine team, and guide the athlete in goal setting. When implementing strategies, it may be helpful for athletic trainers to create a "Next Steps" checklist that reminds them when and how these strategies will be incorporated into the rehabilitation and return-to-participation process. For example, this Next Steps checklist may include the following tasks:

- Guide the athlete on goal setting for each phase of rehabilitation and return to participation.
- Discuss with the coach the role he or she plays to support the athlete in the rehabilitation and return-to-participation process.

- Discuss the biological and psychological implications of stress, and provide the athlete with a relaxation script to listen to during icing times.
- Discuss the implications of a brace and how performance imagery may benefit the transition to wearing a brace.

The process of identifying potential barriers to rehabilitation and return to participation and then identifying and implementing strategies to reduce these barriers is a dynamic process. Ideally, these steps should be revisited at each new phase of rehabilitation. The collaborative nature of this process should be emphasized, and the biopsychosocial perspective should be considered during each of these steps.

EVIDENCE-BASED PRACTICE

Brewer, B. W., Cornelius, A. E., Van Raalte, J. L., et al. (2003b). Age-related differences in predictors of adherence to rehabilitation after anterior cruciate ligament reconstruction. *Journal of Athletic Training, 38*(2), 158–162.

Description of the Study

The purpose of the study was to investigate the moderating effects of age between psychological factors and rehabilitation adherence. Sixty-one participants (40 male, 21 female; mean age 26.03 years, range 14–47 years) were receiving rehabilitation following ACL reconstruction; 57% of participants were competitive athletes, and 41% were recreational athletes. Psychological factors that were examined included self-motivation, social support, athletic identity, and distress. Adherence to home-based rehabilitation activities was measured by participant self-report of home exercise completion and home cryotherapy completion. Adherence was measured in clinic-based rehabilitation activities by attendance ratio and rehabilitation practitioner ratings on the SIRAS.

Results of the Study

For younger participants, athletic identity was positively related to home-based rehabilitation exercise completion and home cryotherapy completion. Alternately, for older participants, self-motivation and social support were positively related to home exercise completion. Age was not found to be a moderator for clinic-based rehabilitation adherence.

Implications for Athletic Training Practice

Athletic trainers should keep in mind developmental issues when working with athletes in rehabilitation. Age should be an important consideration when planning rehabilitation, particularly when prescribing home-based rehabilitation activities.

PSYCHOSOCIAL STRATEGIES

Psychosocial strategies should be implemented throughout the rehabilitation process. This section begins by revisiting the psychosocial strategy intervention model. Next, psychosocial strategies within the phases of rehabilitation are discussed together with their transference from sport to rehabilitation. Finally, specific psychosocial strategies are discussed, including education, motivation, relaxation, and stress management.

Psychosocial Strategy Intervention Model—Revisited

The psychosocial strategy intervention model was introduced in Chapter 3, and it serves as a visual representation of where athletic trainers can intervene with psychosocial strategies related to stress. As the schematic shows, stress contributes to a variety of physical outcomes, such as increased tightness, spasm, and guarding of the muscles. These conditions, in turn, contribute to additional outcomes such as decreased ROM and increased pain. Athletic trainers may recognize the interplay between the spasm and pain as the well-known ***pain-spasm cycle***. Chapter 7 discusses this pain-spasm cycle in detail.

As shown in Figure 8-3, this model can be expanded for use in the rehabilitation context to demonstrate that physical tools (i.e., modalities such as ice, heat, and electrical stimulation) are routinely used to interrupt the pain-spasm cycle. In addition, this model shows the use of a variety of psychological tools or psychosocial strategies to not only

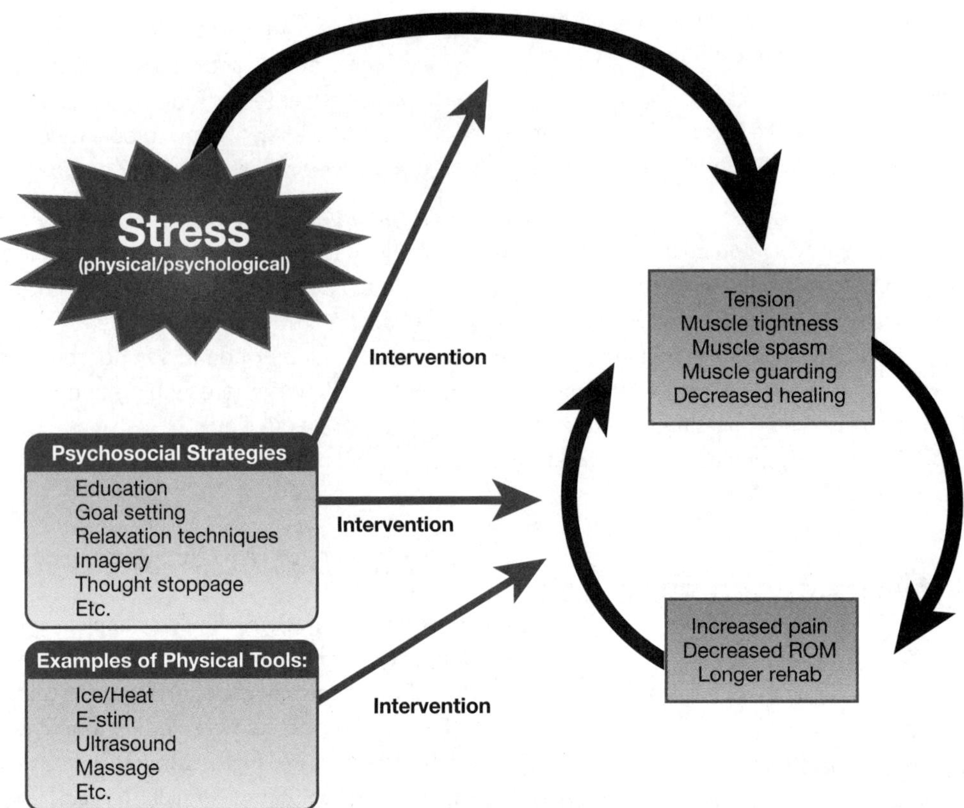

Figure 8-3 | Psychosocial strategy intervention model—revisited. *From Granquist, M.D. (2008). Psychology of injury and clinical practice: an athletic trainer's perspective. Presented at the National Athletic Trainers' Association Clinical Symposium, 2008. Used by permission.*

reduce the incidence of stress that may trigger the pain-spasm cycle, but also to intervene once the cycle has begun.

Psychosocial Strategies Within the Three Phases of Rehabilitation

Athletic trainers should incorporate psychosocial strategies into the rehabilitation process and across the phases of rehabilitation. The three phases of rehabilitation (i.e., inflammatory, fibroblastic, maturation) can call for different psychosocial strategies across phases. Integrated rehabilitation is the practice of not only treating the physical injury of the athlete, but also taking into account the whole athlete (Flint, 1998, 2007). The integrated rehabilitation model (Flint, 1998) is consistent with a biopsychosocial approach to rehabilitation. The model suggests that tissue damage (caused by either ***macrotrauma*** from an acute injury or ***microtrauma*** from an overuse injury) influences responses in three major categories: (a) physical or physiological, (b) psychological and emotional, and (c) sport. As such, athletic trainers can use the integrated rehabilitation model across the three phases of rehabilitation. For each of the phases, the athletic trainer should consider the physical or physiological goals, the psychological goals, and the sport goals.

CLINICAL TIP

Psychosocial strategies (e.g., goal setting, imagery, positive self-talk) that are integrated into rehabilitation may be transferable from the rehabilitation setting to return to participation in the sports setting (and even to life in general). Athletic trainers can guide athletes to use rehabilitation time to learn and practice these strategies.

Transferring Psychosocial Strategies From Sport to Rehabilitation

Athletes use psychological skills (also known as mental skills) as part of their sporting performance. Therefore, it may simply take the athletic trainer explaining this connection to athletes for them to transfer these skills into the rehabilitation setting. For example, when discussing imagery, the athletic trainer may say, "You probably already use this in your sport ... it is also useful in rehabilitation." The athletic trainer can educate the athlete about the purpose and uses of imagery and then provide examples of times when imagery may be integrated into rehabilitation, such as during heating or icing modalities.

As discussed earlier in this chapter, viewing the rehabilitation setting as an extension of the sporting performance may help athletes maintain their motivation throughout rehabilitation. A word of caution should be included here, because overadherence may be detrimental to rehabilitation outcomes. Therefore, education of the athlete should be emphasized to counteract the often-held belief that "more is better."

Education

As discussed throughout this text, educating the athlete is of primary importance. This holds true throughout the rehabilitation process. Increasing athletes' understanding and knowledge of their injury and the rehabilitation process influences their ***cognitive appraisal*** of the situation, which, in turn, influences their emotional responses and behavioral responses.

Education may be particularly essential at the beginning of the rehabilitation, when athletes may be uncertain about the extent of their injury and of their healing and the process of rehabilitation. Throughout the rehabilitation, education may also be important, perhaps particularly to counteract overadherence. Education should be emphasized again at the end of rehabilitation, when athletes may be nearing return to participation. Athletic trainers can enhance the rehabilitation experience for athletes by thoroughly explaining rehabilitation activities, avoiding jargon or slang and overly technical terminology, and being aware of their own nonverbal cues.

CLINICAL TIP

Consistent with an integrated approach to rehabilitation, athletic trainers can use the commencement of each rehabilitation phase as a marker to revisit education, goal setting, and other psychosocial strategies with athletes (Fig. 8-4).

Education is also the first step in increasing the athlete's awareness of psychosocial strategies. When integrating psychosocial strategies into the rehabilitation process, athletic trainers should begin by educating athletes. If athletic trainers introduce imagery, for example, they should describe what imagery is, the purpose of imagery, and the uses of imagery. Educating athletes regarding psychosocial strategies increases their awareness of the skill, and it may enhance their willingness to try and use the skill in rehabilitation. Athletic trainers may consider these tips for integrating psychosocial strategies into practice:

- Emphasize to athletes the idea of rehabilitation as a performance.

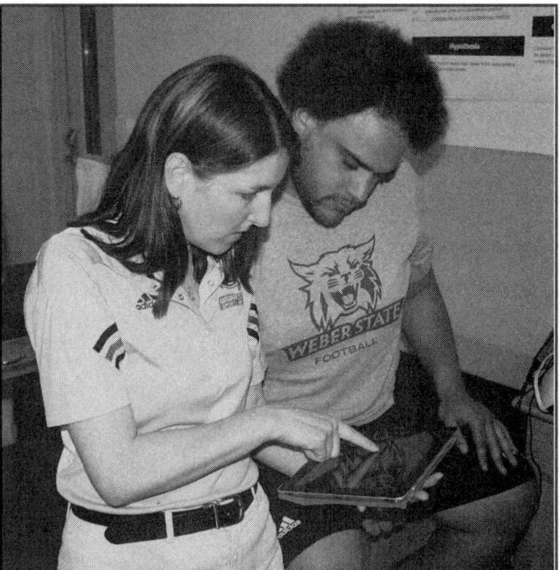

Figure 8-4 | Educating the athlete during the rehabilitation process.

- Explain and demonstrate to athletes that they can use rehabilitation time to learn and practice these strategies.
- Explain to athletes how these strategies are transferable from rehabilitation to sports and to life.

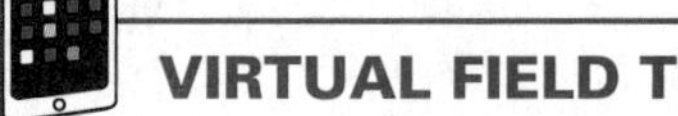

VIRTUAL FIELD TRIP

Listen to a healing imagery script, and a conversation between an athlete and athletic trainer, in Critical Listening Exercise #1 for this chapter.

http://davisplus.fadavis.com

Motivation Strategies

Personal and situational factors as ***rehabilitation antecedents*** influence an athlete's motivation toward rehabilitation. Specifically, goal setting (Scherzer et al, 2001) and positive self-talk (Evans & Hardy, 2002; Penpraze & Mutrie, 1999; Scherzer et al, 2001) are two motivational strategies that may be effective to enhance rehabilitation adherence.

Goal Setting

Consistent with integrated rehabilitation, for each of the phases of rehabilitation, athletic trainers should guide athletes in collaboratively setting goals for the following domains: physical, psychological, and sport performance. In addition, lifestyle goals such as sleep, diet, and overall healthy living should be included. As discussed in Chapter 10, each of these goals should be considered at three different levels: immediate daily goals, medium-term rehabilitation process/stage goals, and ultimate recovery/outcome goals. Goal setting may be a useful strategy for athletes to help maintain their control over their situation; as such, goal setting may serve to enhance motivation. Goal setting may also enhance rehabilitation adherence by providing the athlete with specific, measurable, and realistic points at which to aim.

CLINICAL TIP

When working with athletes in rehabilitation, athletic trainers should be sure to address athlete concerns about losing sport skills and fitness. Athletic trainers should work with athletes on exercises that can be done to maintain or enhance function in unaffected areas. This time is also an opportunity to work on underdeveloped physical skills (e.g., shooting a basketball with a nondominant hand) and psychosocial strategies (e.g., performance imagery, relaxation). By athletic trainers addressing these concerns, athletes may feel less like they are falling behind their teammates. It may also make rehabilitation more dynamic and interesting, and thus increase athletes' motivation for adherence.

Positive Self-Talk

Positive self-talk, or self-affirmations, may increase athletes' ***self-efficacy*** in rehabilitation, which may, in turn, enhance their performance in rehabilitation. Stopping negative, unproductive thoughts and reframing them as positive, productive thoughts is a strategy that athletic trainers can integrate into the rehabilitation process. For example, athletic trainers can explain to athletes that negative thoughts, such as "I'm never going to get better" or "I'm never going to be the player that I was before," are common when coping with an injury; however, they may be counterproductive in rehabilitation and return to participation. Athletic trainers can help athletes reframe these thoughts by providing examples, such as "I'm determined to get better" or "I'm motivated to be the player I was before." Posting positive thoughts on posters around the rehabilitation area may serve as reminders to athletes to stay positive.

CLINICAL TIP

Rehabilitation partners and support groups may enhance the rehabilitation process for an athlete. Athletic trainers should consider working with a sport psychology consultant or their institution's counseling center to establish these groups. This is discussed in detail with social support in Chapter 9. For specific information on establishing performance enhancement groups, see Clement, Shannon, and Connole (2012).

Relaxation and Stress Management

Stress influences physical (e.g., increased muscle tension, decreased healing and repair) and psychological (increased distraction, difficulty focusing, memory impairment, etc.)

responses. Therefore, stress may influence an athlete's motivation toward rehabilitation. Stress-management techniques, such as deep breathing and progressive muscle relaxation, may be used to decrease the stress response (these strategies are discussed in detail in Chapter 10).

When introducing relaxation strategies to athletes, athletic trainers should begin by educating the athletes on the physical and psychological effects of stress. Although it may be uncomfortable for athletic trainers to broach the topic of stress, this should be part of the biopsychosocial approach to rehabilitation. The athletic trainer may open by saying to the athlete, "There are many demands on athletes ... stress is a normal occurrence."

The relaxation strategies that can be used to decrease the stress response can then be explained, and athletic trainers should demonstrate the technique for athletes. Athletes should try these strategies while they are in the rehabilitation session. Finally, athletic trainers should then help athletes identify when the strategy can be used, such as during heating and icing, before sleeping, or to manage pain. Periodically during rehabilitation, the athletic trainer should inquire about how the strategy is working for the athlete; this may serve as a reminder for the athlete to use the strategy and to problem-solve any difficulties the athlete may be having with incorporating it into rehabilitation.

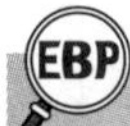

EVIDENCE-BASED PRACTICE

Scherzer, C. B., Brewer, B. W., Cornelius, A. E., et al. (2001). Psychological skills and adherence to rehabilitation after reconstruction of the anterior cruciate ligament. *Journal of Sport Rehabilitation, 10*(3), 165–172.

Description of the Study

Fifty-four participants (37 men, 17 women; mean age 28 years, SD 8.33) were receiving rehabilitation following ACL reconstruction; 28 participants were competitive athletes, and 25 were recreational athletes. The use of goal setting, healing imagery, and positive self-talk during rehabilitation was assessed using the Sports Injury Survey (Ievleva & Orlick, 1991). Rehabilitation adherence was assessed by attendance ratio, the SIRAS, and participant self-report of home rehabilitation exercise completion and home cryotherapy completion.

Results of the Study

Goal setting was a significant predictor of home exercise completion and clinic SIRAS scores. Healing imagery was not found to be significantly related to or predictive of home or clinic rehabilitation adherence. Although only 20 participants reported using self-talk, a significant relationship was found between self-talk and home exercise completion.

Implications for Athletic Training Practice

The introduction of psychological skills by the athletic trainer to the athlete may contribute to better rehabilitation adherence. For example, educating the athlete on the process of healing imagery and positive self-talk may increase the athlete's use of these skills during rehabilitation.

RED FLAG

Particularly with longer rehabilitations and more severe injuries, athletic trainers should be aware of signs athletes may demonstrate that warrant referral to a mental health practitioner. For more information, see Chapter 4 for emotional responses to injury and Chapter 6 for identification of distress and referral.

ATHLETE INSIDER CONCLUSION

After 2 weeks of icing and stretching on his own, José returns to the athletic training room so that the athletic trainer can instruct him on foam-roller exercises. José reports that the pain has subsided some but is still bothering him quite a bit. He is frustrated because he is not able to complete his weekend runs without pain. José shares his concerns with the athletic trainer in hopes that there is a quicker fix for his pain.

Effective Psychosocial Strategies for the Athletic Trainer to Use with José

The athletic trainer can implement the following psychosocial strategies during José's rehabilitation process:

1. Keeping in mind José's age, educate José on the cause of his injury and explain its overuse nature and how it relates to the healing process.
2. Assist José in setting goals that are realistic yet challenging.
3. Teach José relaxation skills, such as deep breathing and progressive muscle relaxation.
4. Introduce José to psychosocial strategies, such as imagery, that he can practice as an alternate for his weekend runs, such that he is working to train his mind while his knee repairs.
5. Teach him how to transfer these strategies to his running to enhance his performance.

CONCLUSION

This chapter provided an overview of factors that influence sport injury rehabilitation adherence from a biopsychosocial perspective. Rehabilitation nonadherence (including underadherence and overadherence) were discussed related to rehabilitation outcomes (e.g., functional ability, strength, ROM, readiness to return to sport, treatment satisfaction, quality of life). Within this chapter, sport injury rehabilitation was described as performance; athletes may not be currently performing in their sport, but they must still perform in rehabilitation; and the psychosocial strategies athletes practice in the sport setting can be applied to rehabilitation.

REFERENCES

Alzate Saez de Heredia, R., Muñoz, A. R., & Artaza, J. L. (2004). The effect of psychological response on recovery of sport injury. *Research in Sports Medicine, 12,* 15–31.

Bassett, S. F., & Prapavessis, H. (2007). Home-based physical therapy intervention with adherence-enhancing strategies versus clinic-based management for patients with ankle sprains. *Physical Therapy, 87*(9), 1132–1143.

Boyce, D., & Brosky, J. A. (2008). Determining the minimal number of cyclic passive stretch repetitions recommended for an acute increase in an indirect measure of hamstring length. *Physiotherapy Theory and Practice, 24*(2), 113–120. doi: 10.1080/09593980701378298

Brewer, B. W. (1999). Adherence to sport injury rehabilitation regimens. In: S. J. Bull (Ed.), *Adherence Issues in Sport and Exercise* (pp. 145–168). Hoboken, NJ: John Wiley & Sons, Inc.

Brewer, B. W. (2004). Psychological aspects of rehabilitation. In: G. S. Kolt & M. B. Andersen (Eds.), *Psychology in the Physical and Manual Therapies* (pp. 39–53). Edinburgh, United Kingdom: Churchill Livingstone.

Brewer, B. W., Andersen, M. B., & Van Raalte, J. L. (2002). Psychological aspects of sport injury rehabilitation: Toward a biopsychosocial approach. In: D. L. Mostofsky & L. D. Zaichkowsky (Eds.), *Medical and Psychological Aspects of Sport and Exercise* (pp. 41–54). Morgantown, WV: Fitness Information Technology.

Brewer, B. W., Avondoglio, J. B., Cornelius, A. E., et al. (2002). Construct validity and interrater agreement of the Sport Injury Rehabilitation Adherence Scale. *Journal of Sport Rehabilitation, 11*(3), 170–178.

Brewer, B. W., Cornelius, A. E., Stephan, Y., & Van Raalte, J. (2010). Self-protective changes in athletic identity following anterior cruciate ligament reconstruction. *Psychology of Sport & Exercise, 11*(1), 1–5. doi: 10.1016/j.psychsport.2009.09.005

Brewer, B. W., Cornelius, A. E., Van Raalte, J. L., et al. (2003a). Protection motivation theory and sport injury rehabilitation adherence revisited. *The Sport Psychologist, 17*(1), 95–103.

Brewer, B. W., Cornelius, A. E., Van Raalte, J. L., et al. (2003b). Age-related differences in predictors of adherence to rehabilitation after anterior cruciate ligament reconstruction. *Journal of Athletic Training, 38*(2), 158–162.

Brewer, B. W., Daly, J. M., Van Raalte, J. L., Petitpas, A. J., & Sklar, J. H. (1999). A psychometric evaluation of the Rehabilitation Adherence Questionnaire. *Journal of Sport & Exercise Psychology, 21*(2), 167–173.

Brewer, B. W., Van Raalte, J. L., Cornelius, A. E., et al. (2000). Psychological factors, rehabilitation adherence, and rehabilitation outcome after anterior cruciate ligament reconstruction. *Rehabilitation Psychology, 45*(1), 20–37. doi: 10.1037/0090-5550.45.1.20

Brewer, B. W., Van Raalte, J. L., Petitpas, A. J., et al. (2000). Preliminary psychometric evaluation of a measure of adherence to clinic-based sport injury rehabilitation. *Physical Therapy in Sport, 1*(3), 68–74.

Byerly, P. N., Worrell, T., Gahimer, J., & Domholdt, E. (1994). Rehabilitation compliance in an athletic training environment. *Journal of Athletic Training, 29*(4), 352–355.

Chan, D. K., Lonsdale, C., Ho, P. Y., Yung, P. S., & Chan, K. M. (2009). Patient motivation and adherence to postsurgery rehabilitation exercise recommendations: The influence of physiotherapists' autonomy-supportive behaviors. *Archives of Physical Medicine & Rehabilitation, 90*(12), 1977–1982.

Christensen, A. J. (2004). *Patient Adherence to Medical Treatment Regimens: Bridging the Gap between Behavioral Science and Biomedicine.* New Haven, CT: Yale University Press.

Clement, D., Shannon, V., & Connole, I. (2012). Performance enhancement groups for injured athletes part 1: Preparation and development. *International Journal of Athletic Therapy & Training, 17*(3), 34–36.

Crossman, J., & Roch, J. (1991). An observation instrument for use in sports medicine clinics. *Journal of the Canadian Athletic Therapists Association,* 10–13.

Daly, J. M., Brewer, B. W., Van Raalte, J. L., Petitpas, A. J., & Sklar, J. H. (1995). Cognitive appraisal, emotional adjustment, and adherence to rehabilitation following knee surgery. *Journal of Sport Rehabilitation, 4*(1), 23–30.

Duda, J. L., Smart, A. E., & Tappe, M. K. (1989). Predictors of adherence in rehabilitation of athletic injuries: An application of personal investment theory. *Journal of Sport & Exercise Psychology, 11*(4), 367–381.

Evans, L., & Hardy, L. (2002). Injury rehabilitation: A goal-setting intervention study. *Research Quarterly for Exercise and Sport, 73*(3), 310–319.

Fields, J., Murphey, M., Horodyski, M., & Stopka, C. (1995). Factors associated with adherence to sport injury rehabilitation in college-age recreational athletes. *Journal of Sport Rehabilitation, 4*(3), 172–180.

Fisher, A. C., Domm, M. A., & Wuest, D. A. (1988). Adherence to sports-injury rehabilitation programs. *The Physician and Sportsmedicine, 16*(7), 47–52.

Flint, F. (1998). *Psychology of Sport Injury: A Professional Achievement Self-Study Program Course.* Champaign, IL: Human Kinetics.

Flint, F. (2007). Matching psychological strategies with physical rehabilitation. In: D. Pargman (Ed.), *Psychological Bases of Sport Injuries* (3rd ed., pp. 319–334). Morgantown, WV: Fitness Information Technology.

Frey, M. (2008). The other side of adherence: injured athletes who are too motivated. *Athletic Therapy Today, 13*(3),13–14.

Granquist, M. D. (2008). Psychology of injury and clinical practice: an athletic trainer's perspective. *Presented at the National Athletic Trainers' Association Clinical Symposium*, 2008.

Granquist, M. D., Gill, D. L., & Appaneal, R. N. (2010). Development of a measure of rehabilitation adherence for athletic training. *Journal of Sport Rehabilitation, 19*(3), 249–267.

Ievleva L., & Orlick T. (1991). Mental links to enhanced healing: an exploratory study. *The Sport Psychologist, 5*, 25–40.

Johnston, L. H., & Carroll, D. (2000). Coping, social support, and injury: Changes over time and the effects of level of sports involvement. *Journal of Sport Rehabilitation, 9*(4), 290–303.

Kolt, G. S., Brewer, B. W., Pizzari, T., Schoo, A. M. M., & Garrett, N. (2007). The Sport Injury Rehabilitation Adherence Scale: A reliable scale for use in clinical physiotherapy. *Physiotherapy, 93*(1), 17–22.

Lampton, C. C., Lambert, M. E., & Yost, R. (1993). The effects of psychological factors in sports medicine rehabilitation adherence. *Journal of Sports Medicine and Physical Fitness, 33*(3), 292–299.

Laubach, W. J., Brewer, B. W., Van Raalte, J. L., & Petitpas, A. J. (1996). Attributions for recovery and adherence to sport injury rehabilitation. *Australian Journal of Science and Medicine in Sport, 28*(1), 30–34.

Levy, A. R., Polman, R. C. J., & Borkoles, E. (2008). Examining the relationship between perceived autonomy support and age in the context of rehabilitation in sport. *Journal of Rehabilitation Psychology, 53*(2), 224–230.

Levy, A. R., Polman, R. C. J., & Clough, P. J. (2008). Adherence to sport injury rehabilitation programs: An integrated psycho-social approach. *Scandinavian Journal of Medicine and Science in Sport, 18*(6), 798–809. doi: 10.1111/j.1600-0838.2007.00704.x

Levy, A.R., Polman, R., Clough, P., Marchant, D., & Earle, K. (2006). Mental toughness as a determinant of beliefs, pain and adherence in sport injury rehabilitation. *Journal of Sport Rehabilitation, 15*, 246–254.

Maehr, M., & Braskamp, L. (1986). *The Motivation Factor: A Theory of Personal Investment.* Lexington, MA: Lexington Books.

Maddux, J. E., & Rogers, R. W. (1983). Protection motivation and self-efficacy: A revised theory of fear appeals and attitude change. *Journal of Experimental Social Psychology, 19*(5), 469–479.

Milne, M., Hall, C., & Forwell, L. (2005). Self-efficacy, imagery use, and adherence to rehabilitation by injured athletes. *Journal of Sport Rehabilitation, 14*(2), 150–167.

Murphy, G. C., Foreman, P. E., Simpson, C. A., Molloy, G. N., & Molloy, E. K. (1999). The development of a locus of control measure predictive of injured athletes' adherence to treatment. *Journal of Science and Medicine in Sport, 2*(2), 145–152. doi: 10.1016/S1440-2440(99)80194-7

Noyes, F. R., Matthews, D. S., Mooar, P. A., & Grood, E. S. (1983). The symptomatic anterior cruciate-deficient knee. Part II: The results of rehabilitation, activity modification, and counseling on functional disability. *Journal of Bone and Joint Surgery, 65*(2), 163–174.

Penpraze, P., & Mutrie, N. (1999). Effectiveness of goal setting in an injury rehabilitation programme for increasing patient understanding and compliance [Abstract]. *British Journal of Sports Medicine, 33*, 60.

Rand, C. S., & Weeks, K. (1998). Measuring adherence with medication regimens in clinical care and research. In: S. A. Shumaker, E. B. Schron, J. K. Ockene, & W. L. McBee (Eds.), *The Handbook of Health Behavior Change* (2nd ed., pp. 114–132). New York: Springer Publishing.

Scherzer, C. B., Brewer, B. W., Cornelius, A. E., et al. (2001). Psychological skills and adherence to rehabilitation after reconstruction of the anterior cruciate ligament. *Journal of Sport Rehabilitation, 10*(3), 165–172.

Taylor, A. H., & May, S. (1995). Physiotherapist's expectations and their influence on compliance to sports injury rehabilitation. In: R. Vanfraechem-Raway & Y. Vanden Auweele (Eds.), *IXth European Congress on Sport Psychology proceedings: Part II* (pp. 619–625). Brussels, Belgium: European Federation of Sports Psychology.

Taylor, A. H., & May, S. (1996). Threat and coping appraisal as determinants of compliance to sports injury rehabilitation: An application of protection motivation theory. *Journal of Sports Sciences, 14*(6), 471–482. doi: 10.1080/02640419608727734

Udry, E. (1997). Coping and social support among injured athletes following surgery. *Journal of Sport & Exercise Psychology, 19*(1), 71–90.

Wiese-Bjornstal, D. M., Smith, A. M., Shaffer, S. M., & Morrey, M. A. (1998). An integrated model of response to sport injury: Psychological and sociological dimensions. *Journal of Applied Sport Psychology, 10*(1), 46–69.

Wittig, A. F., & Schurr, K. T. (1994). Psychological characteristics of women volleyball players: Relationships with injuries, rehabilitation, and team success. *Personality and Social Psychology Bulletin, 20*(3), 322–330. doi: 10.1177/0146167294203010

BOARD OF CERTIFICATION STRATEGIES AND COMPETENCIES

As the Sixth Edition of the Board of Certification's Role Delineation Study outlines, athletic trainers are involved in the treatment and rehabilitation of injury (Domain 4). Specific to the Fifth Edition Athletic Training Education Competencies, strategies for enhancing rehabilitation adherence and outcomes based on a biopsychosocial model supports psychosocial strategies (e.g., goal setting, imagery, positive self-talk, relaxation/anxiety reduction) that athletic trainers can use to motivate athletes during rehabilitation (PS-7) and the integration of psychosocial strategies (e.g., motivation, goal setting, imagery, self-talk, relaxation) into the rehabilitation program (CIP-7).

Board of Certification Style Questions

1. Rehabilitation nonadherence includes (select all that apply):
   a. underadherence.
   b. overadherence.
   c. compliance.
   d. conformity.

2. Which factors have been prospectively linked to and/or predictive of rehabilitation adherence? (Select all that apply.)
   a. Injury severity
   b. Age
   c. Rehabilitation environment
   d. Perceived value of treatment

3. The biopsychosocial model of sport injury rehabilitation includes (select all that apply):
   a. biological factors.
   b. psychological factors.
   c. sociodemographic factors.
   d. social/contextual factors.

END-OF-CHAPTER EXERCISES

1. Explain why a biopsychosocial approach to rehabilitation is important for athletic trainers to keep in mind when working with athletes.
2. Describe how psychosocial considerations affect clinical decision-making in the athletic training setting related to return to participation.
3. Explain the consequences of nonadherence, including underadherence and overadherence.
4. Explain why attendance at rehabilitation sessions is not an adequate measure of rehabilitation adherence.
5. Describe how an athlete's rehabilitation adherence may be measured and monitored.
6. List and describe the psychosocial strategies that the athletic trainer can use to motivate the athlete during rehabilitation and return to participation.
7. a. Based on the example provided in Figure 8-2 related to a biopsychosocial perspective, what else would be helpful for the athletic trainer to know about José from the Athlete Insider case study to help identify possible barriers to rehabilitation?
   b. What additional potential barriers may be encountered with José?
   c. What additional possible strategies could be used to avoid or reduce potential barriers to rehabilitation and return to participation?
8. Consider an athlete whom you are currently observing in rehabilitation. Select and integrate appropriate psychosocial techniques into that athlete's rehabilitation program to enhance rehabilitation adherence, return to play, and overall outcomes.
9. Based on the Athlete Insider case study with José, discuss how his response could be based on the following frameworks:
   a. Personal investment theory (Maehr & Braskamp, 1986)
   b. Protection motivation theory (Maddux & Rogers, 1983)
   c. Integrated model of psychological response to sport injury (Wiese-Bjornstal et al, 1998)

Chapter 9

Social Support and the Athletic Trainer

Megan D. Granquist with Stephanie A. Stadden

CHAPTER OUTLINE

KEY TERMS

Active listening Communication technique that requires the listener to feed back what is heard by restating or paraphrasing; to confirm what was heard and to confirm the understanding of both parties.

Athlete-centered care Providing individualized care to an athlete.

Empathy Being sensitive to and vicariously experiencing the feelings, thoughts, or motives of another person.

KEY TERMS *continued*

Help-seeking Involves the willingness to ask for assistance from identified resources, such as those with whom athletes feel comfortable seeking help and advice.

Matching hypothesis Involves matching the available social support to the social support needs of the athlete.

Rapport The harmonious or synchronous relationship of two or more people who relate well to each other.

Self-efficacy Confidence in one's ability to perform a particular task in a specific situation.

Social support Includes the feeling or sense of being supported by others, the act of supporting others, and social integration.

Sport ethic Socially defined criteria for consideration as an athlete in competitive sports.

CHAPTER OBJECTIVES

After reading this chapter, you will be able to:

1. Identify and describe types of social support.
2. Describe the relationships between help-seeking tendencies and social support.
3. Explain the importance of matching athletes' social support needs with the provision of social support.
4. Describe the role the athletic trainer plays in the provision of social support.
5. Explain the importance of educating athletes, their parents/guardians, and others regarding their injury condition to enhance the athletes' well-being.
6. Implement psychosocial strategies into athlete care before and after injury to enhance the athlete's perception and availability of social support.

ATHLETE INSIDER

Kate is competing in her freshman season of collegiate soccer when she experiences a torn anterior cruciate ligament. Kate moved across the country to the Southeastern United States to attend school and to play NCAA Division II soccer. Although she has made friends with teammates and classmates, and is familiar with the athletic training staff through their regular interactions and from her coursework, her family and friends with whom she is most comfortable are on the West Coast. To complicate things, her insurance requires her to have the surgery performed in her hometown for it to be covered, which requires significant logistical considerations by all involved. Fortunately, winter break is approaching, and her surgery is scheduled during her trip home for the holidays. Upon her return to campus, she is adherent to her rehabilitation plan and often finds herself doing rehabilitation at the same time as a baseball player who is returning from an ulnar collateral ligament reconstruction surgery (also known as Tommy John surgery). They become "rehab buddies" of sorts, as they find themselves working next to each other day after day and week after week.

INTRODUCTION

Athletic trainers, particularly in the more traditional athletic settings, have the significant advantage of being able to get to know the athletes with whom they work extremely well. Many times, these relationships will not only develop throughout the season but will build from season to season throughout the athletes' sporting careers.

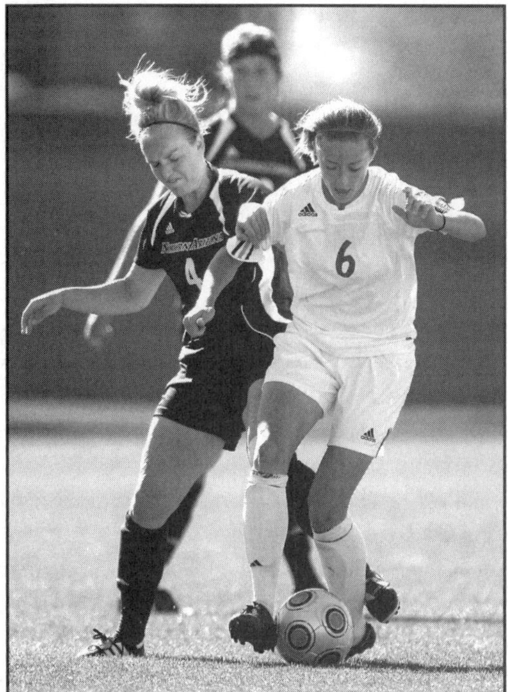

Figure 9-1 | Athlete Insider *(Courtesy of Weber State University Athletics)*

Such relationships may involve not only management of their athletes' health care, but will likely also involve knowing which classes are giving their athletes the biggest problems in any given semester or hearing about recent relationship status changes in their lives. Athletic trainers are in the position to be able to see and get to know their athletes before they become injured. Athletic trainers are able to see athletes perform before the occurrence of injury, through the injury recovery process, and as they are returning to participation. Because of this steadiness and stability, it is no wonder that athletes often feel comfortable turning to their athletic trainers during difficult times.

Social support includes the feeling or sense of being supported by others, the act of supporting others, and social integration. There is a positive relationship between the amount of and satisfaction with social support that one receives and that person's well-being. This is also true with athletes as the recipients of social support. Athletic trainers are in a prime position to offer such support to the athletes with whom they interact. Therefore, this chapter focuses on the use of social support as a coping resource in response to injury, the types of social support commonly seen in the athletic training setting throughout the injury recovery process, and strategies athletic trainers can use to enhance the injury recovery process for their athletes by serving as social support providers.

Social Support as a Coping Resource

Coping is defined as "constantly changing cognitive and behavioral efforts to manage specific external and/or internal demands that are appraised as taxing or exceeding the resources of the person" (Lazarus & Folkman, 1984, p. 141). Because of its dynamic nature, coping is a process that constantly changes throughout one's exposure to a stressor, and addressing the context in which the coping is occurring is essential (Kerr & Miller, 2001). This can be particularly true in working with athletes who are experiencing prolonged rehabilitation from injury. An athlete who has undergone a surgical repair for a labral tear in the shoulder, which limits activity for months, will likely require different coping strategies than an athlete with an acute ankle sprain faced with a week of limited activity. However, this may not always be the case, because responses to injury can be as diverse as the injuries sustained. It is important to understand that, after experiencing an injury, regardless of the severity, athletes will likely use a variety of coping resources and strategies because their thoughts, emotions, and physical demands change throughout the injury recovery process. Just as athletes have been taught physical skills to perform at their best on the field of play, they may need assistance in identifying appropriate and effective coping strategies after injury to enhance and ultimately optimize their recovery. Specifically, the identification and seeking of social support can be one such coping strategy.

Coping resources are identified in the models discussed in Chapters 3 and 4 that address injury risk (stress injury model; Williams & Andersen, 1998) and injury response (integrated model of response to sport injury; Wiese-Bjornstal, Smith, Shaffer, & Morrey, 1998). The stress injury model specifies three coping resources, including general coping behaviors, social support systems, and stress-management and mental skills. In the integrated model of response to sport injury, coping resources and use of social support are viewed as influencing injury occurrence and the emotional and behavioral response to injury. This is consistent with the health and wellness benefits related to being part of a social group as described by Cohen and colleagues (2001). As suggested by these models, social support and social integration may play a role in the risk for injury. In the biopsychosocial model of sport injury rehabilitation (Brewer, Andersen, & Van Raalte, 2002), as discussed in detail in Chapter 8, social support is listed as one of the social/contextual factors that influence both psychological responses and immediate and overall rehabilitation outcomes. These models that describe factors that contribute to injury, injury responses, and rehabilitation outcomes demonstrate the importance of social support as a coping resource throughout the injury process.

However, research that examines the relationship between injury and coping resources, including social support, has resulted in mixed findings. Williams, Tonymon, and Wadsworth (1986) found low levels of coping resources to be a significant predictor of injury in college volleyball players, whereas Blackwell and McCullagh (1990) found injured athletes had higher scores on life stress and competitive anxiety, and lower scores on coping resources than uninjured athletes. A strong relationship was reported between negative life events and injury outcome for those with low social support and low coping resources only (Smith, Smoll, & Schutz, 1990). In addition, coping resources were also found to influence injury frequency and injury severity (Hanson, McCullagh, & Tonymon, 1992). Hardy and Crace (1990) found athletes who reported high levels of social support had a lower incidence of injury, whereas those with low levels of social support experienced more injuries. However, no relationship between level of social support and injury risk was found by Lavallée and Flint (1996).

Shumaker and Brownell (1984) described social support as "an exchange of resources between at least two individuals perceived by the provider or the recipient to be intended to enhance the well-being of the recipient" (p. 73), and it is believed to influence injury risk and rehabilitation through a number of mechanisms. Social support is believed to provide protection or a buffering effect on stressors. This buffering effect is believed to decrease the strength of the stress response, thus decreasing the associated cognitive, emotional, and behavioral responses. Another influence of social support involves its direct effect, or main effect. A third mechanism of influence for social support was presented by Albrecht and Adelman (1987), who suggested social support may provide benefits through the reduction of uncertainty. Supportive communication may reduce "ambiguity, complexity, and unpredictability—sources of uncertainty—and thus provides the support recipient with increased feelings of personal control" (Robbins & Rosenfeld, 2001, p. 279). Regardless of the mechanism, it is important to remember that, for social support to be effective, the support needs of the recipient must coincide with the support the provider is willing and able to provide. Without this match, sometimes referred to as the ***matching hypothesis***, the satisfaction with and effects of social support will likely be impaired.

Nixon (1994) examined the role of what he termed the "sportsnet" (specifically coaches, teammates, and sports medicine personnel) in athletes' responses to injury. Nixon found approximately two thirds of athletes reported having avoided coaches or attempted to hide their pain and injuries from their coaches when they were hurt. He also found that nearly half of the athletes reported feeling pressure from their coaches to play hurt. Interestingly, Nixon indicated the greatest determinant in whether an athlete would report injury to an athletic trainer was found to be the athletic trainer's expression of sympathy or caring toward the athlete reporting the injury. Based on this finding, athletic trainers should take care to establish positive ***rapport*** with athletes before injury, with the aim of being approachable to athletes if they become injured and enhancing their ***help-seeking*** behaviors.

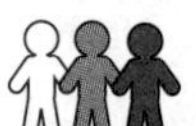

SPECIAL CONSIDERATIONS

Athletes with high levels of stress and athletes with low levels of stress have been found to be similar with respect to their social support networks (Rosenfeld, Richman, & Hardy, 1989). Therefore, athletic trainers should help athletes identify their social support needs, identify individuals within their social support network who can meet these identified needs, and then develop strategies for seeking the needed social support.

Help-Seeking Tendencies and Social Support

Help-seeking involves the willingness of an individual to ask for assistance from identified resources, such as those with whom athletes feel comfortable seeking help and advice. In the athletic training context, help-seeking may involve an athlete's willingness to go to an athletic trainer with a particular injury for assistance in identifying the nature and severity of the injury, but it may also involve seeking advice or just an empathetic ear for emotional issues he or she may be experiencing. Within the context of sport, it may be easier for athletes to seek assistance for physical pain associated with injury than it may be to seek assistance for the cognitive and emotional issues related to that same injury. Because of their accessibility and rapport with the athlete, athletic trainers are in the prime position to be able to assist athletes with both their physical and their psychological issues related to injury. One way athletic trainers can provide this assistance is by intentionally offering social support.

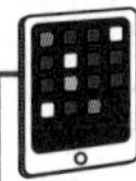

VIRTUAL FIELD TRIP

The Association for Applied Sport Psychology website offers resources related to sport injury and rehabilitation. Go to http://davisplus.fadavis.com for a link to access the article "With a Little Help from My Friends: Using Your Social Support Network When Dealing With Injury."

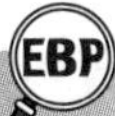

EVIDENCE-BASED PRACTICE

McCrea, M., Hammeke, T., Olsen, G., Leo, P., & Guskiewicz, K. (2004). Unreported concussion in high school football players: Implications for prevention. *Clinical Journal of Sport Medicine, 4*(1), 13–16.

Description of the Study

This retrospective study was conducted to examine the frequency of unreported concussion and to estimate the overall rate of concussion in high school football players. Participants (n = 1532) for this study were recruited from 20 high schools in the upper Midwest region of the United States. All participants completed a questionnaire on history and frequency of previous concussion at the time they agreed to participate in the study at the beginning of the football season. At the completion of the football season, players completed a questionnaire inquiring whether they had experienced a concussion during the current football season based on a concussion definition provided in the questionnaire. For this study, concussion was defined as a "blow to the head followed by a variety of symptoms that may include any of the following: headache, dizziness, loss of balance, blurred vision, 'seeing stars', feeling in a fog or slowed down, memory problems, poor concentration, nausea, or throwing up. Getting 'knocked out' or being unconscious does *not* always occur with a concussion" (p. 14). In addition, participants were asked whether they had reported their injury, to whom it was reported, and reasons they did not report a concussion.

Results of the Study

At the completion of the football season, 229 participants (15.3%) reported having experienced a concussion based on the provided definition during the current football season. Of the participants who reported experiencing a concussion, only 47.3% indicated they reported the concussion to appropriate personnel. Most often, those who reported concussions indicated they advised the athletic trainer providing coverage of the incident (76.7%). Participants indicated with less frequency reporting the concussion to coaching staff (38.8%), parents (35.9%), or teammates (27.2%). For those who indicated they did not report the concussion, most participants (66.4%) revealed they did not report the concussion because they did not believe it was serious enough to seek

Continued

medical attention. Additional reasons for not reporting the concussion were the desire to not be withheld from participation (41%) and a lack of knowledge about the signs of concussion (36.1%). Twenty-two percent of participants indicated they did not report the concussion because they did not want to let down their teammates.

Implications for Athletic Training Practice

The findings of this study support the need for education regarding concussion for those involved in sport at all levels of play. Although the study addressed high school football, it is likely the underreporting of concussion occurs at all levels and in all activities. This underreporting places participants at significant risk for potentially catastrophic and long-term disability. The clear lack of understanding about the signs and symptoms of concussion, and belief the signs and symptoms being experienced were not severe enough to seek medical attention are major concerns for athletic training professionals. Although athletic trainers commonly witness the mechanism of injury to increase suspicion of concussion, it is impossible to witness all potential traumas. This makes it critical for the overall health care of the athletes that they are able to understand the nature of concussion and be willing to seek medical assistance when they are experiencing key signs and symptoms. From this study, it is clear that athletes do not engage in help-seeking behaviors related to concussions and need to be better educated about the signs and symptoms of a concussion, and the importance of their responsibility to report accompanying signs and symptoms to appropriate personnel. It is also important to educate athletes about the potentially significant negative consequences of participating in sport with concussion-like symptoms (e.g., second-impact syndrome). It is somewhat reassuring that the majority of participants who reported injury told their athletic trainers about it. Coaches were second to athletic trainers as the ones to whom participants reported their concussions, making it equally important for coaches to be educated about the signs and symptoms of the condition, negative consequences of participating with a concussion, and the expected procedure in reporting concussion-like symptoms to medical personnel.

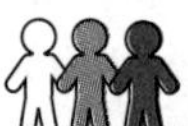

SPECIAL CONSIDERATIONS

Gender differences have been found in the use of coping strategies and social support. In general, Carver, Scheier, and Weintraub (1989) and Ptacek, Smith, and Zanas (1992) found females to be more likely to seek social support and use more emotion-focused coping than males. Specific to sport, Crocker and Graham (1995) found that females reported higher levels of seeking social support for emotional issues than males. These gender differences may be because of the different ways in which the types and levels of stress are perceived by the genders, but they may also be associated with socialization with the gender-role stereotypes and expectations learned by each gender. As athletes reach higher levels of performance, it may be likely to see more similarities than differences between the genders. Greater differences in support-seeking tendencies may be found within teams than necessarily compared by gender. To best serve their athletes, it is important for athletic trainers to make an attempt to understand the various issues that may be influencing each athlete's emotional, cognitive, and behavioral responses, regardless of gender.

TYPES OF SOCIAL SUPPORT

Social support may come from a variety of people who surround the athlete and can serve as providers. Social support sources include:

- Teammates
- Coaches
- Family
- Friends
- Significant others
- Sports medicine team (athletic trainer, physician, nutritionist, sport psychology consultant, etc.)

Of the potential sources of social support available, as already mentioned, athletic trainers are in a unique position to provide such support because of the amount of time they will spend with the athlete during their athletics involvement and rehabilitation process, and athletic trainers may become trusted confidants because of the quantity and quality of interactions.

Richman, Rosenfeld, and Hardy (1993) identified eight categories of social support (see Table 9-1 for examples of types of social support). These include:

- Listening support
- Emotional support
- Emotional challenge
- Reality confirmation
- Task appreciation
- Task challenge
- Tangible assistance
- Personal assistance

Taking these eight types of social support into account, athletic trainers are in a key position to provide support. Examples in each of these eight areas of social support that

TABLE 9-1 **Types of Social Support**

Type of Social Support	Description
Listening support	Involves the perception by the athlete that the other person is listening without giving advice or being judgmental
Emotional support	Involves the perception by the athlete that another person is providing comfort and caring, and indicating that he or she is on the athlete's side
Emotional challenge	Involves the perception by the athlete that another person is challenging him or her to evaluate his or her attitudes, values, and feelings
Reality confirmation	Involves the perception by the athlete that another person, who is similar to the athlete and who sees things the same way the athlete does, is helping to confirm the athlete's perspective on the world
Task appreciation	Involves the perception by the athlete that another person is acknowledging the athlete's efforts and is expressing appreciation for the work he or she does
Task challenge	Involves the perception by the athlete that another person is challenging the athlete's way of thinking about a task or an activity to stretch, motivate, and lead the athlete to greater creativity, excitement, and involvement
Tangible assistance	Involves the perception by the athlete that another person is providing him or her with financial assistance, products, and/or gifts
Personal assistance	Involves the perception by the athlete that another person is providing services or help, such as running an errand or driving the athlete somewhere

From Richman, J. M., Rosenfeld, L. B., & Hardy, C. J. (1993). The social support survey: A validation study of a clinical measure of the social support process. Research on Social Work Practice, *3(3), 288–311.*

can be provided by the athletic trainer are described in Table 9-2.

The research supports the role of the athletic trainer as a key social support provider. Clement and Shannon (2011) found athletes were significantly more satisfied with the social support provided by athletic trainers and indicated the support received from athletic trainers was "more satisfying, more available, and contributed more to their overall well-being" (p. 464). (See the Evidence-Based Practice special feature later in this chapter for more details on this study.) In addition, researchers have found athletes' perceived social support from athletic trainers increased following injury as athletes reported relying on athletic trainers more for social support after injury and were also more satisfied with their postinjury social support from athletic trainers (Yang, Peek-Asa, Lowe, Heiden, & Foster, 2010). (See the Evidence-Based Practice special feature in this chapter for more details on this study.)

During rehabilitation, injured athletes have reported that they perceive their athletic trainers' social support, specifically listening, task appreciation, task challenge, and emotional challenge, as more important to them than support from their coaches (Robbins & Rosenfeld, 2001). Thus, as athletic trainers are likely to have a better understanding of the injury recovery process, it may be beneficial for them to play a mediating role between athletes and coaches, including educating coaches about the psychosocial effects of injury (Robbins & Rosenfeld, 2001).

One specific type of social support, tangible assistance, which involves providing money or gifts, is obviously not feasible for an athletic trainer. However, it has been reported that perceived tangible assistance, such as providing a brace or support for the injury or scheduling a physician's office visit, significantly influenced the athlete's view of treatment efficacy (Bone & Frye, 2006). It is important for the athletic trainer to consider the stage of recovery and individual needs of the athlete to provide the appropriate and necessary type and amount of support.

TABLE 9-2 Examples of Social Support Athletic Trainers Can Provide

Type of Social Support	Athletic Trainer's Demonstration
Listening support	Athletic trainer actively listens to the athlete without giving advice or being judgmental.
Emotional support	Athletic trainer comforts the athlete and indicates he or she is on the athlete's side and cares about the athlete.
Emotional challenge	Athletic trainer challenges the athlete to evaluate his or her attitudes, values, and feelings.
Reality confirmation	Athletic trainer who is similar to the athlete, or sees things the way the athlete does, helps to confirm the athlete's perceptions about and perspectives on the world, and helps the athlete keep things in focus.
Task appreciation	Athletic trainer acknowledges the athlete's efforts and expresses appreciation for the work the athlete has done.
Task challenge	Athletic trainer challenges the athlete's way of thinking about his or her activity to stretch, motivate, and lead the athlete to greater creativity, excitement, and involvement in that activity.
Tangible assistance	Athletic trainer provides the athlete with products or equipment.
Personal assistance	Athletic trainer provides the athlete with services or help.

From Richman, J. M., Rosenfeld, L. B., & Hardy, C. J. (1993). The social support survey: A validation study of a clinical measure of the social support process. Research on Social Work Practice, *3(3), 288–311.*

INTEGRATING SOCIAL SUPPORT WHEN WORKING WITH INJURED ATHLETES

Being aware of the dynamic and individualized psychological response to injury is important in providing appropriate support. Just as athletes perform physical training and conditioning for their bodies in preparation for sport participation, it is important for these athletes to be equally prepared to handle the psychological, emotional, and social issues that may arise during participation in sport. Teaching and providing participants with various, and most importantly appropriate, coping strategies may help to not only prevent some injuries from occurring, but may also be beneficial during the injury recovery process. Determining a strong social support network is just one of the coping strategies that should be incorporated before one actually needs the support. Athletes who develop strong relationships with a variety of people to meet their ever-changing needs and to provide various forms of support may help to buffer whatever stress responses those athletes experience should an injury occur.

It is important for athletic trainers to work with other members of the sports medicine staff to educate athletes about their injuries and about the anticipated injury recovery process. This education may also be necessary with others in athletes' social support networks, such as parents, friends, significant others, teammates, and coaches. Figure 9-2 describes individuals who are part of athletes' social support networks. Rosenfeld et al (1989) found teammates and coaches to be the primary sources of technical-type social support, but they were not sought out for emotional-type social support. Rather, emotional support was sought from friends and family, who may not be as knowledgeable about athletic injuries and who may actually overprotect the athletes, produce anxiety about the severity of the injury, or potentially avoid any discussions about the injury process itself because of lack of knowledge (Petitpas, 1999).

Athletic trainers should become familiar with the various types of support that may be warranted in given situations and then take steps to either provide that support

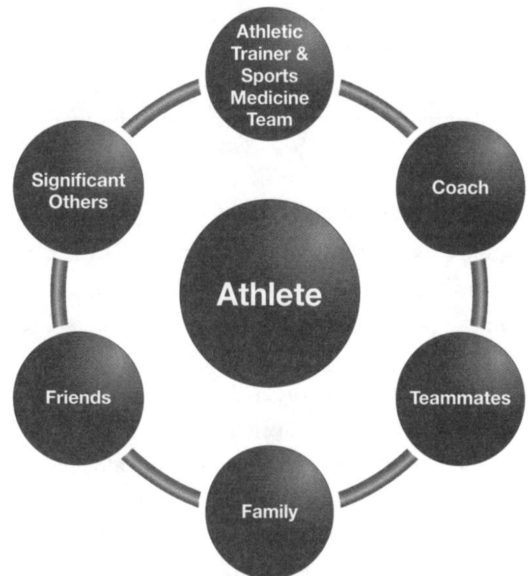

Figure 9-2 | An athlete's social support network.

themselves or to assist athletes in identifying other sources for the desired support. Barefield and McCallister (1997) found athletes expressed expectations to receive listening support and task appreciation from athletic trainers and athletic training students, and subsequently reported receiving mostly these types of support. In contrast, athletes reported receiving tangible and personal assistance least often, although also least expecting to receive these types of support from staff and athletic training students. Athletic trainers should make an effort to use ***active listening*** techniques, as discussed in Chapter 5, when interacting with athletes. Overall, it is important for athletic trainers to create a positive, nonthreatening environment where athletes feel comfortable seeking various forms of support.

SOCIAL SUPPORT NEEDS

It is important to recognize that there are multiple dimensions to social support and that social support is dynamic; therefore, an athlete's social support needs may change on injury, throughout the rehabilitation process, and as return to participation progresses. As discussed throughout this chapter, athletic trainers and other members of the sports medicine team, coaches, teammates, family, friends, and significant others may all serve as social support providers for athletes. But what are athletes' needs when it comes to the type, amount, and timing of social support?

Identifying Social Support Needs

An athlete's social support network includes the athletic trainer and members of the sports medicine team, coaches, teammates, family, friends, and significant others. Each of these social support providers can contribute positively, and negatively, to injury risk, response, rehabilitation, and return to participation following injury.

Social support is multidimensional, and athletes' social support needs may vary based on their personal characteristics (e.g., age, gender, psychological factors) and situational characteristics (e.g., time of season, rehabilitation environment). Based on the matching hypothesis, it is important for athletic trainers to identify and match the social support needs of the athletes with whom they interact. Because social support needs are dynamic, the demands of a prolonged rehabilitation and/or recovery may cause the athlete to have a variety of social support needs. One way to identify an athlete's social support needs at the beginning of and throughout rehabilitation is with a formal inventory measure. Examples of measures are provided in the Measuring Social Support section later in this chapter. By identifying the social support needs of the athlete, the athletic trainer can work to best match these needs and also help the athlete identify people who can help meet those needs.

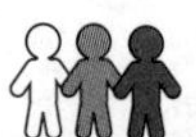

SPECIAL CONSIDERATIONS

Research shows that severity of injury and an athlete's social support needs are related. Bone and Fry (2006) found a significant relationship between perceived social support and beliefs about effectiveness of rehabilitation in only those with severe injuries. Athletes who experienced more severe injuries indicated they felt the athletic trainer was "on their side and cared for them," likely resulting from the increased time and interaction involved. However, no significant relationship was found for those experiencing less severe injuries. In addition, listening support was reported to be the most important type of social support received by athletes across injury severities (Bone & Fry, 2006).

As previously mentioned, in addition to athletic trainers, athletes' teammates, coaches, family, friends, and significant others can be social support providers. When comparing teammates, coaches, and athletic trainers, athletes have reported they were most satisfied with the social support received from their athletic trainers and that social support was most available from their athletic trainers (Clement & Shannon, 2011). Although this demonstrates the important role athletic trainers play in supporting injured athletes, many types of social support do not require special expertise. Athletic trainers can encourage athletes' teammates, coaches, family, and significant others to be supportive as well. These individuals may provide different types of support to better meet the overall social support needs of the athlete.

Athletes' satisfaction with the available social support, including the type of social support and the amount and timing of that support, is of prime importance. Athletic trainers should keep in mind that the inconsistent provision of social support may negatively affect athletes' well-being (Corbillon, Crossman, & Jamieson, 2008). Different types of social support in different amounts may be optimal throughout the injury and rehabilitation process. Athletic trainers should keep the type, amount, and timing of social support in mind when working with athletes (see Fig. 9-3).

Measuring Social Support

A general measure of social support that can be used in the athletic training setting is the Social Support Behaviors Survey–Clinical Form, more commonly known as the Social Support Survey (SSS; Richman et al, 1993). This measure contains eight subscales: listening support, task appreciation, task challenge, emotional support,

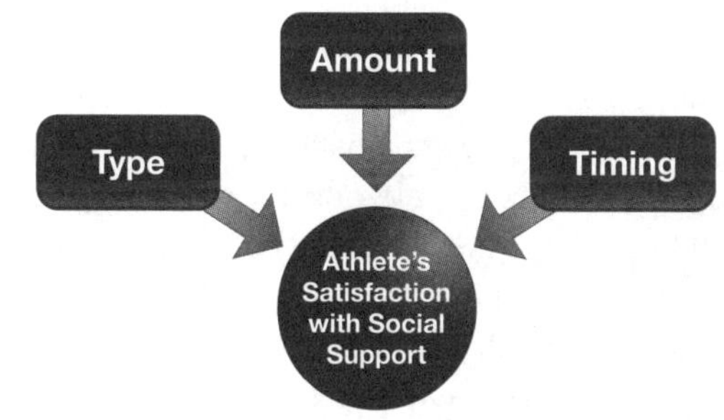

Figure 9-3 | Social support satisfaction.

emotional challenge, reality confirmation, tangible assistance, and personal assistance. This measure provides athletes with a definition of each type of social support and asks participants to identify individuals who provide that specific type of social support. For example, regarding listening support, the survey asks, "Write the initials of all the individuals who provide you with listening support. If no one provides you with this support, please indicate 'no one.' After each person, indicate the relationship you have with her or him (for example, friend, co-worker, spouse, parent, brother, or sister)" (p. 306). For each of the eight types of social support, the measure then asks respondents to rate their satisfaction with the quality of this support, how difficult it would be to obtain more of this type of social support, and the importance of this type of social support.

Athletic trainers could use the SSS as a tool to help identify an athlete's social support needs. This measure takes approximately 20 minutes to complete and could be filled out by the athlete in the early stages of rehabilitation during a heating or icing session, for example. Further, this measure could be used as a basis for a discussion between athletes and their athletic trainers to help determine from whom within their social support network they can receive specific types of social support. For example, during this discussion, a social support identification worksheet can be completed (see Fig. 9-5 later in this chapter).

A population-specific measure of social support is the Social Support Inventory for Injured Athletes (SSIIA; Mitchell, Rees, Evans, & Hardy, 2005). The SSIIA is a 16-item self-report inventory that assesses perceived social support in four major areas: emotional (such as providing moral support or listening), esteem (such as reassurance and motivation), tangible (such as financial help and transportation), and information (such as decision making and advice). For each of the 16 items, the athlete is asked, "To what extent do you have someone who provides [type of support]," and the athlete rates the item from 1 (not at all) to 5 (a lot) on a Likert-type scale.

Athletic trainers could use the SSIIA in a similar fashion described in the use of the SSS. The advantages of using the SSIIA rather than the SSS is that the SSIIA was specifically designed to capture the social support needs of athletes who are injured, and it takes only about 5 minutes to complete.

Social Support Needs Before Injury

Sport injury risk has been hypothesized to be positively related to stress (including life stress, daily hassles, and previous injury history; Williams & Andersen, 1998) and negatively related to available coping resources. Therefore, social support as a means to buffer stress by way of modifying an athlete's cognitive appraisal of the stress, as well as serving as a coping resource, may be important in reducing injury risk (Udry, Gould, Bridges, & Tuffey, 1997).

Being socially connected may play a role in reducing the risk for injury by serving as a buffer from stress. Current social support research has shown us that the quality rather than the quantity of relationships is related to the athlete's satisfaction with social support, and thus is important to health and well-being. Therefore, athletes who are more socially integrated and satisfied with the social support they are receiving may be better equipped to deal with stressors.

Social Support Needs After Injury

Athletes' beliefs regarding rehabilitation—including their susceptibility to future injury, treatment efficacy, ***self-efficacy***, value of recovery, and severity of injury—are influenced by their perceptions of the social support they receive from their athletic trainer (Bone & Fry, 2006). In addition, athletes who engage in longer rehabilitation may form stronger relationships with their athletic trainer, and thus social support may have a greater influence on their recovery.

As previously discussed, social support can serve a protective role by buffering rehabilitation-related stressors, and it can also serve a direct role in improving rehabilitation (Mitchell, Wadey, Neil, & Hanton, 2007). Social support may influence an athlete's response to injury by buffering the associated stress or by serving directly as a coping resource. During postinjury, when an athlete may have much fear of the unknown and concerns about the future, the athletic trainer can serve as an emotional challenge. As the athlete demonstrates emotions such as anger or frustration, the athletic trainer can provide listening support and emotional support. As perceived stressors change throughout the rehabilitation process, athletes' social support needs, their seeking of support, and their satisfaction with support may also change. This dynamic process is verified in the research literature.

Johnston and Carroll (2000) found that the perceived *amount* of support did not change across the rehabilitation process; however, significant decreases were seen for seeking support. In addition, satisfaction was significantly lower at the beginning of the rehabilitation process than in the middle or at the end. The researchers also found that women were significantly more satisfied with emotional and practical support at the beginning of rehabilitation and with practical support at the end of rehabilitation than their male counterparts. This demonstrates the premise of the dynamic nature of preferred and received social support throughout the rehabilitation process. Henert (2001) found that male athletes recovering from minor-to-moderate injuries reported increased focus on their emotional response immediately following injury but decreased focus as they progressed through the rehabilitation process, whereas female athletes were found to be more consistent in their emotion-focused coping throughout the rehabilitation process. Despite the differences, both males and females stated that having emotional support available to them was very important throughout the rehabilitation process.

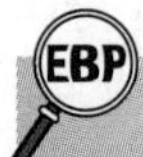

EVIDENCE-BASED PRACTICE

Yang, J., Peek-Asa, C., Lowe, J. B., Heiden, E., & Foster, D. T. (2010). Social support patterns of collegiate athletes before and after injury. *Journal of Athletic Training, 45*(4), 372–379.

Description of the Study

This prospective observational study examined the preinjury and postinjury social support patterns among male and female collegiate athletes. The study involved 256 athletes who participated in NCAA Division I–sponsored sports at a Big Ten Conference institution. Participants represented 13 sports, including baseball, women's basketball, women's cross-country, football, men's and women's golf, women's field hockey, men's gymnastics, women's rowing, men's tennis, women's track, coed spirit squad, and wrestling. A repeated-measure design was used in this study. Initial contact was made with prospective participants at the beginning of their respective sport seasons, at which time baseline data were collected on those athletes who chose to participate, including demographic characteristics, sports experience, history of injury, sources of social support, and satisfaction with social support. Social support was measured using the modified six-item Social Support Questionnaire, which addressed both quantity of and satisfaction with social support. Injury incidence for participants in this study was tracked using an electronic injury surveillance system, which was maintained by team athletic trainers. Participants (n = 42) experiencing injuries were contacted 3 months after their injury onset, at which time data addressing social support during the injury recovery period were collected.

Results of the Study

Descriptive statistics were calculated for baseline data, including average number of social support sources and satisfaction with social support based on gender. Statistical analyses were performed to examine differences in social support sources and satisfaction with social support. Statistical analyses were also performed to examine changes in social support sources and satisfaction before and after injury for those who experienced injuries during the period of study. In all, baseline data were collected on 256 participants (male = 167; female = 89) representing 13 sports. Results indicated family (96%) and friends (93%) were the primary sources of social support for participants. Satisfaction with social support provided from family was found to be 5.7 of 6 (93%) and 5.4 of 6 (90%) for social support from friends. Researchers also found female participants relied more on friends for social support than their male counterparts, but they reported higher levels of satisfaction from all social support sources, except from coaches. Male participants were found to rely on coaches, athletic trainers, physicians, and counselors more for social support than did female participants. More than half of the participants (53.1%) reported having experienced at least one athletic injury in the previous 12 months. With regard to changes in sources of social support and satisfaction with social support before and after injury, participants who had experienced injury during this study (n = 42) reported greater reliance on coaches, athletic trainers, and physicians after being injured than at their baseline measurements. In addition, participants also reported higher postinjury satisfaction with social support from friends, coaches, athletic trainers, and physicians. Male and female participants indicated greater reliance on athletic trainers for social support after injury and reported greater satisfaction with this support following injury as compared with baseline. Female participants reported greater satisfaction with social support provided by friends, coaches, and physicians following injury, whereas male participants reported greater satisfaction with the social support received from physicians following injury but decreased satisfaction with support from their families.

Implications for Athletic Training Practice

Consistent with previous research that examined social support, results from this study suggest it is important to consider not only the perceived sources or quantity of social support, but also athletes' satisfaction with the social support received. The study examined and found athletes likely experience changes in both their perceived sources of social support and their satisfaction with social support during the injury recovery process. More participants reported receiving social support from their athletic trainers following injury and also reported increased satisfaction with the social support received from athletic trainers. As has been discussed throughout this chapter, it is important for athletic trainers to develop relationships with their athletes based on trust so athletes feel comfortable not only reporting injuries to their athletic trainers, but also using them as sources of social support both before and, possibly most importantly, after injuries. For social support to be effective and for athletes to be satisfied with the social support they receive, the desired type of social support must match the social support provided. It is important for athletic trainers to be aware of how their athletes are responding and to be willing to be flexible with the types of support needed throughout the injury-management and recovery process.

SPECIAL CONSIDERATIONS

Social support has been found to serve as a positive influence on psychological responses to sport injury. However, with high-performance individuals (participating in sport at the national or international levels), high levels of social support have been found to have main effects on negative psychological responses (such as

Continued

devastation and dispiritedness, whereas with low-performance individuals (participating at the collegiate or recreational levels), such levels of support acted as a buffer against stress (Rees, Mitchell, Evans, & Hardy, 2010). Although social support may be operating under different conditions based on individual athlete differences, social support should be viewed by athletic trainers as important to the physical and psychological well-being of both recreational and elite-level athletes.

Generally, studies have found that social support provided to athletes by their coaches is lacking during rehabilitation. Specifically, during rehabilitation, injured athletes have reported that task challenge support that was provided by their coaches made a significantly greater contribution to their well-being than that provided by their teammates. Reality confirmation support and emotional support were provided significantly more by teammates than by coaches. It has also been reported that nonstarters, athletes with more experience, and athletes who sustained more injuries reported receiving less social support (Corbillon et al, 2008; Robbins & Rosenfeld, 2001). As noted by Cohen and colleagues (2001), being socially connected and part of a group positively contributes to health and well-being. In the case of injured athletes, disconnection from their team (including teammates, coaches, and support staff) may be the source of distress during their injury recovery and rehabilitation process.

Postinjury athletes may also receive the news that they will need surgery for their injury. During this time, athletes may be in disbelief or denial. Athletic trainers can provide informational support by educating athletes on the process of surgery and associated rehabilitation; this may decrease their worry and anxiety. Tangible support in the form of goal setting may also be beneficial. For athletes who are facing season-ending or career-ending injuries, emotional support may be of prime importance as feelings of anger, sadness, frustration, loss, and self-pity may be salient (Udry, Gould, Bridges, & Beck, 1997). As discussed in Chapter 6, referral may be warranted for athletes who are experiencing reactions that are interfering with normal functioning.

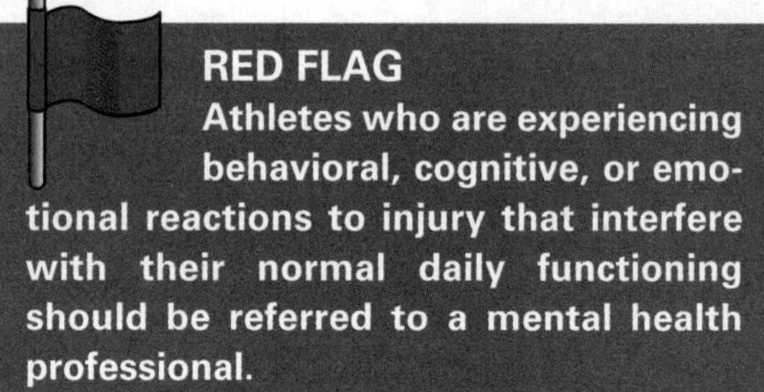
RED FLAG
Athletes who are experiencing behavioral, cognitive, or emotional reactions to injury that interfere with their normal daily functioning should be referred to a mental health professional.

Athletes have noted that their coach may play a negative role when dealing with injury. As one athlete noted, "He [coach] never called me ... nothing. So I sort of got this idea that he didn't care, that he was of the school of thought that if you were injured, it was your problem. . . ." (Udry, Gould, Bridges, & Tuffey, 1997, p. 385). Athletes may perceive that, now that they are injured, their coach no longer values them. The athletic trainer might talk with the coach to recommend positive interactions with the athlete, such as staying in touch and emotionally connected with the athlete, being involved in the rehabilitation process, and providing encouragement and support.

Social factors, including social support, are known to influence athletes' pain and injury experiences (Nixon, 1994). ***Sport ethic*** and an expectation of toughness encourage athletes to play through pain and injury, and may also influence injury reporting and subsequent treatment (Nixon, 1994). (See Chapter 7 for a discussion of pain and reporting of pain.) Therefore, appropriate social support from the athletic trainer, as well as from the athletes' social support network, is important to ensure a trusting relationship, so the athlete feels comfortable reporting pain and injury. Athletes have reported they are more likely to talk to athletic trainers and coaches who express sympathy and caring toward them (Nixon, 1994). Therefore, athletic trainers should build a rapport based on trust with the athletes with whom they work and encourage coaches to do the same.

Early Rehabilitation

During the early phases of rehabilitation, when pain and swelling may be at their peak, athletes' stress may also be at peak levels. Often, athletes cope with stress by engaging in physical activity; if activity is limited, athletes may struggle with stress management. In these cases, the athletic trainer can provide task challenge and suggest alternate methods of stress management. Athletes may also feel isolated from their teammates, and athletic trainers can provide emotional support during this time. Athletic trainers can also provide tangible support in the form of crutches, wraps, and ice packs. In addition, athletes may feel like their injury and rehabilitation are out of their control. In such cases, athletic trainers can assist by providing emotional challenge and task challenge in helping athletes identify areas in which they are in control, including their thoughts and behaviors.

Also during this time, athletes are faced with the transition from performing on the playing field to performing in the rehabilitation setting. This transition may be more difficult for athletes who highly identify themselves as athletes. Corbillon and colleagues (2008) reported that athletes may desire more emotional support immediately after being injured. In these cases, athletic trainers can provide emotional and listening support by allowing athletes to vent their feelings, as well as task support in the form of goal setting. Athletic trainers can also provide emotional challenge to assist with reframing the perceived obstacles in rehabilitation.

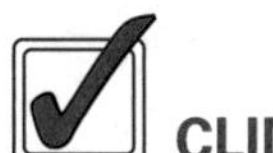

CLINICAL TIP

Adjusting an athlete's rehabilitation appointment time to better accommodate his or her schedule is an example of personal assistance support. Although this individual appointment approach may not be realistic in some traditional athletic training environments, efforts should be made to provide ***athlete-centered care***.

Depending on the type and severity of injury, in the early stages of the injury and rehabilitation process, athletes will likely need personal assistance support in the form of help with tasks of daily living (e.g., providing assistance in the cafeteria, providing transportation to and from classes), as well as personal assistance support specifically related to their injury, such as transportation to and from medical appointments. Family, friends, and teammates may be in a good position to assist athletes with this type of support; the athletic trainer can discuss this with them and help them identify those within their social support network who may provide this support. Also, in the early stages of injury and rehabilitation, it is important for the social support network to provide emotional support; family and teammates may be in a good position to provide this type of support (Udry, Gould, Bridges, & Tuffey, 1997).

In addition, with limited function, athletes may be bored by their situation; in these cases, it may be especially important for the athletic trainer to provide task appreciation and task challenge support, such as goal setting to keep the athlete motivated and enhance rehabilitation adherence. Task support is particularly important during this early phase to enhance motivation, and thus rehabilitation adherence.

Midrehabilitation

During both midrehabilitation and late rehabilitation, athletic trainers may allow athletes to work more independently, because they have learned the appropriate rehabilitation exercises. A word of caution should be noted here, however, because individuals in the rehabilitation environment, including the athletic trainer or rehabilitation partner, serve as important social support providers for the rehabilitating athlete. Although athletes may desire to work independently, they may also feel more isolated and may have a decline in motivation.

Especially for long rehabilitations and in cases where the athlete may not be able to see the end in sight, it is important for the athletic trainer to provide task support in the form of goal setting; this is crucial for the athlete's maintenance of rehabilitation adherence. As Evans, Hardy, and Fleming (2000) suggest, emotional support may be most important to athletes who have a long rehabilitation, have experienced setbacks with rehabilitation, or have life stress weighing on them.

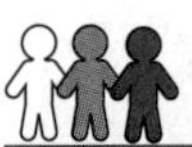

SPECIAL CONSIDERATIONS

During rehabilitation, gender differences have been reported with athletes' perceptions of social support, with females reporting significantly higher on the emotion subscale (with items such as providing moral support and listening) and the esteem subscale (with items such as reassurance and motivation; Mitchell et al., 2007). Therefore, athletic trainers should be aware that males and females seek different types of support, and thus may cope differently with injury.

Late Rehabilitation and Return to Participation

As rehabilitation benchmarks are either reached or not reached, the athlete's goals may need to shift. If an athlete has not reached the desired outcomes, it is important for athletic trainers to provide listening support as the athlete talks about his or her situation, emotional support as the athlete shares feelings and frustrations, emotional challenge when exploring the obstacles that may be facing the athlete, and task support that includes goal setting to help the athlete refocus and stay motivated to complete rehabilitation (Evans et al, 2000). Particularly with rehabilitation setbacks, task support may be used to enhance self-efficacy.

CLINICAL TIP

Coaches may be of particular importance during later rehabilitation and return to participation. Athletic trainers can encourage coaches to provide social support to their athletes during these times.

PSYCHOSOCIAL STRATEGIES

Social support is one of the psychosocial strategies that athletic trainers can use when working with both injured and noninjured athletes. In addition, athletic trainers should encourage those around athletes to provide support. Coaches, teammates, family, significant others, and other members of the sports medicine team, including physicians and sport psychology consultants, should be part of the social support network.

Based on Cohen and colleagues' (2001) intervention model, interventions should be targeted at two areas: increasing the athlete's perception of social support and increasing the availability of social support. Athletic trainers should take into account the athletic training environment and how this environment contributes to athletes' perceptions and to the availability of social support. Consistent with Gottlieb (2000), social support interventions should take several factors into consideration, including the characteristics of the athlete (e.g., coping style, beliefs and attitudes about help-seeking, social support needs) and characteristics of the support (e.g., scope, duration, dosage). As such, this section provides an overview for the athletic trainer to use general counseling skills, to educate the athlete on the importance of receiving social support and identifying social support needs and sources, and to facilitate rehabilitation partners and support groups.

General Counseling Skills

Social support is considered a foundational counseling skill. The rapport built between the athlete and athletic trainer serves as the basis for a trusting relationship. The use of active listening, demonstrations of ***empathy***, and a nonjudgmental demeanor by the athletic trainer are important ways to provide social support to the athlete. Chapter 5 provides detailed information regarding communication strategies between the athletic trainer and the athlete.

Education

Because athletic trainers are viewed as having expertise related to athletic injury, the athlete may particularly rely on them for informational support. Athletic trainers must not assume that athletes understand their injury and rehabilitation process. Athletic trainers may make the mistake of neglecting to fully educate the athlete and assume that the athlete understands the situation; therefore, care should be taken to meet athletes at their level of understanding. As discussed in Chapter 5, injury education is of prime importance to reduce the athlete's uncertainty related to the injury and rehabilitation process, and to ultimately boost the athlete's ownership of and motivation toward rehabilitation (Fig. 9-4).

In addition to educating the athlete on the injury and rehabilitation process, the athletic trainer can teach athletes about the importance of their social support networks. As discussed earlier in the chapter, using a social support identification worksheet, such as shown in Figure 9-5, athletes can identify individuals who can provide them with specific types of support. This worksheet can serve as the basis for implementing psychosocial strategies that can assist athletes in developing their social support networks to meet their desired social support needs. This worksheet may also be used in conjunction with one of the social support measures, such as the SSS (Richman et al, 1993) or the SSIIA (Mitchell et al, 2005), previously described in the Measuring Social Support section.

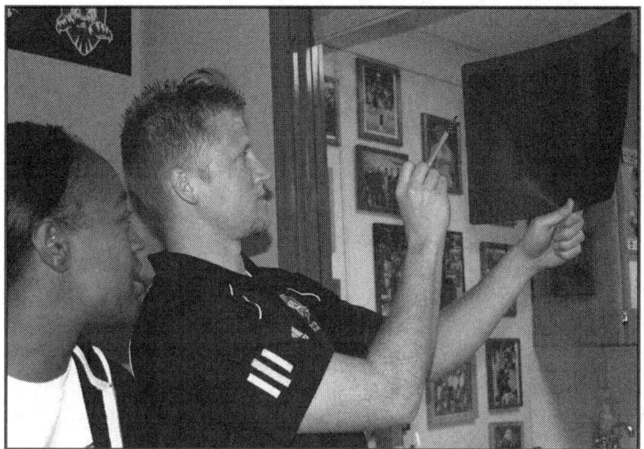

Figure 9-4 | Providing education as a means of social support.

Who are your support providers?

Tangible Support (such as financial and personal assistance)	
Informational Support (such as information about your injury, rehabilitation, and your playing status)	
Emotional Support (such as listening and showing care)	

Figure 9-5 | Social Support Identification Worksheet.

As rehabilitation progresses and an athlete's social support needs change, a social support identification worksheet and social support surveys could be revisited during the later stages of rehabilitation and return to participation.

Rehabilitation Partners and Support Groups

Rehabilitation partners and support groups are widely used in medical settings (e.g., persons with cancer, multiple sclerosis, heart disease, diabetes). These sources of social support can also be valuable in athletic training settings, particularly during rehabilitation when existing social ties may be compromised.

Rehabilitation partners (also referred to as rehab mentors, rehab buddies, etc.) can be facilitated by the athletic trainer. The rapport that can be built between people can enhance the perceived availability of social support to the injured athlete. Partners may include athletes who are similar in nature (e.g., at similar stages in rehabilitation, experiencing similar injuries) or who are in more of a mentor–mentee role, such as an athlete who is at a later stage in rehabilitation or has successfully returned to participation. In addition, depending on the setup of the athletic training program, beginning athletic training students may serve a key role by partnering with athletes who are undergoing rehabilitation. This can serve the dual purpose of providing social support to the athlete and providing the athletic training student with practical ways to offer social support.

Support groups may also be a good resource for providing social support for athletes during rehabilitation. As an example, Clement, Shannon, and Connole (2011) describe performance enhancement groups for use with injured athletes specifically as a means of providing social support. They suggest that groups be no larger than 10 members because an increase in numbers decreases group cohesion. As noted by Clement et al (2011), group composition, absences, and adherence may be issues with support groups. In addition, they advocate cofacilitation of the group by an athletic trainer and an individual competent in sports psychology. Although a sports psychology consultant may not be available at all settings, an institution's counseling center may be able to assist in this support group.

RED FLAG

A word of caution here for both rehabilitation partners and support groups: social comparison has been noted as a source of stress for many athletes. Although social comparison models can have positive effects on athletes, they may also have negative effects. Therefore, care should be taken to get feedback from athletes as to how they view the partner or group process related to their own individual rehabilitation progress and their own individual social support needs.

EVIDENCE-BASED PRACTICE

Clement, D., & Shannon, V. R. (2011). Injured athletes' perceptions about social support. *Journal of Sport Rehabilitation, 20,* 457–470.

Description of the Study

The study was conducted to examine injured athletes' perceptions of satisfaction, availability, and contribution of social support by teammates, coaches, and athletic trainers following injury. In all, 49 collegiate student–athletes (27 men, 22 women) from NCAA Division II and III institutions in the Mid-Atlantic region participated in the study. The mean age for participants was 20.1 years (SD 1.26 years). All participants had recently experienced injuries, whereas 44 of the 49 participants reported never having experienced an injury before the current injury or had experienced one or two previous injuries. Most of the participants represented the sports of football, volleyball, basketball, baseball, and soccer. Participants in this study completed an instrument packet including demographic questions and a modified version of the SSS (Corbillon et al, 2008; Richman et al, 1993). The 72-item survey was used to assess participants' satisfaction with, availability of, and contribution to overall well-being of eight types of social support, including listening support, emotional support, emotional-challenge support, reality confirmation, task appreciation support, task challenge support, tangible support, and personal assistance. Participants were asked to evaluate the perceived social support provided by teammates, coaches, and athletic trainers.

Results of the Study

Repeated-measures multivariate analyses of variance were performed to compare satisfaction with support, availability of support, and contribution of support from the three sources (teammates, coaches, and athletic trainers) for the eight types of social support. The 3×8 repeated-measures multivariate analyses of variance found significant main effects for type of support and for the three sources of support based on satisfaction with social support, availability of social support, and contribution from social support. In relation to satisfaction, pairwise comparisons between sources of social support indicated participants were more satisfied with social support provided by athletic trainers than by teammates or coaches. In terms of satisfaction and type of support, pairwise comparisons found participants expressed greater satisfaction with listening support than with reality-confirmation support from any of the sources of social support. Pairwise comparisons for availability of social support indicated participants reported significantly greater availability of social support from athletic trainers than from teammates or coaches. No significant pairwise comparisons were found for availability of social support based on types of social support. Lastly, in terms of contribution of social support, pairwise comparisons found significantly greater contributions of social support were provided by athletic trainers than by teammates and greater contributions from listening support, emotional support, reality-confirmation support, and task-appreciation support than tangible support from any of the sources.

Implications for Athletic Training Practice
Results from this study demonstrated the importance of the relationship between the athletic trainer and the athlete. It appears that injured athletes commonly turn to athletic trainers for various types of social support in managing and dealing with their injuries. In general, participants reported greater satisfaction with the social support provided by their athletic trainers than from their teammates or coaches, and they also reported greater availability of social support from their athletic trainers. Overall, the injury-related social support received from their athletic trainers was reported to contribute more to athletes' overall well-being compared with the support received from their teammates or coaches. It is important for athletic trainers to be aware of the important role they play in athletes' recovery, beyond the management of the physical pain and injury. It may also be beneficial for athletic trainers to work with athletes and coaches to educate them about the role of social support following injury, so athletes who experience injury may feel more supported and perceive greater support from those with whom they have the most regular contact—their teammates and coaches.

ATHLETE INSIDER CONCLUSION

Fast forward a year and Kate experiences another injury—a labral tear in her shoulder—and the process begins again. This time, she has a much better understanding of what is ahead, even though it is a completely different surgery. Although she is a couple of thousand miles away from home, she is very familiar with all of the athletic training staff members and many of the athletic training students from her previous experiences. As she did with her knee, she is adherent with her rehabilitation and goes on to complete her final two seasons of eligibility without significant injury.

Effective Psychosocial Strategies for the Athletic Trainer to Use with Kate

As discussed in this chapter, the athletic trainer could use the following psychosocial strategies with Kate to enhance her social support:

1. Educate Kate about her injury, surgery, and the rehabilitation and return-to-participation process.
2. Assist Kate in identifying her social support needs using the SSS (Richman et al, 1993) or SSIIA (Mitchell et al, 2005).
3. Help Kate identify people within her social support network using the Social Support Identification Worksheet (Fig. 9-5).
4. Facilitate a rehabilitation partner or group support in which Kate can be involved.

CONCLUSION

This chapter highlighted the use of social support as a coping strategy related to injury, rehabilitation, and return to participation, and examined the role the athletic trainer plays in the social support of athletes. More specifically, the types of social support were described, the identification of social support needs was discussed, examples of measuring social support were provided, and psychosocial strategies related to enhancing social support were presented.

REFERENCES

Albrecht, M. B., & Adelman, T. L. (1987). Communication networks as structure of social support. In: T. L. Adelman & M. B. Albrecht (Eds.), *Communicating Social Support* (pp. 40–64). London: SAGE Publications.

Barefield, S., & McCallister, S. (1997). Social support in the athletic training room: Athletes' expectations of staff and student athletic trainers. *Journal of Athletic Training, 32*(4), 333–338.

Blackwell, B., & McCullagh, P. (1990). The relationship of athletic injury to life stress, competitive anxiety, and coping resources. *Athletic Training, 25,* 23–27.

Bone, J. B., & Fry, M. D. (2006). The influence of injured athletes' perceptions of social support from ATCs on their beliefs about rehabilitation. *Journal of Sport Rehabilitation, 15,* 156–167.

Brewer, B. W., Andersen, M. B., & Van Raalte, J. L. (2002). Psychological aspects of sport injury rehabilitation: Toward a biopsychosocial approach. In: D. I. Mostofsky & L. D. Zaichkowsky (Eds.), *Medical and Psychological Aspects of Sport and Exercise* (pp. 41–54). Morgantown, WV: Fitness Information Technology.

Carver, C. S., Scheier, M. F., & Weintraub, J. K. (1989). Assessing coping strategies: A theoretically based approach. *Journal of Personality and Social Psychology, 56,* 267–283.

Clement, D., & Shannon, V. R. (2011). Injured athletes' perceptions about social support. *Journal of Sport Rehabilitation, 20,* 457–470.

Clement, D., Shannon, V. R., & Connole, I. J. (2011). Performance enhancement groups for injured athletes. *International Journal of Athletic Therapy & Training, 16*(3), 34–36.

Cohen, S., Gottlieb, B. H., & Underwood, L. G. (2001). Social relationships and health: Challenges for measurement and intervention. *Advances in Mind-Body Medicine, 17,* 129–141.

Corbillon, F., Crossman, J., & Jamieson, J. (2008). Injured athletes' perceptions of the social support provided by their coaches and teammates during rehabilitation. *Journal of Sport Behavior, 31*(2), 93–107.

Crocker, P. R. E., & Graham, T. R. (1995). Coping by competitive athletes with performance stress: Gender differences and relationships with affect. *The Sport Psychologist, 9,* 325–338.

Evans, L., Hardy, L., & Fleming, S. (2000). Intervention strategies with injured athletes: An action research study. *The Sport Psychologist, 14,* 188–206.

Gottlieb, B. H. (2000). Selecting and planning support interventions. In: S. Cohen, L. G. Underwood, & B. H. Gottlieb (Eds.), *Social Support Measurement and Intervention: A Guide for Health and Social Scientists* (pp. 195–220). New York: Oxford.

Hanson, S. J., McCullagh, P., & Tonymon, P. (1992). The relationship of personality characteristics, life stress, and coping resources to athletic injury. *Journal of Sport & Exercise Psychology, 14,* 262–272.

Hardy, C. J., & Crace, R. K. (1990). Dealing with injury. *The Sport Psychology Training Bulletin, 1,* 1–8.

Henert, S. (2001). Gender differences in coping with injury. *Athletic Therapy Today, 6*(2), 26–27.

Johnston, L. H., & Carroll, D. (2000). Coping, social support, and injury: Changes over time and the effects of level of sports involvement. *Journal of Sport Rehabilitation, 9*(4), 290–303.

Kerr, G. A., & Miller, P. S. (2001). Coping strategies. In: J. Crossman (Ed.), *Coping with Sports Injuries: Psychological Strategies for Rehabilitation* (pp. 82–102). Oxford: Oxford Press.

Lavallée, L., & Flint, F. (1996). The relationship of stress, competitive anxiety, mood state, and social support to athletic injury. *Journal of Athletic Training, 31*(4), 296–299.

Lazarus, R. S., & Folkman, S. (1984). *Stress, appraisal, & coping.* New York: Springer.

McCrea, M., Hammeke, T., Olsen, G., Leo, P., & Guskiewicz, K. (2004). Unreported concussion in high school football players: Implications for prevention. *Clinical Journal of Sport Medicine, 4*(1), 13–16.

Mitchell, I. D., Rees, T., Evans, L., & Hardy, L. (2005). The development of the social support inventory for injured athletes. Paper presented at: The Association for the Advancement of Applied Sport Psychology Conference; October 27, 2005; Vancouver, BC.

Mitchell, I. D., Wadey, R., Neil, R., & Hanton, S. (2007). Gender differences in athletes' social support during injury rehabilitation. *Journal of Sport and Exercise Psychology, 29,* S189.

Nixon, H. L. (1994). Social pressure, social support, and help seeking for pain and injuries in college sports networks. *Journal of Sport & Social Issues, 18,* 340–355.

Petitpas, A. J. (1999). Providing the right support. *Athletic Therapy Today, 4*(5), 61–62.

Ptacek, J. T., Smith, R. E., & Zanas, J. (1992). Gender, appraisal, and coping: A longitudinal analysis. *Journal of Personality, 60*(4), 747–770.

Rees, T. J., Mitchell, I., Evans, L., & Hardy, L. (2010). Stressors, social support and psychological responses to sport injury in high- and low-performance standard participants. *Psychology of Sport and Exercise, 11*(6), 505–512.

Richman, J. M., Rosenfeld, L. B., & Hardy, C. J. (1993). The social support survey: A validation study of a clinical measure of the social support process. *Research on Social Work Practice, 3*(3), 288–311.

Robbins J. E., & Rosenfeld, L. B. (2001). Athletes' perceptions of social support provided by their head coach, assistant coach, and athletic trainer, pre-injury and during rehabilitation. *Journal of Sport Behavior, 24*(3), 277–297.

Rosenfeld, L. B., Richman, J. M., & Hardy, C. J. (1989). Examining social support networks among athletes: Description and relationship to stress. *The Sport Psychologist, 3*(1), 23–33.

Shumaker, S. A., & Brownell, A. (1984). Toward a theory of social support: Closing conceptual gaps. *Journal of Social Issues, 19,* 71–90.

Smith, R. E., Smoll, F. L., & Schutz, R. W. (1990). Conjunctive moderator variables in vulnerability and resiliency research: Life stress, social support and coping skills, and adolescent sport injuries. *Journal of Personality and Social Psychology, 58,* 360–369.

Udry, E., Gould, D., Bridges, D., & Beck, L. (1997). Down but not out: Athlete responses to season-ending injuries. *Journal of Sport & Exercise Psychology, 1,* 229–248.

Udry, E., Gould, D., Bridges, D., & Tuffey, S. (1997). People helping people? Examining the social ties of athletes coping with burnout and injury stress. *Journal of Sport & Exercise Psychology, 19,* 368–395.

Wiese-Bjornstal, D. M., Smith, A. M., Shaffer, S. M., & Morrey, M. A. (1998). An integrated model of response to sport injury: Psychological and sociological dynamics. *Journal of Applied Sport Psychology, 10,* 46–69.

Williams, J. M., & Andersen, M. B. (1998). Psychosocial antecedents of sport injury: Review and critique of the stress and injury model. *Journal of Applied Sport Psychology, 10,* 2–25.

Williams, J. M., Tonymon, P., & Wadsworth, W. A. (1986). Relationship of stress to injury in intercollegiate volleyball. *Journal of Human Stress, 12,* 38–43.

Yang, J., Peek-Asa, C., Lowe, J. B., Heiden, E., & Foster, D. T. (2010). Social support patterns of collegiate athletes before and after injury. *Journal of Athletic Training, 45*(4), 372–379.

BOARD OF CERTIFICATION STRATEGIES AND COMPETENCIES

The Fifth Edition Athletic Training Educational Competencies (2011) includes knowledge and skills in the content area of Psychosocial Strategies and Referral (PS), and within this content area, knowledge and skills related to social support are included. Specific to this content area, this chapter has described social interactions as they affect athletes (PS-1), as well as reinforced effective interpersonal communication between the athlete and members of their social support network (PS-4). Theories of social support were discussed (PS-5) and education was emphasized as a psychosocial strategy (PS-6). Although these competencies do not use the term *social support*, they each are aimed at providing the athlete with the feeling or sense of being supported by others. The athletic trainer plays a primary role as support provider, and the athletic trainer must also facilitate others in the athlete's social support network to provide for the needs of the athlete.

Board of Certification Style Questions

1. An example of tangible social support is (select all that apply):
   a. providing education about the injury.
   b. providing information related to the rehabilitation process.
   c. providing crutches and ice packs.
   d. providing a ride to the physician's office.
2. Which of the following people is likely part of an athlete's social support network? (Select all that apply.)
   a. Athletic trainer
   b. Coach
   c. Teammates
   d. Significant others
3. Which of the following describes the agreement of available social support with the social support needs of the athlete?
   a. Matching hypothesis
   b. Social support hypothesis
   c. Network hypothesis
   d. Needs hypothesis

END-OF-CHAPTER EXERCISES

1. Identify and describe types of social support. How could the athletic trainer provide these types of social support to the athlete?
2. Describe the relationship between help-seeking tendencies and social support. What considerations may be made for different athletes? In your response, consider their level of play, severity of injury, and gender.
3. Explain the importance of matching an athlete's social support needs with the provision of social support. How might an athletic trainer demonstrate this with an athlete?
4. List and describe psychosocial strategies that can be incorporated into athlete care before and after injury to enhance the athlete's perception and availability of social support.
5. Have an athlete complete the SSS or the SSIIA. What do the scores indicate?
6. Complete the Social Support Identification Worksheet (Fig. 9-5) with an athlete who is currently injured or is participating in sport injury rehabilitation, or both.

Chapter 10

Psychosocial Strategies: Effectiveness and Application

Jennifer Jordan Hamson-Utley with Monna Arvinen-Barrow and Megan D. Granquist

CHAPTER OUTLINE

CHAPTER OUTLINE *continued*

KEY TERMS

Affirmation Statement(s) made to the self to encourage, motivate, and improve self-worth.

Athletic identity The degree to which a person identifies the self as an athlete.

Clinical trial Research involving tests that generate safe-use data for health interventions by comparing existing and new drugs or procedures that change a participant's health/behavior.

Cognitive relaxation A relaxation method that includes verbal and visual cues, which lead individuals to a relaxing time and place.

Cognitive restructuring A cognitive behavioral strategy used to identify and replace irrational or maladaptive thoughts that often occur in anxiety-provoking situations.

Coping skills Mechanisms that promote the ability to cope with a stressor or situation; built from experience or learned.

Evidence-based practice A methodology that combines clinical expertise and the best available systematic research evidence when making decisions about patient care.

Extrinsic motivation Behavior that is driven by a desire to attain a specific outcome; motivation from an outside source.

Healing imagery Focusing attention on a target visual stimulus to produce a specific physiological change that can promote healing.

Holistic Related to healing; a holistic approach includes all parts of the healing system—the mind and the body—in the healing process.

Intrinsic motivation Behavior that is driven by an interest or enjoyment in the task itself (e.g., personal best).

Meta-analysis A research method that takes data from a number of independent studies and integrates it using statistical analysis.

Nonresponse bias A research term that describes a situation in which the answers of respondents differ from the potential answers of those who did not answer.

Pain-management imagery Focusing attention on a target visual stimulus to produce specific images to promote pain-management strategies (e.g., visualizing the pain flying away or lying in a meadow free of pain).

Performance imagery The creation or re-creation of an experience in the mind from memory or quasi-experience using a combination of the five senses with the goal of improving an aspect of a performance in sport or rehabilitation.

Positive affirmation A positive declaration of truth; used in rehabilitation and healing to improve mind-set and to motivate.

Psychological skills Mental skills, techniques by which the individual can use the mind to control the body or to create an outcome.

Psychosocial strategies A term typically used to describe a range of psychosocial skills and techniques athletes can use to control their thoughts, emotions, and behaviors.

Psychosocial techniques Methods athletes can use to rehearse, improve, and maintain their psychological skills.

Rehabilitation-process imagery Focusing attention on a target visual stimulus to produce specific images of different aspects of the rehabilitation process.

Relaxation Release of tension in the body; return to equilibrium.

KEY TERMS *continued*

Self-talk Internal and/or external statements to the self, multidimensional in nature, that have interpretive elements associated with their content; it is dynamic and serves at least two functions (instructional and motivational).

Somatic relaxation A relaxation method that leads the participant to a relaxed state through focus on the breath and breathing patterns.

Systematic review A research method that provides a comprehensive and detailed summary of literature relevant to a research question.

Thought stopping A psychological strategy that allows the athlete to gain control over the thought process, changing negative thoughts to more productive positive thoughts.

CHAPTER OBJECTIVES

After reading this chapter, you will be able to:

1. Identify psychosocial strategies that athletic trainers can use in athletes' treatment, rehabilitation, and return to participation.
2. Describe the psychosocial strategies that athletic trainers can use to motivate athletes during treatment, rehabilitation, and return to participation.
3. Describe the use of goal setting to increase motivation and facilitate athletes' adherence in rehabilitation.
4. Describe the use of imagery in athletes' treatment, rehabilitation, and return to participation.
5. Describe cognitive and somatic relaxation techniques that athletic trainers can use with athletes' treatment, rehabilitation, and return to participation.
6. Describe the psychosocial strategies that athletic trainers can use to facilitate athletes' pain management during rehabilitation.
7. Implement appropriate psychosocial strategies into athletes' treatment or rehabilitation programs to enhance rehabilitation adherence, return to participation, and overall rehabilitation and recovery outcomes.

ATHLETE INSIDER

'A'amakua (AH ah MAH kooah) has played football ever since he can remember; it is *who* he is. He finished his second year at a medium-sized Division I university with top honors. Since his family is from Hawaii, they don't get to watch him play; however, they read press releases and the university's website to stay on top of his performances. Football is central to 'A'amakua's life and, like most who achieve success in college ball, he envisions supporting his family by going on to the NFL. Two games into his junior season, he tears a labrum in his shoulder and has surgery, keeping him out only 7 weeks. 'A'amakua set high, yet achievable goals and worked hard to make it back for the final regular season game; then he reinjured his shoulder and missed the conference championship game and the bowl game that year. In his last year of eligibility, he was chronically injured, with shoulder instability, patellar tendinopathy, and muscle strains; he underwent another surgery, this time on the opposite shoulder. He felt lost. All that he had going for him was gone. He kept asking his athletic trainer, "How could this be happening to me? Why is my body falling apart? Why now?" His mother

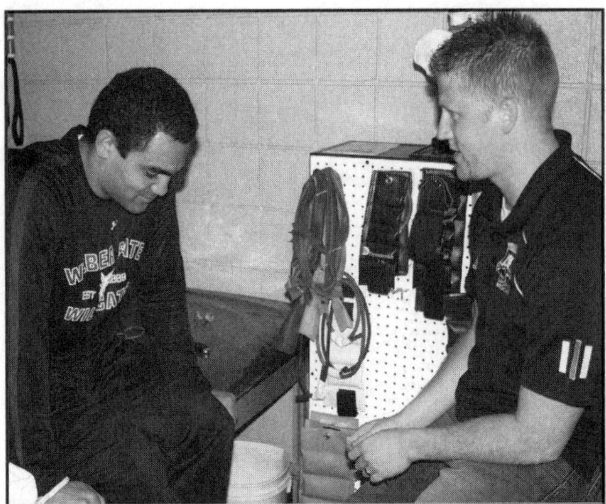

Figure 10-1 | Athlete Insider

demanded he return home so that she could "nurse him to health." His athletic trainer advised against returning home and educated 'A'amakua on the importance of repairing his body by completing his rehabilitation on campus. He missed his family and wanted to go home. His mind wouldn't rest; he kept wondering, *Do I still have a shot at the NFL? Should I give up and go home?*

INTRODUCTION

Psychosocial strategies (e.g., ***self-talk***, imagery, ***relaxation*** techniques, and goal setting) are identified by the Commission on Accreditation of Athletic Training Education as essential skills that athletic trainers should know about and be proficient in using. In addition, athletic trainers and sports medicine physicians have endorsed using psychosocial strategies as a way to positively influence the rehabilitation process. This chapter introduces and provides details of various psychosocial strategies that can be used in the context of sport injury prevention, rehabilitation, and return to participation. This chapter also provides details to assist the athletic trainer in introducing these ***coping skills*** to athletes and educating them regarding practice and use of the skill. An important aspect of this chapter is the inclusion of practical implementation of the psychosocial strategies within the athletic training context (i.e., when and how). Both cognitive (e.g., self-talk, imagery) and somatic (e.g., deep breathing, ***cognitive relaxation***, and ***somatic relaxation***) skills, as well as the process of using goal setting during rehabilitation, are discussed. The discussion of the use and effectiveness of psychosocial strategies is evidence-based, drawing from both current research and historical mind–body literature.

Understanding the important role that psychosocial strategies play in the athletic training context is valuable to the ***holistic*** care of the athlete. The field of athletic training is uniquely situated to provide care to others besides injured athletes. Today, athletic trainers work in diverse settings including hospitals, orthopedic and physical therapy clinics, universities, colleges, high schools, physicians' offices, corporations, and government settings. Although this chapter focuses on the care of injured athletes and highlights the importance of athletic trainers in the psychosocial care of injured athletes, many strategies presented and discussed are valuable for use across settings and patient populations. This chapter presents examples in which strategies can be applied outside of sport/athletic settings and the special considerations that may be involved in these settings. In addition, this chapter uses red flags to point out times when introducing a strategy may not be appropriate or when it may warrant special procedures (i.e., with a minor).

As stated earlier, the main aim of this chapter is to stress the importance of the role of athletic trainers in athletes' psychosocial care. Because the locations and populations served in the field of athletic training are unique, the athletic trainer is also in a key position to assist athletes on a daily basis. What other allied health-care professional works with injured athletes every day? As it is, the athletic trainer has the opportunity to *positively influence* the injury situation from the on-field evaluation to the return to play. The athletic trainer can monitor daily progress both physically and mentally, gathering pieces of the puzzle each day to increase their understanding and improve their ability to empathize with injured athletes; time spent with any other allied health-care provider just does not match up. Thus, it is important that the athletic trainer be familiar with and comfortable in implementing *best practices* of care, including how to support athletes emotionally, mentally, and socially during this stressful period. This chapter also discusses athletes' expectations of their health-care providers and presents research that has established a set of "essentials" for athlete care, making the already stressful experience of being injured and away from their comfort zone (the playing field) a better one.

IMPORTANCE OF PSYCHOSOCIAL ASPECTS OF INJURY

Consistent with a holistic approach to the care of athletes, psychosocial aspects of injury are part of the athletes' integrated care. As discussed in this chapter, athletic trainers can teach psychosocial strategies to athletes who can use them to help reduce the risk for injury and reinjury, enhance the rehabilitation process and outcomes, and aid return to participation.

Addressing psychosocial aspects of injuries is important for two main reasons. First, psychosocial factors often contribute to injury events. As outlined in Chapter 3, injury risk is influenced by athletes' stress response to a situation. This stress response can be modified to reduce the risk for injury by using coping resources that include ***psychological skills***. Relaxation is one of the primary psychological skills that athletes can use to decrease their response to stress, and thus decrease injury risk. Second, it has been documented that, because of advances in medical technology, many athletes have the potential to recover to their preinjury level of performance (or higher) but fail to do so because of psychosocial factors. For example, an athlete may not adhere to rehabilitation because of lack of motivation (***intrinsic motivation*** or ***extrinsic motivation***) or feelings of depression. These issues can be addressed by using psychosocial strategies. As discussed in Chapter 8, use of goal setting during rehabilitation may play a primary role in the overall development and execution of the treatment plan. Specific to rehabilitation adherence, goal setting may also be effective to increase adherence and home exercise completion. Moreover, athletes' preparation for returning to sport after injury can be hindered because of psychosocial factors. If athletes are experiencing reinjury anxiety or feelings of self-doubt about being able to play again, they can use psychosocial strategies such as imagery and self-talk as part of a preperformance routine to assist with their return to participation.

Understanding Psychosocial Aspects of Athletic Injury and Prevention

As demonstrated earlier, understanding the cyclical nature of psychosocial aspects of the sport injury process (from injury onset, through rehabilitation, to return to sport) is important in providing effective care to athletes. Often psychosocial strategies are seen as tools to be primarily used in rehabilitation. Yes, this is a great time to use these strategies and skills; however, using such strategies to reduce the risk for injury should be of prime importance.

More specifically, when considering the implementation of psychosocial skills, athletic trainers should understand the underpinning theories that explain the psychosocial process of sport injury and rehabilitation from injury onset to recovery. According to the integrated model of response to sport injury (Wiese-Bjornstal, Smith, Shaffer, & Morrey; 1998), and adapting from the earlier work by Andersen and Williams (1988), a number of preinjury antecedents (i.e., personality, coping resources, previous history of stressors, and use of interventions) can impact athletes' responses to a stressful situation and their subsequent stress response (Williams & Andersen, 1998). This stress response, as explained in Chapter 3, will, in turn, impact the likelihood of injury occurrence. The earlier mentioned antecedents along with the actual injury will then, in turn, have an impact on how an individual responds to the injury and the rehabilitation process. When injured, athletes often experience a range of thoughts (i.e., cognitive appraisal of the injury), emotions, and feelings (i.e., emotional response), which can have either a positive or a negative effect on their behavior (i.e., behavioral response) during rehabilitation. The integrated model proposes that this interaction is a dynamic and bidirectional cyclic process, which, in turn, will impact the overall physical and psychosocial injury recovery outcomes. Moreover, these responses are seen as being influenced by a range of personal factors (e.g., individual differences) and situational factors (e.g., sports medicine team influences, including the athletic trainer; Fig. 10-2).

Understanding the Relationship Between Cognitive Appraisals and Emotional and Behavioral Responses to Athletic Injury

Athletes have both emotional and behavioral responses to athletic injury that are influenced by their cognitive interpretation. Both preinjury and postinjury factors influence responses to athletic injury (Wiese-Bjornstal et al, 1998). Athletes' responses are dynamic; cognitive, emotional, and behavioral responses continuously interact and influence injury recovery. For example, athletes whose self-identity is wrapped up with their ***athletic identity*** may perceive the injury as a partial loss of self. Their cognitive appraisal of the situation would therefore be negative, and they might

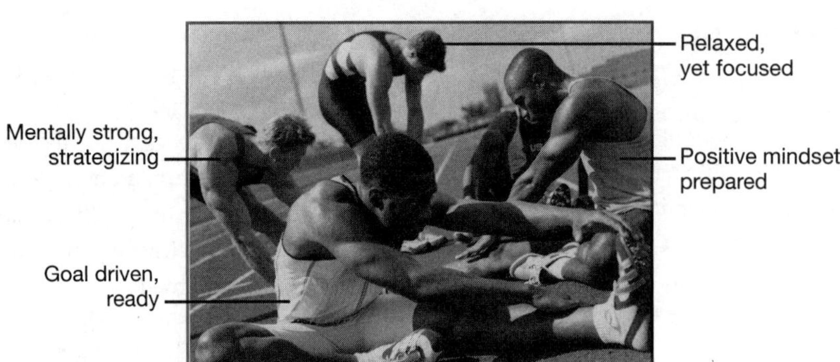

Figure 10-2 | Factors associated with injury rehabilitation.

consider themselves to be "less of a person" as a result of the injury. Thus, their emotional responses to injury may include sadness, anger, and frustration. This can then lead to negative behavioral responses such as withdrawal, hypervigilance, and irritability. The use of psychosocial strategies could be beneficial to assist athletes. For example, athletes who have cognitively appraised their situation as negative and perceive their self-worth as lower can use self-talk in the form of ***cognitive restructuring*** or ***positive affirmations*** to assist in improving outlook, leading to positive, functional behavior. In a similar manner, such athletes could take ownership of the rehabilitation process by involving themselves in setting goals for rehabilitation. Being more involved can facilitate their feelings of self-worth and subsequently change their appraisal of the situation. This will, in turn, have an impact on their behavior and emotions, and therefore impact their overall rehabilitation and recovery outcomes. The athlete may better adhere to their rehabilitation program, be less frustrated and more content with the process, and as a result, overall outcomes may be enhanced.

Why Athletic Trainers Should Address Psychosocial Aspects of Sport Injury

Medical professionals such as athletic trainers are an important source of emotional first aid to athletes during injury recovery. Along with physical treatment, athletic trainers should be using a range of psychosocial strategies with injured athletes. Given the close nature of the relationship injured athletes typically have with their athletic trainers, it seems fitting for them to be responsible for the athletes' psychological support. Research tends to suggest that sports medicine professionals are best positioned to provide psychological assistance for injured athletes for four main reasons: (1) They typically are the primary treatment providers who work with injured athletes on a day-to-day basis (Larson, Starkey, & Zaichkowsky; 1996); (2) the techniques athletic trainers use in injury rehabilitation typically involve touch, and that can facilitate athletes opening up about psychological issues in their recovery (Nathan, 1999); (3) research tends to suggest that psychological issues related to injury are often discussed in conjunction with physical aspects of rehabilitation (Kolt, 2003); and (4) existing studies suggest that athletes themselves feel that athletic trainers are in an ideal position to address the psychological aspects of injury (Larson et al, 1996; Wiese & Weiss, 1987; Wiese, Weiss, & Yukelson, 1991). Athletes' expectations of such support may vary because of gender and previous athletic training experience. These expectations are explained in greater detail in the following paragraphs.

Athletic trainers are trained to recognize a range of psychological reactions experienced by injured athletes and to have the skill set to intervene (i.e., use basic psychosocial strategies) and refer when necessary. More importantly, athletic trainers should have the basic understanding of the theories underpinning psychosocial reactions to injury, and as such, they should also be adequately trained to identify which psychosocial strategy would be most appropriate to address the source of the problem, not just the symptoms of the problem.

In addition to the above, competent athletic trainers should also possess appropriate skills to refer an athlete on to relevant professionals when necessary (discussed in

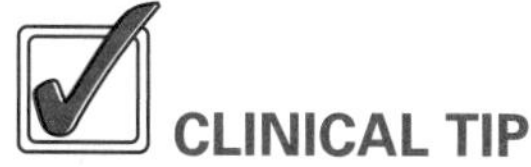

CLINICAL TIP

An athlete may show signs of nonadherence, which typically would be a symptom of lack of motivation, and as such, this may be addressed through the use of goal setting. However, lack of adherence could also be a symptom of increased levels of reinjury anxiety possibly because of recurrent pain; therefore, the most appropriate intervention may be the use of relaxation techniques and cryotherapy to alleviate pain rather than simply trying to get the athlete to "re-adhere" by setting goals.

detail in Chapter 6). For example, in cases involving clinical issues (e.g., depression, substance abuse, and eating disorders) that influence the rehabilitation, having adequate referral procedures and a network of relevant professionals in place is very important. Athletic trainers should be encouraged to build relevant networks around them and, at the start of the athlete's rehabilitation, identify which professionals and significant others will be an integral part of a successful recovery.

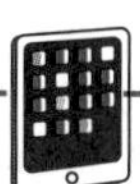

VIRTUAL FIELD TRIP

Athletic trainers should consider seeking assistance from certified sports psychology consultants to learn specific psychosocial skills or to assist athletes with performance-enhancement issues following returning to play. The Association for Applied Sport Psychology certifies sports psychology consultants; athletic trainers can find contact information for certified consultants via the Association for Applied Sport Psychology website: The Davis*Plus* website (http://davisplus.fadavis.com) provides a link for this site.

ATHLETES' EXPECTATIONS OF THEIR HEALTH-CARE PROVIDER

Those who deliver care possess a variety of characteristics and, possibly most important, many personalities. In the case of providing care to injured athletes in need, it is the role/job of the athletic trainer to see that *all of the athletes' needs* are met or to take a holistic approach to athlete care. This is often the area of rehabilitation that receives the least amount of focus or energy from athletic trainers because they are likely trained to heal the physical rather than the mental side of injury.

SPECIAL CONSIDERATIONS

Recent research on academic preparation of the athletic training student confirms that this set of competencies is often lumped in with other course content as an afterthought or taught in one lecture or one week (three 50-minute lectures); less often, a course is dedicated to delivery of the content and titled something like "Psychological Aspects of Athlete Care" or "Psychology of Sport, Injury, and Rehabilitation." During the 1990s, graduating athletic training students were likely educated on the mental aspects of injury through a "Psychology of Coaching" course or a "Sports Psychology" course, neither of which may directly address the psychosocial aspects of athletic injury and return to play. What's more, it is likely that the aforementioned preparation courses teaching the Psychosocial Strategies and Referral content area of the Fifth Edition of the Education Competencies in Athletic Training to aspiring athletic training students are not taught by certified athletic trainers trained in the psychology of sport injury and rehabilitation who apply these strategies with athletes on a daily basis. Herein lies the quandary; the importance of the psychosocial aspects of athlete care is often underemphasized in the instruction of future athletic training professionals because of an undereducated instructor (fault may not be their own). The consideration of this, or acknowledging that continuing education is needed in the case of the undereducated athletic trainer, is the responsibility of the athletic trainer. Engaging in continuing education offerings related to the psychosocial

Continued

strategies and referral content area will undoubtedly improve the holistic care provided to injured athletes. Of additional concern are the institutional confines within which the athletic training program operates; it might not be an option to "add a course" to cover the Psychosocial Strategies and Referral content area.

It is the athletic trainer's job to treat athletes professionally and in a way that is perceived by athletes as caring about their needs and having empathy for their situation. Also of importance is the athletic trainer's knowledge about the injury or limitation athletes face. In the supporting literature, the topic of being "a good athletic trainer" arises and is often not discussed. A good athletic trainer or Allied Health Care Professional is someone who is professional, thoughtful, knowledgeable, and patient-centered in delivering care. Are there some individuals who just shouldn't enter a caring field? Do you know people like this? What are they lacking? Table 10-1 outlines factors that may affect the ability of a provider to deliver effective care. How many of these do you possess? Are some more important than others?

Following injury, athletes are dealing with physical limitations along with many new stressors associated with being injured and the inability to return to participation (see Chapter 3 for a review on stressors). As rehabilitation begins, they may find themselves in a foreign environment—the athletic training room. Many athletes may try to avoid the athletic training room because it means to them that they are dented, broken, or no longer athletes. For first-time injured athletes, this is especially true, and athletic trainers need to recognize when an athlete is experiencing angst about "just being here" in the athletic training room. Signs and symptoms might include appearing lost, uncomfortable, unusually quiet or shy when otherwise not so, and anxious about treatments and the recovery process (Table 10-2). Athletes might also miss appointments and exhibit other nonadherent behaviors, such as malingering, not putting forth effort on exercises, or questioning the use of treatments and exercises (i.e., overall negative attitude about being present in the athletic training room). In addition, those who have been injured before and sought help may avoid the athletic training room as they recall its connection with being held out of competition.

The athletic trainer plays many roles in the care of the athlete, from prevention of injury (e.g., protective taping, stretching) all the way through to return to play (e.g., on-field testing, confidence building). The concept that one individual assists throughout the entire process places focus on the salient role of that individual and the expectations that athletes may have while receiving care from that individual. Furthermore, athlete expectations are important, as they have been linked to rehabilitation outcomes. Knowing what athletes expect will allow the athletic trainer to mold or change the environment, and possibly their own practices, to better meet the needs of injured athletes (Table 10-3).

TABLE 10-1 **Factors That Affect Care Delivery**

Personality Traits of Care Provider	Situational Traits of Setting	Situational Traits of Injury
Happy ("always smiling"), pleasant to be around, helpful, supportive	One-on-one interaction, quality time, connection/bonding	Can explain the injury and educate at a level that is easily understood
Conversational, displays interest in the patient beyond the injury	Affords private conversation, free of judgment	Knowledgeable about care options and presents all options, free of bias
Loves what he or she does, enjoys being an athletic trainer and providing care to all athletes	Convenient time and place to receive care, convenient scheduling of care/communication about care	Supportive when setbacks occur, educates on chronic and acute injury situations

TABLE 10-2 **Observable Signs and Symptoms of Psychological Distress in the Athletic Training Room**

Stressor(s)	Resulting Athlete Behavior in ATR
Dealing with pain	Skipping treatments, avoiding AT, negative attitude or outlook, malingering behaviors (e.g., reporting to be ill when not ill to avoid therapy)
Not being with team	Looking sad, not motivated to be at treatment or to do any exercises, moving sluggishly, less eye contact, less conversation, negative attitude
Giving up on returning to play	Resistant to suggestions by AT, questioning of AT recommendations, uses outside resources to determine own timeline for return to play, consulting other medical professionals to ensure receiving best-practice care
Not invested in goals set by AT	Not motivated by things that were once motivating, skipping treatment, atypical negative attitude, questioning every suggestion by the AT, appears depressed (lacking hygiene, no eye contact, little to no communication compared with normal behavior)

AT, athletic trainer; ATR, athletic training room.

TABLE 10-3 **Differences in Athlete–Patient Expectations Based on Gender and Prior Experience with Athletic Trainers**

Males	Males with Prior AT Experience	Males without Prior AT Experience	Females	Females with Prior AT Experience	Females without Prior AT Experience
Lower personal commitment expectations than females	Highest expectations of AT expertise in the treatment and education process	Lowest personal commitment expectations	Higher personal commitment expectations on the part of the AT as compared with males	Least likely to have realistic expectations of AT in the care setting	Highest personal commitment expectations
Higher expectations that ATs would provide a facilitative environment		Lowest expectations of ATs as providing a facilitative environment	Higher expectations that ATs would provide a facilitative environment		Highest expectations of ATs as providing a facilitative environment
		Lowest expectations of AT expertise			

AT, athletic trainer.
Adapted from Clement, Hamson-Utley, et al. (2012).

EBP EVIDENCE-BASED PRACTICE

Russell, H., & Tracey, J. (2011). What do injured athletes want from their health care professionals? *International Journal of Athletic Therapy & Training, 16*(5), 18–21.

Description of the Study

Taking a holistic approach to rehabilitation of athletic injury is important to athletes. This study examined what athletes want from their health-care providers in an attempt to guide the services that athletic trainers and physiotherapists provide during rehabilitation from injury. Participants were both varsity (n = 20) and recreational athletes (n = 3) recruited from health-care clinics (N = 27; mean age 21.48 years; range 19–29 years) with injuries that kept them out of sport for at least 7 days (defined as "moderate-to-severe injury"). Male (n = 10) and female (n = 13) participants were asked to complete an online survey following care received as a result of their injury. Questions on the survey asked the participants to identify what they wanted their care provider to do or to offer to address the psychological aspects of injury. Health-care professionals included athletic trainers (56.6%), physical therapists (60.9%), and sports medicine physicians (47.8%).

Results of the Study

Two main themes emerged from the qualitative analysis of the survey data: education and atmosphere. Regarding education, athletes reported they wanted education about their injury, the rehabilitation process, and guidelines for return to play. Athletes reported that, when they received education, they felt it was helpful and that it reduced their anxiety about the unknown. Related to education, one athlete reported, "The worst part for me was the lack of understanding I had with my injury. I would show up and get treatment and then leave. I felt that I could have used more info on the injury" (p. 19). The second theme, atmosphere, outlined four main aspects of this factor: (1) opportunity to ask questions, (2) social support, (3) time spent with the care provider, and (4) positive comments and interactions. Athletes valued the relationship with the care provider when they felt comfortable to ask any question that they had about treatment or rehabilitation; a number of athletes indicated not feeling welcome to ask questions. As one athlete said, "It would be helpful if he (i.e., a sports medicine physician) actually had a conversation with me. He simply told me the diagnosis and what to do or not to do and left. He seemed frustrated with me when I even asked or questioned him" (p. 19). In addition, athletes wanted the health-care provider to ask them how they were doing with the injury emotionally and psychologically; the majority reported that it would be unlikely for them to start a conversation about psychological issues related to their injury. Also, in terms of the environment theme, athletes noted that, when the care provider spent time with them, they felt more "important" and that the athletic trainer had a "vested interest" in their recovery. Athletes said they appreciated the relationship with the care provider; for example, "her athletic trainer chat[ted] when I needed someone to talk to and understood what I was going through" (p. 20). One athlete reported that her athletic trainer "took on the role of psychological supporter because I saw her on a daily basis" (p. 20). Last, regarding the positive nature of the environment that athletes expect from their care providers, one athlete reported, "The mental aspect of injury can be just as debilitating as the injury itself. It's very easy to lose your confidence and start to believe you will never get better—they need to keep you on track both physically and emotionally" (p. 20). Athletes want the rehabilitation environment to be positive and supportive, reassuring them that they will eventually return to their sport.

Implications for Athletic Training Practice
Injured athletes want athletic trainers to be educators in the rehabilitation and return-to-sport process. They expect that athletic trainers will provide detailed information about their injury and surgical procedures, which leads to a reduction in the athlete's anxiety about the unknown. Injured athletes also expect that athletic trainers "spend time" with them, support them, and notice when they are uncertain or feeling defeated and provide positive reassurance that "they will overcome this hurdle." Potentially the most important aspect of this research to the practice of athletic training is that athletes are unlikely to start a conversation about the psychological struggles they are experiencing surrounding their injury. Athletic trainers must feel comfortable with and competent in starting this conversation with the injured athlete, and not wait for it to "surface." Furthermore, athletic trainers must be able to see signs of distress that warrant a referral to a mental health professional and then be competent in making the referral.

Paying attention to athletes' expectations stands to improve the overall process of injury rehabilitation facilitated by the athletic trainer. The focus of current literature in educational pedagogy suggests that students are requesting more technology in the classroom to foster their education and that they are more satisfied when they receive education through technology. Because many athletes are also students, this expectation will likely expand, if not already, into other areas of their lives, including injury care and rehabilitation in the athletic training room. There are many ways that technology can be incorporated into the injury-care and rehabilitation process to foster the readiness to return to play. Athletes today, like students, are entering college equipped with a mobile device that can access and use applications, digital media, and online support groups or social media that can play an important role in the recovery process (Fig. 10-3). The research on patient satisfaction suggests that being satisfied with the care provided is related to rehabilitation outcomes, so much so that making sure patients are satisfied with their care could be the leading predictor of a successful outcome (see the following Evidence-Based Practice feature).

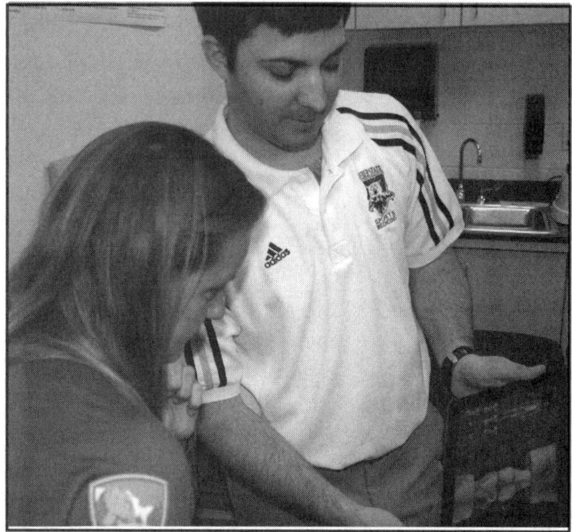

Figure 10-3 | Using mobile technology with the athlete.

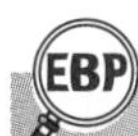

EVIDENCE-BASED PRACTICE

Taylor, A. (1995). Development of a Sports Injury Clinic Athlete Satisfaction Scale for auditing patient perceptions. *Physiotherapy Theory and Practice, 11*(4), 231–238.

Description of the Study
An athlete's perception of the quality of care received during rehabilitation from injury may be a key factor in predicting rate of recovery and adherence to the assigned program. This study developed and evaluated a survey to assess patient satisfaction by administering a 16-item survey to patients (n = 160; 63% male, 37% female; mean age 33 years) at five sports injury clinics in the United Kingdom. The survey was created by an extensive literature review

Continued

and by interviewing injured athletes and the physiotherapists who provide their care.

Results of the Study

Three themes were revealed: Evaluation of Empathy, Information Given, and Competence, which explained 41.7%, 7.7%, and 5.8% of the variance, respectively. Survey evaluation revealed acceptable reliability and construct validity. Regarding the satisfaction of the recreational and competitive athletes in this study, they were most satisfied with the Competence of their health-care professional. Potentially more interesting, females and athletes with high athletic identity were least satisfied with Information Given. Finally, those who were most recently injured were least satisfied with Evaluation of Empathy or a situational understanding shown by the physiotherapist.

Implications for Athletic Training Practice

Although this study was published in 1995, it stands as a historical occurrence and measure of expectations that athletes have of their health-care providers. Athletic trainers must function outside of the capacity to heal a physical injury and enter the realm of holistic healing of the injured athlete. This study suggests that athletic trainers should gain or reinforce the understanding of "what is good care?" of the injured athlete. Consistent with current research, injured athletes want empathy or a discussion that allows them to express how they feel and a response from the athletic trainer illustrating emotional support and understanding. Injured athletes also require a solid base of information, offered by the athletic trainer, to establish a new reality in a foreign environment otherwise called "rehabilitation." Athletic trainers are teachers in the rehabilitation setting; teaching should be both practical and appropriate for the educational maturity level of the athlete. This can pose a challenge as teaching should be both up to date and evidence based, and may require extra work or time to provide. Athletic trainers also need to be aware of gender differences in injured athlete expectations; female athletes may require more social support, one-on-one time, and encouragement than male athletes.

CLINICAL TIP

The field of physical therapy also plays a role in rehabilitation of the injured athlete. Physical therapy services often include musculoskeletal therapies and are usually postsurgical situations for athletes. These therapies may include specific modalities, specialized equipment, and often a 1:1 practitioner-to-athlete ratio. Not every athletic training room is equipped to offer these services; in addition, they might be too busy to attend to the vast rehabilitation needs of various injured athletes, especially if the 1:1 ratio is required. Services provided by physical therapists are highly similar, if not equal, in the early phases of rehabilitation. Most common in the high school setting, athletes will attend a physical therapy clinic to perform rehabilitation and will return to the athletic training room to make the return-to-sport transition. Research on patient satisfaction is prevalent in physical therapy scholarship and should be examined in relation to satisfaction literature in athletic training.

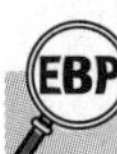

EVIDENCE-BASED PRACTICE

Hush, J., Cameron, K., & Mackey, M. (2010). Patient satisfaction with musculoskeletal physical therapy care: A systematic review. *Physical Therapy, 91,* 25–36.

Description of the Study

The study conducted a ***systematic review*** of the literature and examined factors associated with satisfaction with musculoskeletal physical therapy care. ***Clinical trials***, observations, surveys, and qualitative designs were accepted wherein patient satisfaction was evaluated in receiving physical therapy services; the systematic review search located 3790 citations, while

15 studies met the inclusion criteria. The United States, Ireland, United Kingdom, and Northern Europe were represented in the final data set.

Results of the Study

A ***meta-analysis*** of patient satisfaction revealed a pooled estimate of 4.44 (range 3.5–4.67; 95% confidence interval, 4.41–4.46) on a 5-point scale where 5 indicated high satisfaction. Interpersonal attributes of the treating therapist (communication, friendliness, approachability) and the process of care (informational, professional, organizational) were found to be key determinants of patient satisfaction. In addition, patients with more acute injuries reported higher levels of satisfaction as compared with those with chronic injuries; females reported higher levels of satisfaction as compared with males. The authors noted that ***nonresponse bias*** could limit study findings.

Implications for Athletic Training Practice

Because a systematic review is a combined look at a topic or problem, the meta-analysis (or analysis of that review) can be very powerful in the information that it provides as it informs ***evidence-based practice*** (Fig. 10-4). In this case, parallels can be drawn between the physical therapy clinic, which treats various types of patients of all ages and activity backgrounds, to the athletic training room, which generally treats competitive athletes. It appears that the key determinants of satisfaction (easy to communicate with, approachable, friendly, positive, and informative about the injury) found in the study are highly similar to those found in competitive athlete studies (positive environment, spending time, and education). The message, then, to athletic trainers is to be mindful to spend time with injured athletes and provide a sense of connection and support. The athletic trainer should use daily interactions with injured athletes to educate them on their injury and recovery process, questioning often for understanding and to promote a comfortable environment.

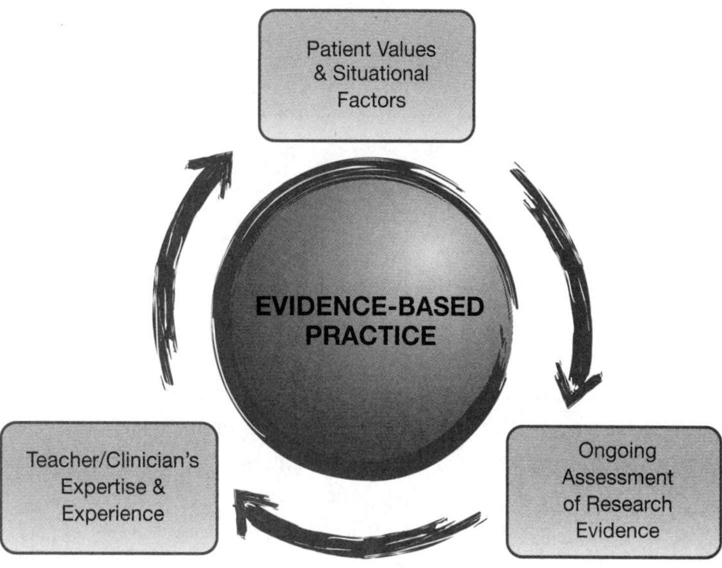

Figure 10-4 | Evidence-based practice (EBP) flow sheet.

Identifying what injured athletes expect and what things relate to patient satisfaction are crucial to the delivery of effective care for these athletes. Developing strategies or processes to identify or predict specific needs and ways to meet those needs is the starting place for implementation of quality care. From the earlier evidence-based practice features, the following expectations of care are viewed as essential to meeting the needs of injured athletes: education and atmosphere.

Athletes expect that the athletic trainer will educate them on their injury and what to anticipate during the rehabilitation and return-to-play process. Looking for the right time and place is usually not the problem, as the athlete may present with question after question. The athletic trainer must be ready to educate and have a plan of attack that can be used with each injury occurrence and be modifiable with each athlete. Having charts and models ready, as well as three-dimensional anatomy applications, will make for a highly effective education session with the athlete.

VIRTUAL FIELD TRIP

Apps can be an effective tool to use with injured athletes, as the majority of student-athletes have a smart phone and iTunes or Google Play accounts. This resource (available at http://davisplus.fadavis.com) provides a list of over 100 apps, most of which are free, that can be implemented based on the specific needs of the injury rehabilitation or athlete.

This educational discussion often includes a return-to-play timeline, which is difficult to discuss because of many unknowns. Unknowns may include rehabilitation setbacks or changes in pain tolerance or motivation. When athletes ask when they will return to play, it is customary for an athletic trainer to say, "I'm not exactly sure," or "It's too early to tell." However, these responses have limited effect in pacifying or educating athletes. It is common for the athletic trainer to want to be supportive and uplifting to athletes by telling them what they want to hear: "You'll make it back by playoffs." However, this can cause more stress and discouragement when that goal is left unmet. It is important to be factual with the athlete and present data that suggest the injury's typical recovery time, whereas also mentioning that there are many individual differences that affect the calculation. By providing evidence and estimates of recovery times, the athlete will have something realistic to set goals around in their quest to return to play. For example, in the case of the athlete who wants to begin to jog following an anterior cruciate ligament (ACL) repair, the athletic trainer should point out the typical timeline or reference the rehabilitation protocol outlining when that activity is appropriate. The athletic trainer can get information from the team physician and from various reputable journals, including *Journal of Athletic Training* and *The Physician and Sportsmedicine*, to guide the athlete to a realistic recovery timeline.

RED FLAG

Comparing athletes' progress with their peers' may seem useful and even motivating, but it is often a mistake; even though they may be the same gender, same sport, and have exactly the same injury, they may recover in completely different ways.

During the rehabilitation process, education remains important and is often a daily occurrence. Educating athletes about the progress of rehabilitation will keep them on track and may motivate them to continue attending rehabilitation sessions and to work hard (for more on psychosocial aspects of rehabilitation, see Chapter 8). Finally, during the rehabilitation process, athletes will commonly encounter pain. Education about what causes pain and the difference between "good" and "bad" pain is the role of the athletic trainer. When athletes experience pain, they may think more damage is being done to the injured area and fail to understand the efficacy of the prescribed exercise.

For example, one athletic trainer is working on knee flexion after ACL reconstruction. The process of getting to 90 degrees of range of motion (ROM) is extremely painful for the athlete. Thus, the athlete deduces that the athletic trainer is hurting the repaired ACL and begins to question his or her knowledge and the care being provided. This example is a perfect opportunity for the athletic trainer to educate the athlete by explaining that:

> *"Obtaining full range of motion is very important to returning the knee to full functional capacity. The pain that you are experiencing is not damaging your ACL or your surgical repair in any way. It is painful because we are breaking up scar tissue that has already begun to form and also, due to swelling in the area, making your knee feel tight. Both of these things are normal occurrences post-surgery, and it is essential to move your knee to facilitate healing. Again, we are not damaging your knee but improving the chances for it to heal appropriately."*

This example should lead the athletic trainer into a discussion with the athlete regarding education on the physiological and psychological aspects of pain and associated pain-management strategies that may reduce any discomfort experienced while attempting to achieve the prescribed ROM goals. These strategies may include relaxation techniques and pain association/disassociation techniques. These pain-management strategies are discussed at length in the next section of this chapter and reinforce the content discussed in Chapter 7.

CLINICAL TIP

Providing feedback is an important part of the perceived support often sought out by athletes from the athletic trainer and can be as simple as using text messaging. The athletic trainer can send daily messages to athletes to encourage and motivate them to come to rehabilitation; messages can also be used as appointment reminders and focusing cues for the athlete before rehabilitation. Goal setting can also happen via the use of mobile apps or mobile messaging. Considering the athletes of today, using the device at the center of their life (e.g., their iPhone or other smartphone) seems like a wonderful way to communicate with them. Athletes expect communication, approachability, and friendliness in an organized, professional, caring atmosphere.

The second important expectation of athletes is that, following injury, they will be spending time rehabilitating in an atmosphere that will be supportive, encouraging, and comfortable. Creating that atmosphere and meeting athletes' expectations has been shown to be related to patient satisfaction and recovery. So, how does the athletic trainer create this atmosphere in a chaotic, loud, busy athletic training room? Sometimes athletes who are sensitive to a busy environment can be scheduled for rehabilitation in the morning or at a less busy time for the athletic trainer. This might be more important in the early phases of rehabilitation when athletes are still learning how to function in their new role as injured athletes. Fostering a caring, open, and supportive atmosphere can be a challenge; however, an effective care provider stays focused and motivated in providing quality care by dedicating time and energy to the situation. The athletic trainer may benefit from trying the following three techniques to foster the environment: weekly and/or daily goal setting to improve focus and motivation and provide feedback to athletes, rehabilitation "menus" where athletes select their exercises for the day, and involving teammates in the rehabilitation sessions.

CLINICAL TIP

As part of an integrated approach to injury prevention and rehabilitation, posters can be placed on the walls in the athletic training room to remind athletes to use psychosocial strategies. For example, one could read, "What's your positive thought for today?"; another could say, "Got goals?"

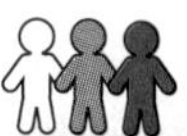

SPECIAL CONSIDERATIONS

Gender differences also play a role in effective care and patient satisfaction. Male and female athletes have varied needs when it comes to the rehabilitation setting, and the athletic trainer should be aware of these differing needs to best serve each gender. Research by Clement and Arvinen-Barrow et al. (2012)

Continued

found that the female athlete requires more time with the care provider and seeks a relationship and social support from the athletic trainer. The male athlete, in contrast, seeks education and leadership from the athletic trainer in the rehabilitation process. This research also suggests that the athletic trainer should provide special guidance and education to the first-time injured male athlete about the role he plays in the care process because this athlete often struggles with adherence and motivation in the rehabilitation setting.

ROLE OF PSYCHOSOCIAL STRATEGIES IN FACILITATING RECOVERY FROM ATHLETIC INJURY

Athletic trainers are educated on the selection and use of psychosocial strategies during the rehabilitation of athletic injury (Fifth Edition Athletic Training Education Competencies). Because the rehabilitation process is both physical and mental, it is the responsibility of the athletic trainer to notice when the athlete is struggling in rehabilitation and, when appropriate, to select an appropriate psychosocial strategy to manage the stressor. Because of the relationship between the athlete and athletic trainer, the athletic trainer is likely to know what the athlete may need even before the rehabilitation process begins. For example, if the athletic trainer is aware of the athlete's need for a lot of attention, they will schedule the rehabilitation sessions when the athlete can have the trainer's undivided attention (for a detailed description of the process of identifying potential barriers to rehabilitation, and identifying and implementing strategies to avoid or reduce these barriers, see Chapter 8). Making this adjustment to the schedule in advance shows the athlete that they are of importance and may be the key to the entire rehabilitation process.

The selection and use of psychosocial strategies should be guided by the phases of rehabilitation model. During the Reaction to Injury, phase 1, the athlete is likely to be panicked, in pain, and experiencing physical limitations. This phase includes immediately following injury (or surgery) up to the point of elimination of edema and achieving full ROM. Useful psychosocial strategies for phase 1 include relaxation techniques and ***healing imagery*** to manage pain, and goal setting and injury education to map out the rehabilitation plan.

Phase 2 of the rehabilitation process is the strengthening phase where the athlete must regain function and proprioception in preparation for return to play. Setting rehabilitation goals and maintaining motivation are key in this phase, especially for a longer (or surgical) rehabilitation. Self-talk and cognitive reframing/***thought stopping*** are also useful and easy to employ. ***Rehabilitation-process imagery*** can be useful if athletes are struggling with a specific aspect of rehabilitation or a certain exercise, and ***performance imagery*** can be used to help athletes maintain their sport-specific skills, particularly if they have long-term injuries.

Lastly, phase 3 of the rehabilitation process includes the fine-tuning of muscles and joint receptors with sport-specific exercises. Stressors surrounding a successful return to play are prominent in this phase and, if not managed, may lead to reinjury. Examples of stressors experienced by injured athletes preparing to return to play include worry about performance from coaches, team members, or bystanders; confidence in the rehabilitated limb; and the ability to execute new plays or strategies that happened in their absence. Useful psychosocial skills include performance imagery and self-talk to build self-confidence; self-talk can also be used in focusing routines to prepare the athlete mentally for "game day." More about each of these phases of rehabilitation is presented in Chapter 8.

As demonstrated earlier, these stressors can be grouped by phases of rehabilitation; however, they are often a daily occurrence in the process of rehabilitation. The athlete may worry about returning to play; meeting the expectations of coaches, parents, and teammates; regaining confidence in the injured limb; or managing the time demands of rehabilitation, practice, classes, work, and personal life. When these stressors are occupying athletes' minds, they have a harder time focusing on the goals of rehabilitation. Getting athletes to "leave their life at the door" when they come into the rehabilitation session is harder than it seems. The athletic trainer often serves as a sounding board for these stressors and acts in the role of social supporter. Following the listening phase, it might be effective to provide an exercise that focuses the athlete on the rehabilitation goals of the day. A summary of common athlete stressors paired with examples of useful psychosocial strategies is presented in Table 10-4; this table should serve as a starting point for the athletic trainer, keeping in mind that each athlete's stressors will be different and that athletes will respond to stressors and strategies in different ways. Do not be discouraged when the first strategy is not the answer to dissolving the stressor. There will also be cases where the athlete is resistant to the use of psychosocial strategies. In these cases, education about the effectiveness and use of the strategy may lessen the resistance and provide an opportunity for the athlete to experience a reduction in stress, resulting in a better rehabilitation experience.

Notice that each of the suggested strategies in Table 10-4 is supported by empirical evidence. One of the main reasons that psychosocial strategies rarely have been used in prior decades by athletic trainers and physical therapists is that there was much doubt about the effectiveness of such techniques. Providing the athlete with the benefits associated with using psychosocial strategies may improve effectiveness, ultimately improving rehabilitation outcomes. For example, if an athlete is struggling with pain associated with forced knee flexion, the athletic trainer may offer somatic relaxation during the ROM exercises. This psychosocial strategy assists in facilitating a relaxation response in the body (a reduction in cortisol), thereby reducing heart rate, breathing rate, and muscle spasm, as well as the sensation and perception of pain. Before implementing the strategy, the athletic trainer should educate the athlete on the benefits associated with a relaxed state, such as pain reduction and decreased muscle tension.

Acting almost as a salesperson, the athletic trainer should educate athletes on potential benefits of the strategy to guide the behavioral response that follows its use. The "experimenter effect," or the power of the athletic

TABLE 10-4 **Common Athlete Stressors and Effective Psychological Strategies**

Stressor	Psychosocial Strategy	Evidence
Pain in rehabilitation	Somatic or cognitive relaxation	Dawson, Hamson-Utley, et al (2014)
Negative self-talk	Thought stopping, cognitive reframing, positive affirmations, positive self-talk	Tod, Hardy, & Oliver (2011)
Intrinsic motivation issues	Goal setting, positive affirmations	Goal setting (e.g., Clement, Arvinen-Barrow, et al, 2012; Clement, Granquist, & Arvinen-Barrow, 2013)
Extrinsic motivation issues	Social support (coaches, teammates routed into the athletic training room)	Gillet, Vallerand, Amoura, & Baldes (2010) Mageau & Vallerand (2003)
Apprehension about the future	Education, communication, social support	Russell & Tracey (2011)
Balancing coursework and social activities with rehabilitation and attending practice	Time management App, goal setting, identifying priorities	Goal setting (e.g., Clement, Arvinen-Barrow, et al, 2012; Clement et al, 2013)
Managing setbacks	Education, goal setting, imagery, relaxation	Goal setting (e.g., Clement, Arvinen-Barrow, et al, 2012; Clement et al, 2013) Relaxation (Dawson, Hamson-Utley, et al (2014) Imagery (Walsh, 2005)

trainer's position as guide in the rehabilitation process, works almost as a placebo in this case. If it fails to work, nothing is lost, and another strategy could be selected and implemented. However, the athletic trainer should be careful in the selection of the first few strategies because athletes may lose confidence in the psychosocial strategies or the athletic trainer, or both. The next few sections outline the main psychosocial strategies and illustrate where they would be most effective in the rehabilitation setting.

PSYCHOSOCIAL STRATEGIES

As demonstrated earlier, both theoretical and empirical evidence exists in support of the usefulness of psychosocial strategies in benefiting injured athletes. For example, the integrated model of psychological response to sport injury (Wiese-Bjornstal et al, 1998) posits that use of psychosocial strategies (i.e., a behavioral response) can have an impact on how injured athletes cognitively appraise the injury (i.e., how they perceive the injury), as well as their emotional responses to the injury (i.e., how they feel about the injury). (For more details on this model, see Chapter 4.)

CLINICAL TIP

One of the first studies examining psychological care of the injured athlete found that use of psychosocial strategies during rehabilitation had an impact on the overall healing rate. In this study, "fast-healing" athletes were more likely to use psychosocial strategies such as self-talk, imagery, and goal setting than their "slow-healing" counterparts (Ievleva & Orlick, 1991). Athletic trainers should move to a holistic care model of the injured athlete, including both mind and body exercises to facilitate healing.

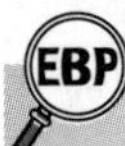

EVIDENCE-BASED PRACTICE

Evans, L., Hardy, L., & Fleming, S. (2000). Intervention strategies with injured athletes: An action research study. *The Sport Psychologist, 14,* 188–206.

Description of the Study

Guided by Action Research methodology, the study sought to longitudinally investigate psychological interventions with injured athletes during rehabilitation. Participants in this study were three elite-level rugby players, all of whom had sustained serious injuries (e.g., shoulder dislocation, tibia-fibula fracture, ACL rupture) while participating in their sport. Psychological skills interventions were provided by a sports psychologist during both in-person and phone consultations. Data were collected from consultations with the participants, consultations with the physiotherapist, participants' diaries, consultation case notes, and semistructured interviews on conclusion of the study.

Results of the Study

The common psychological skills that were used with these athletes were social support, goal setting, imagery, and, to a lesser degree, simulation training and verbal persuasion. Social support was provided in the forms of emotional support and task support, with goal setting serving as a form of task support. In the early phases of rehabilitation, the development of process goals (as opposed to outcome goals) was most helpful to the athletes, particularly as pain and swelling were less predictable in the early stages. The goals specified met the standard goal-setting principles (i.e., specific, measurable, challenging but realistic), yet were flexible in that the athletes could base the goals on their fluctuating pain levels. In addition, reframing barriers or obstacles into challenges served as a basis for goals. The loss of athletic identity was an issue for these athletes, and performance and process goals were used to reinforce behaviors that were necessary to complete rehabilitation and return to participation. As rehabilitation progressed, goal setting continued to play a role in rehabilitation adherence. However, pain and healing setbacks were barriers to goal setting during this phase of rehabilitation. During the late stages of rehabilitation and return to participation, psychological skills to increase the athletes' confidence were viewed as crucial in their successful return to sport. During this time, the primary psychological skills used were simulation training and imagery. The role of the coaching staff should be emphasized in structuring practice sessions to help athletes regain confidence in their rehabilitated body part, particularly in the later stages of rehabilitation.

Implications for Athletic Training Practice

In addition to providing social support, goal setting for motivation and confidence in the injured body part on return to participation are two areas in which athletic trainers can focus psychological skills training. For example, having athletes perform a 1-minute single-leg stand brings their attention to the successful performance of this rehabilitation exercise. In addition, having athletes focus on foot action in walking and jogging brings their attention to the ambulation process. To increase athletes' confidence in their injured body parts, athletic trainers can use functional progression testing (e.g., jogging, running, figure eights). Athletic trainers can also encourage athletes to use imagery to visualize themselves performing successful plays (e.g., tackling in soccer, sliding in softball). Loss of athletic identity may be very salient for athletes who are facing a long rehabilitation; athletic trainers can help frame rehabilitation as a performance that requires effort, focus, and commitment similar to performing on the field. Finally, if sport psychology consultants are available and are part of the sports medicine team, athletic trainers should encourage athletes to work with consultants as a resource to learn psychological skills that can be beneficial in both rehabilitation and return to participation and then continued into their sporting career.

Other benefits of using psychosocial strategies during rehabilitation include (but are not limited to): increased feelings of personal control over rehabilitation (Durso-Cupal, 1996), assistance in coping with stressful situations, and improved communication between the individuals involved in the rehabilitation process. All of these factors can be regarded as important for successful recovery. For example, athletes who feel they are "in charge" of their rehabilitation tend to take greater levels of ownership of the rehabilitation process; subsequently, their motivation and adherence to a rehabilitation program will be amplified. Also, having the ability to cope effectively with the injury and stressful situations is vital for successful rehabilitation, because rarely is any injury recovery process stress-free, linear, and uncomplicated. Almost all athletes will face setbacks and challenges during the injury-rehabilitation process; however, with high levels of dedication and necessary coping skills, successful recovery is a likely outcome. In a similar manner, good communication between medical professionals and injured athletes can also facilitate athletes' greater understanding of the actual injury and injury process, and subsequently affect the positive recovery outcomes.

As discussed in Chapter 8, the psychosocial strategies and skills that athletes learn as part of their athletic experience are transferrable to the rehabilitation setting (Fig. 10-5). Rehabilitation can simply be viewed as another performance domain, and the rehabilitation period can serve as an opportunistic time to learn new psychological skills that can be transferred back to the playing field.

However, despite many athletes of all levels reporting frequent use of the earlier mentioned strategies for performance enhancement and the apparent benefits within sport injury rehabilitation, it appears athletes seldom transfer these skills from the performance-enhancement setting to rehabilitation. In their research exploring athletes' use of psychosocial strategies during injury rehabilitation, Clement and Hamson-Utley et al. (2012) found that less than a third of athletes indicated using mental skills during sport injury rehabilitation; however, of those who did, nearly two thirds reported that these skills helped them recover more quickly. Moreover, less than a third of the athletes stated that mental skills were taught by a sports medicine professional such as an athletic trainer or

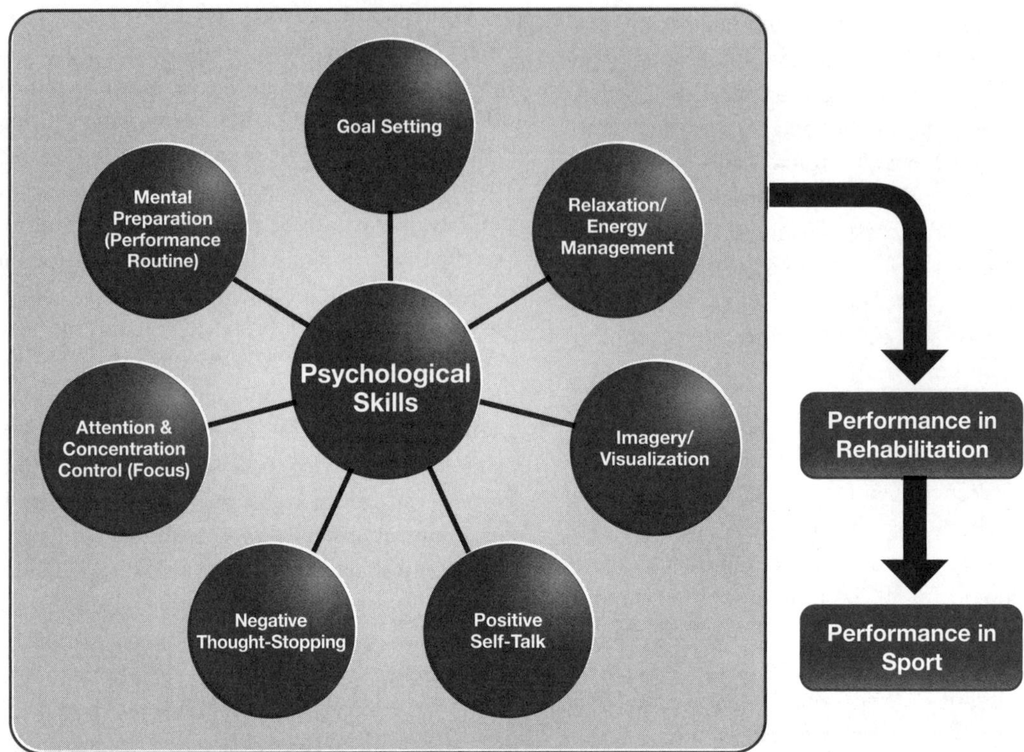

Figure 10-5 | Common psychological skills.

a physiotherapist, rather than a sports psychology professional. Therefore, this is an area that athletic trainers can and should address when working with athletes during rehabilitation. The following section discusses psychosocial strategies that athletic trainers can incorporate into athletes' rehabilitation.

Psychosocial Strategies During Rehabilitation: Strategies to Meet the Individual Athlete's Needs

Thus far, a number of psychosocial interventions have been proposed as useful during the rehabilitation process (refer to Table 10-4). Drawing from the literature on what sports medicine professionals think are important characteristics in distinguishing which athletes cope well with their injuries, the most commonly identified characteristics include adherence/nonadherence with rehabilitation; having a positive/negative attitude; level of motivation; presence of negative mood such as stress, anxiety, or depression; and level of understanding and knowledge of the injury. As such, the introduction and description of the key psychosocial strategies (i.e., positive self-talk, imagery, relaxation techniques, and goal setting) believed to be useful for athletic trainers to use during sport injury rehabilitation are described in relation to the key characteristics for successful rehabilitation as outlined earlier. This does not mean that such strategies are useful only when dealing with the issues with which they are associated in this chapter; they could be beneficial in other ways too. What is presented in this section is merely an example and demonstration of how these psychosocial strategies could be used in rehabilitation. It should be used as a guideline rather than a "prescription" that fits all injured athletes.

Using Self-Talk to Change the Mind-Set and Ways of Thinking

One of the key defining characteristics of an athlete who copes successfully with injuries is an ability to remain positive during the rehabilitation and recovery process.

Indeed, because injuries are typically seen as negative, often the conversations athletes have with themselves are negative, and therefore potentially harmful. Existing theoretical frameworks indicate that these thoughts can influence their emotions and behaviors, as well as subsequent overall rehabilitation and recovery outcomes. Two main self-talk techniques can be used to assist athletes in changing their mind-set from debilitative to facilitative: thought stopping and reframing.

Thought Stopping

Thought stopping in the context of sport injury can be seen as an activity aimed at deliberately assisting injured athletes with shaping the sport injury and rehabilitation-related thinking (Fig. 10-6). The basic principle behind thought stopping is two-fold: (1) to stop an inappropriate thought, and (2) to allow that thought to be replaced by a more functional and purposeful thought. For example, an athlete may think, *I am never*

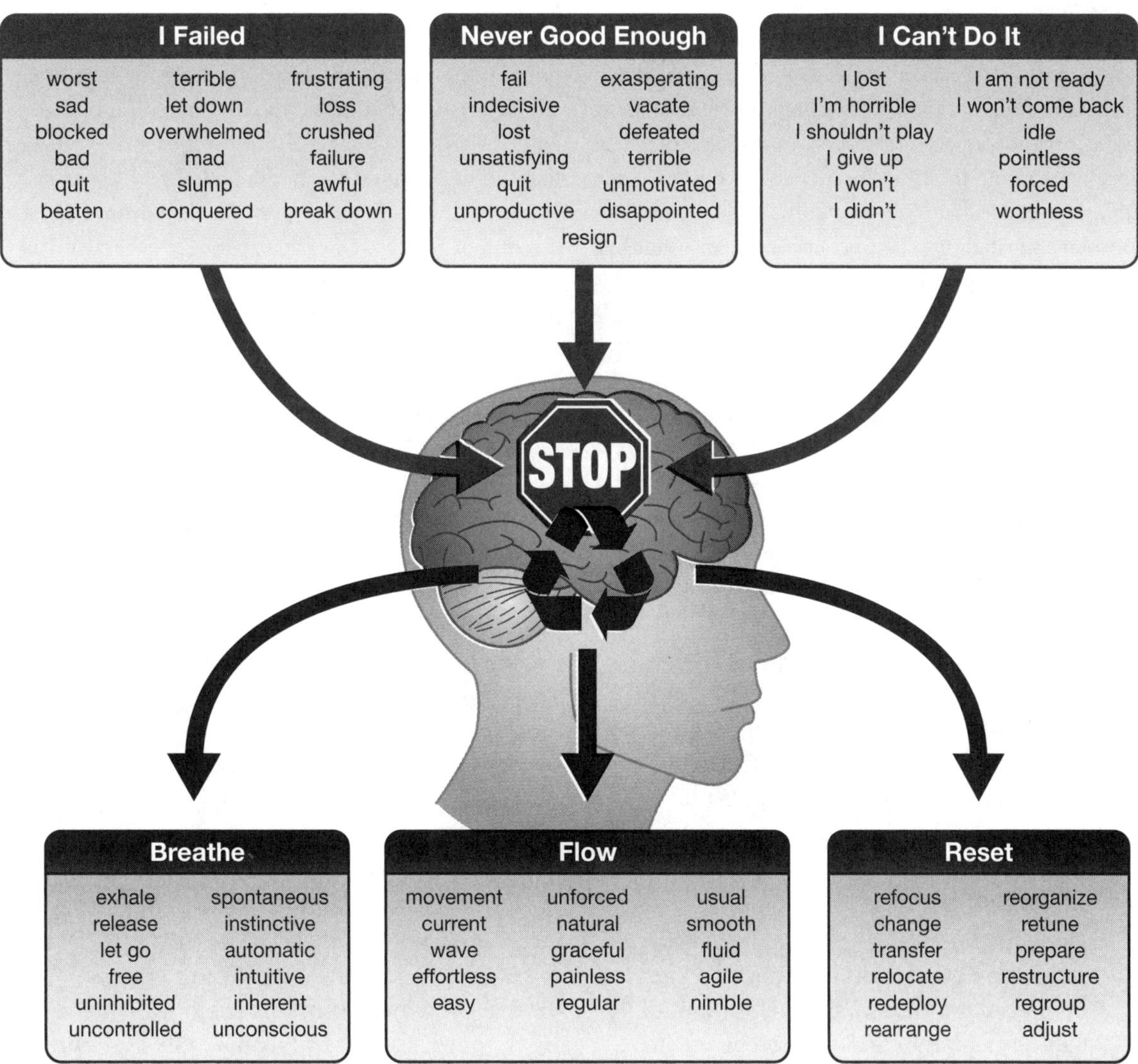

Figure 10-6 | Thought stopping.

going to get back to the level of fitness I was before I got injured. This can then have an impact on the athlete's overall mood, feelings toward the injury and rehabilitation, as well as motivation. By changing the thought into *By doing these exercises, I am now focusing on areas I would not normally have time to focus on. When I return to sport, I will be stronger than I was before I got injured,* the athlete can refocus on areas of rehabilitation that he or she can control, and thus provide a more positive and "purposeful" rehabilitation environment.

Reframing

Another way to influence athletes' thinking during sport injury rehabilitation is through reframing. As noted earlier, many athletes experience feelings of stress, anxiety, and depression as a result of sport injuries, all of which have been found to influence successful coping. When athletes are faced with a potentially stress- or anxiety-provoking situation, or they experience depressive thoughts about their injury and rehabilitation situation, there is a need to challenge their thinking. The basic principle behind reframing is not to try and change the athlete's situation but, rather, to change the ways in which the athlete appraises it. In other words, if athletes appraise the upcoming rehabilitation as "time wasted away from their sport," reframing their thinking into seeing rehabilitation as an "excellent opportunity to focus on building core strength and stamina to be better at sport" can have a positive impact on athletes' overall mood, behavior, and recovery outcome (Box 10-1).

Using Imagery for Maintaining Focus and Being Positive

The abilities to stay positive and to focus on the rehabilitation and the task at hand have also been found to be key characteristics of athletes who are successful in coping with their injuries. One of the psychosocial strategies that can help injured athletes in both aspects is imagery. Imagery in the context of sport has been defined as "the creation or re-creation of an experience generated from memorial information, involving quasi-sensorial, quasi-perceptual, and quasi-affective characteristics, that is

BOX 10-1 | Things to Consider When Implementing Self-Talk with Injured Athletes

1. The key to successful implementation of self-talk is to identify the type of self-talk athletes are currently engaging in and whether this self-talk is indeed harmful or beneficial in their recovery.
2. Once the athletes' existing use of self-talk has been identified, it is important to identify the purpose and desired outcome of the self-talk used. More specifically, the function of self-talk (motivational vs. instructional) needs to be identified to design appropriate self-talk statements.
3. Once the purpose and function of self-talk have been identified, attention should be placed on the actual development of self-talk statements. Research seems to suggest that self-determined self-talk will offer more motivational benefits for athletes than self-talk assigned by another person such as an athletic trainer (Hardy, 2006).
4. It is also imperative to pay attention to the actual wording of the self-talk. That is, sometimes athletes may use so-called negative self-talk to psych themselves up, and as such it may be beneficial.
5. Once athletes have identified the self-talk statements, focus should be placed on the way in which these statements are implemented. Some athletes appear to prefer to talk to themselves in a very overt manner (i.e., talk aloud to themselves), whereas others prefer to engage in more covert self-talk (i.e., talk to themselves through an inner dialogue).

under the volitional control of the imager, and which may occur in the absence of the real stimulus antecedents normally associated with the actual experience" (Morris, Spittle, & Watt, 2005, p. 14). In sport injury rehabilitation, this can be seen as an activity in which the athlete can create images of the following (but not limited to): the healing process, the injured body part fully healed and restored to normal levels of functioning, the rehabilitation setting, successfully completing rehabilitation exercises, and successfully dealing with pain and any emotions associated with the injury and recovery process. Typically, injured athletes feel vulnerable and confused about their situation and have uncertainties about their future. These feelings can be exacerbated by tiredness, which is typically caused by a lack of sleep—often a consequence of physical pain and increased levels of worry and anxiety. By imagining different aspects of the injury, rehabilitation, and healing process, athletes can be helped to regain their focus and, as a consequence, to be motivated and positive during the rehabilitation process. Four main types of imagery may be beneficial to injured athletes: (1) healing imagery, (2) ***pain-management imagery***, (3) rehabilitation-process imagery, and (4) performance imagery.

Healing Imagery

Healing imagery is typically used to visualize the internal processes and anatomical/physical healing that take place during rehabilitation (e.g., imagining a broken bone becoming healed). For healing imagery to be effective, it is important for athletes to have a good understanding of their injury, possess an ability to recreate a realistic picture of the injured area, and have an awareness of the anatomical healing process. They should also understand the treatment modalities used and have a clear knowledge of what the injured body part should look like once healed. Such knowledge and understanding can be facilitated by the athletic trainer, mainly in the form of educating athletes about their injuries, as well as showing them pictures and possibly videos about the injured area at different stages of rehabilitation. However, given the complexity of the human body, it can be assumed that engagement in successful healing imagery requires not only knowledge and training, but also a great deal of time commitment from both injured athletes and their athletic trainers.

> **VIRTUAL FIELD TRIP**
>
> Using existing Internet resources is an effective approach for a busy athletic trainer who cannot create healing imagery scripts for injured athletes. These scripts, or podcasts, function as education and positive guides to the healing process. See examples of healing imagery scripts at http://davisplus.fadavis.com.

Pain-Management Imagery

Pain-management imagery is typically used to assist injured athletes in better coping with pain, alleviating pain, subsequently remaining more positive, and ultimately, coping with their injuries. In pain-management imagery, injured athletes will create images of themselves free of pain. Useful pain-management imagery techniques for sport-injury rehabilitation include pleasant imagining (seeing yourself lying on the grass free from pain), pain association (the pain is seen as having physical properties such as color, size, shape, sounds, and feelings), and dramatized coping (pain seen as part of a challenge and subsequently reframed as a motivational tool). Dissociative and associative strategies for pain management (such as pain-management imagery) are discussed in detail in Chapter 7.

Rehabilitation-Process Imagery

Rehabilitation-process imagery is typically used at different stages of rehabilitation and should be an integral part of any sport injury rehabilitation program. The main aim of rehabilitation-process imagery is to help injured athletes to maintain or regain focus on rehabilitation and to cope with the challenges and setbacks that come during rehabilitation. Rehabilitation-process imagery can have two main functions: either to instruct (e.g., help athletes in completing specific tasks and skills successfully) or to motivate (e.g., help athletes to see themselves completing required exercises, overcoming setbacks and obstacles, and dealing with rehabilitation-related challenges).

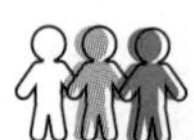

SPECIAL CONSIDERATIONS

It is important for athletic trainers to know their athletes before suggesting they pair with other athletes who are undergoing rehabilitation from injury. If athletes have low self-esteem or are likely to feel less accomplished when paired with someone who is "bigger, faster, stronger" than they are, the pairing of athletes should be avoided. Being cautious about pairing athletes or creating rehabilitation teams during the recovery process because of the potential for unhealthy competition may limit exercise role modeling and motivation opportunities. Athletic trainers can turn to rehabilitation-process imagery to assist athletes who may not do well in the face of competition while injured.

Performance Imagery

Performance imagery is typically used to help injured athletes get back to play, particularly to have the confidence to return to sport. As with rehabilitation-process imagery, performance imagery can also take two main forms: to instruct (i.e., rehearse sport-specific skills and strategies) and to motivate (i.e., see themselves back in the podium and back at play performing successfully and injury free). Because athletes often perceive their injuries as an unnecessary time away from their sport, performance imagery can also be useful in allowing athletes to recognize gains in other areas of performance, which has the potential to increase their motivation and improve the rehabilitation process (Box 10-2).

Managing Pain Through Relaxation Techniques

Particularly in the early stages of rehabilitation, pain can be the leading cause of many psychosocial "dysfunctions" and act as a hindrance to the rehabilitation progress.

BOX 10-2 | Things to Consider When Implementing Imagery with Injured Athletes

1. The key to successful imagery implementation is to identify the purpose of the imagery intervention and the desired outcome. According to Arvinen-Barrow and colleagues (2013), this can be done by using a sound theoretical approach to determine the desired outcome and, as such, the type of imagery required to reach the outcome.
2. Next, identify the athletes' current use of imagery. More specifically, the function of imagery (i.e., instructional, motivational, or healing) needs to be identified to design appropriate imagery scripts.
3. Once the purpose and function of imagery have been identified, attention should be placed on the actual development of the imagery script. Giving the athlete ownership of the content of the images is likely to result in more committed athletes, thus making the imagery intervention more effective.
4. It is also imperative to pay attention to the perspective of the athletes' preferred imagery. This could mean taking into consideration all senses (e.g., visual, kinesthetic, and olfactory), as well as whether the images are best viewed from an internal (seeing from within) or external (like watching oneself from a television) perspective.
5. The earlier actions should then be followed by a step-by step approach to train and implement the imagery into the rehabilitation program (for more details, see Arvinen-Barrow et al, 2013).

As identified earlier, the key characteristics in distinguishing athletes who cope well or do not cope well with their injuries include adherence/nonadherence to rehabilitation; having positive/negative attitude; level of motivation; and presence of negative moods such as stress, anxiety, and depression. All of these characteristics can be a direct or indirect result of pain; athletes can become nonadherent to rehabilitation when pain becomes too much to bear, and attitude can become negative because of lack of sleep and increased levels of irritation resulting from pain, which, in turn, can affect motivation. More importantly, pain can also lead to a range of negative mood disturbances, including (but not limited to) anxiety, irritation, frustration, and depression. To assist athletes in coping with pain, two common relaxation techniques can be used; these are deep breathing and progressive muscle relaxation (PMR).

Deep Breathing

Having the ability to breathe correctly is central to human functioning and informs the core of our physical and psychological functioning. Unfortunately, many of us are unable to breathe correctly, particularly during times of distress. When an individual is distressed, the sympathetic nervous system is activated; as a result, normal breathing patterns are altered, thus making breathing shorter. Often individuals will "forget how to breathe in" and, as a result, inhale less oxygen, subsequently further amplifying the feelings of stress and anxiety. Focusing on breathing normally (i.e., deeper and in a regular pattern) can assist athletes both cognitively and somatically. Focusing on the correct breathing can act as a distraction from worrying thoughts, and increased oxygen intake can relieve muscle tension and other physiological symptoms of distress. Several breathing techniques can be used with injured athletes. Research advocates the use of diaphragmatic and ratio breathing as the most easily applicable techniques during sport-injury rehabilitation.

Diaphragmatic Breathing

The aim of diaphragmatic breathing is for athletes to become aware of how their rib cage moves (expand-recoil) as they inhale and exhale. Often this is best achieved while lying down rather than standing up. To fully engage in diaphragmatic breathing, athletes should be educated about how the lungs and diaphragm work. Use of diaphragmatic breathing can be most beneficial in helping athletes to regain their focus on the task at hand (e.g., different rehabilitation exercises, the rehabilitation session, and tasks that require great attention to detail).

Ratio Breathing

Ratio breathing aims to direct athletes' focus away from distracting thoughts and feelings of distress (e.g., pain) to their breathing by purposefully altering the length of inhalations and exhalations. In ratio breathing, focus the athlete on the number of inhalations (count to four or five) in comparison with exhalations (typically count to seven). It would be beneficial for injured athletes to understand the arousal–nervous system relationship, particularly the role of ratio breathing in activating the parasympathetic nervous system to assist them in regaining a relaxed state. Ratio breathing can easily be applied to a range of situations, and it works well both lying down and standing up. This technique can be extremely useful for athletes engaging in negative self-talk and for those experiencing high levels of cognitive and somatic anxiety, negative arousal, or pain.

Both diaphragmatic and ratio breathing are underpinned by a few basic principles and procedures. Most importantly, all breathing should be based on the principle of *breathe in through the nose and out from the mouth.* In terms of the process of implementing deep breathing, the athletic trainer should teach the technique using a series of steps (Box 10-3).

Progressive Muscle Relaxation

In a sporting context, PMR (Jacobson, 1938) is said to be the most commonly used and taught technique. The aim of PMR is to teach athletes awareness of their body becoming tense by teaching them how to relax different muscle groups. The basic principle underlying PMR is tensing and relaxing different muscle groups sequentially, by first tensing one group, holding the tension (usually for a count of 7 to 10), releasing the tension, and then proceeding to the next muscle group. This procedure is used on every muscle group throughout the body. When initially learning PMR, this process of tensing-relaxing the muscle groups across the body can take up to 30 minutes to complete; however, over time, the time needed to relax the whole body can vary

BOX 10-3 | Steps to Follow When Implementing Relaxation Techniques with Injured Athletes

1. Identify athletes' current understanding and experience of using deep-breathing techniques.
2. Depending on their current need, athletes should be educated about the principles and benefits of deep breathing.
3. Next, identify the purpose and desired outcome of relaxation techniques. More specifically, select an appropriate breathing technique to match the desired outcome.
4. Choose your preferred position for the relaxation training. Many of the deep-breathing exercises can be done either standing up (e.g., ratio breathing) or lying down (e.g., diaphragmatic breathing), depending on the athletes' preference and relaxation skill level.
5. When implementing deep-breathing techniques, the aim is to facilitate athletes' awareness of their regular breathing patterns.
6. Mastering deep breathing will take time. For deep-breathing training to be effective, it is important to consider the practicalities of incorporating it into athletes' routines.

from 30 seconds to 20 minutes. PMR can be beneficial for injured athletes, particularly when they are experiencing high levels of pain and anxiety. By focusing on raising awareness of tenseness in the body, athletes can recognize sources that make them tense, thus becoming more in control of their own situation, which ultimately leads to reduced levels of anxiety and discomfort (Box 10-4).

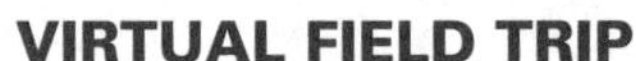

VIRTUAL FIELD TRIP

PMR scripts can be created by the athletic trainer or accessed online. Examples are available at http://davisplus.fadavis.com.

Using Goal Setting to Increase Motivation and Facilitate Adherence

Of all the psychosocial strategies presented in this chapter, goal setting appears to be the most used technique among athletic trainers and athletes alike. Because many athletes experience varying levels of motivation during the different phases of rehabilitation, goal setting can be a useful tool in helping them remain focused and motivated, and subsequently to adhere better to their rehabilitation. In addition to the above, setting goals during rehabilitation is important because it allows injured athletes to regain control of their situation. Sport injury, due to its nature, is something that athletes were not expecting or wanting to experience, and as such, they typically feel they have lost control of their situation and often rely solely on their rehabilitation professional to help them get better. When setting goals for rehabilitation, there are four main types of goals to consider: (1) physical, (2) psychological, (3) performance, and (4) lifestyle goals. Consider each of these goals at three different levels: (1) immediate daily goals, (2) medium-term rehabilitation process/stage goals, and (3) ultimate recovery/outcome goals (Fig. 10-7).

Physical Goals

In the context of injury rehabilitation, physical goals can include goals related to a number of physical parameters such as ROM, strength, stamina, stability, flexibility, and coordination. These are typically relatively easy to establish and often best set with the athletic trainer, because they are the experts in physical aspects of the healing process. By setting physical goals, athletes can gain a sense of control and ownership over the rehabilitation, which

BOX 10-4 | Things to Consider When Implementing Relaxation Techniques with Injured Athletes

1. **Physical location.** The key to successful implementation of relaxation training is to ensure the physical space used is favorable to relaxation. Make sure the environment is warm, quiet, and comfortable, to allow athletes to fully focus on getting relaxed and not be distracted by others. Thus, factors in relation to location, body position, and clothing should be considered. Once athletes master the relaxation, then the importance of physical location becomes less significant.
2. **Education.** Relaxation is a skill, and it needs to be practiced and learned for it to be effective (Flint, 1998). If the athletes you are working with have difficulty relaxing, and, by trying to relax, they appear to be more agitated, then consider not implementing relaxation during rehabilitation. Because being injured already provokes anxiety, there is no need to ask athletes to start practicing something that will increase levels of anxiety even further.
3. **Timing of relaxation practice.** Using relaxation techniques for a few minutes at the start of the rehabilitation can be beneficial. When entering rehabilitation sessions, athletes typically come in straight from daily hassles, and their mind may be preoccupied with a number of thoughts not related to the process of recovery (e.g., thoughts about life in general, anxieties about getting better, or feelings of pain). Deep-breathing techniques at the start of the rehabilitation session can help athletes regain their focus and hence perform better during the session.
4. **Level of relaxation.** According to Crossman (2001), there are three levels of relaxation: symbolic level (breathing comes deeper and slower), mental level (feelings of sense of calm and a shift in focus toward reasserting control over the body), and physical level (learned over time). Depending on the desired outcome of the relaxation (i.e., to help athletes regain focus on rehabilitation or to assist them in reducing pain they are experiencing), the desired relaxation level can vary. Typically in a sport injury setting, the aim of relaxation should be to reach symbolic level and potentially aspects of mental-level relaxation.

will, in turn, facilitate feelings of "being in the know." Goal setting should be a collaborative process, where the athletes and athletic trainers set goals together as a shared task. This will, in turn, assist athletes in their appraisals of the injury (e.g., "I know how serious this is and how to get better."), as well as their emotional (e.g., ability to control changes in mood) and behavioral coping (e.g., adherence). Physical goals are beneficial for all athletes throughout the rehabilitation process and beyond.

Psychological Goals

Psychological goals can have many functions during injury rehabilitation. Often psychological goals can be used to address issues with motivation, adherence, confidence, and levels of arousal. These goals should always be used in conjunction with physical goals, and often some of the physical aspects of rehabilitation are intertwined with psychological goals. For example, if the aim is to increase confidence, athletes' ability to "see" progress can be an

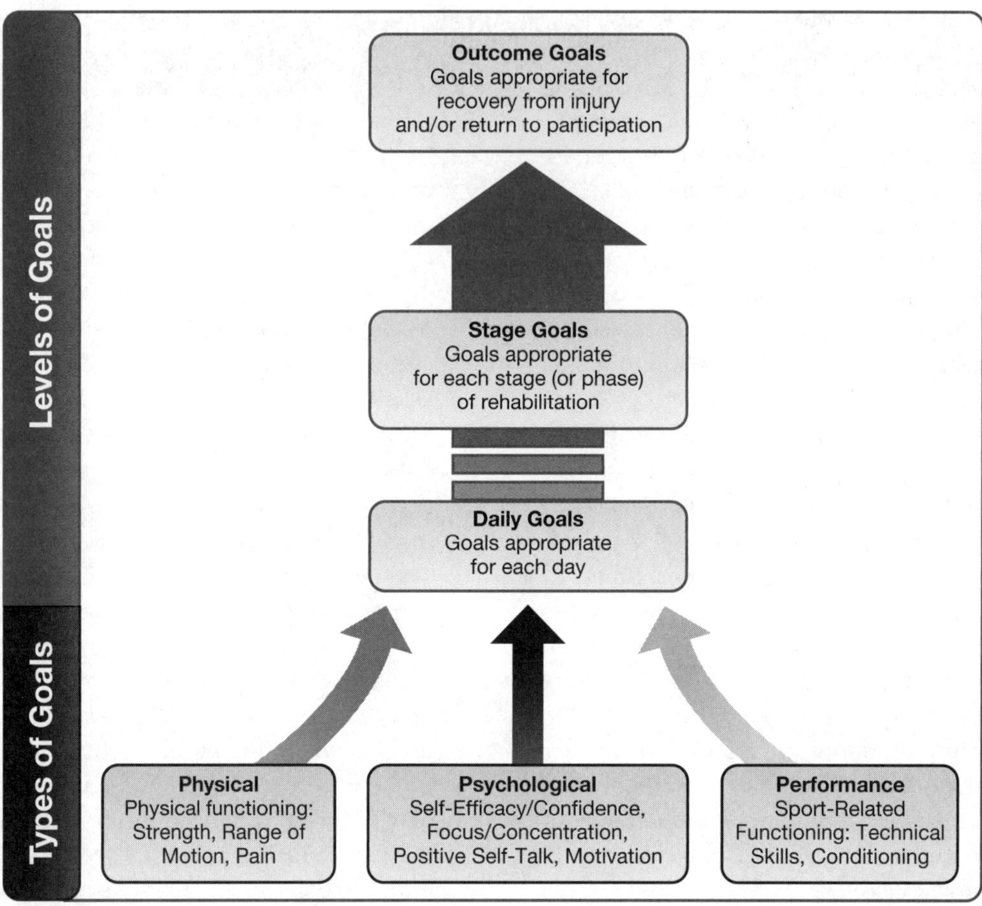

Figure 10-7 | Goal setting chart.

excellent facilitator of confidence. As such, the physical goals should be set in such a way as to help athletes regain their confidence (i.e., small, manageable, and short-term goals). As with physical goals, psychological goals are vital throughout the rehabilitation process to ensure athletes' cognitive appraisals and emotional and behavioral responses are favorable toward successful recovery (Box 10-5).

Performance Goals

Performance goals are ones that athletes may set together with their athletic trainer, a number of other allied health professionals, and the coach during rehabilitation in hopes of improving areas of performance they may not typically have "time for" but which they now, because of their injury, have an excellent opportunity to address. Setting performance goals may mean that professionals such as a strength and conditioning coach, biomechanist, or sports psychologist need to be consulted to ensure the goals set and implemented are the right kind and are implemented appropriately. For example, athletes may typically have poor stress-management skills during competitions; these stress-management techniques could be rehearsed during rehabilitation (and would also help the rehabilitation). Or, athletes may need some adjustment of their technique, and therefore use of their coach would be a benefit. Performance goals could be used throughout rehabilitation, particularly with the aim of assisting athletes in returning to sport.

BOX 10-5 | Issues to Consider When Setting Goals for Rehabilitation

1. Athletes should be educated about the process of goal setting in rehabilitation (Arvinen-Barrow & Hemmings, 2013).
2. Next, their personal and physical needs for successful rehabilitation and recovery should be identified and assessed. This process should be done in cooperation with the athlete, athletic trainer, and potentially, coaches. It would also be important to establish the need for setting lifestyle goals (because sometimes athletes already know what to do, these may not need to be specifically set, but they should be addressed).
3. After identifying the areas to address during rehabilitation, appropriate physical, psychological, and performance goals should be identified and set. Goals set should be appropriate for the purpose and should follow basic principles of goal setting (for more details, see Arvinen-Barrow & Hemmings, 2013).
4. Following the identification and setting of goals, possible factors that affect goal-setting effectiveness need to be considered. These can include (but are not limited to) issues with adherence, goal acceptance, and goal monitoring.
5. This should then be followed by step-by-step implementation of goals in the rehabilitation process.
6. When setting goals during rehabilitation, this should be a joint process between the athlete and the rehabilitation professional. Often this process can and should also involve other important stakeholders such as coaches and a range of allied health professionals. Typically, research seems to suggest that, although medical professionals are good at setting "targets" for rehabilitation, they often fail to include the athlete in the process (Arvinen-Barrow, Penny, Hemmings, & Corr, 2010).

CLINICAL TIP

Active rest is a term used to describe a safe activity that athletes can complete while injured. This typically involves activity of body parts other than those immediately adjacent to the injury. For example, athletes can lift weights with the upper body (guided by the strength coach) while they have a walking cast on a stress-fractured foot. This enablement of athletes to engage in physical activity is connected to fostering self-esteem and bolstering confidence in their return to participation.

Lifestyle Goals

Given that injury rehabilitation is typically a lifestyle-changing event, it is important to consider a number of lifestyle goals. These will typically consist of goals in relation to sleep, diet, and overall daily living. Athletes who are accustomed to training in excess of 10 to 20 hours a week will have to make adjustments in their daily routines and diet to ensure their overall fitness and health do not suffer because of long-term injury. When setting lifestyle goals, it is often appropriate to include Registered Dietitians (RDs) or individuals with sports nutrition expertise. To ensure successful implementation of lifestyle goals throughout rehabilitation, it is also important to include athletes' significant others in the process, because they will typically have a role in a range of aspects of athletes' lives.

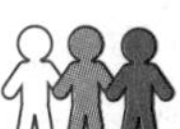

SPECIAL CONSIDERATIONS

When athletes are removed from sport because of injury, it is important for their athletic trainers to watch for signs of them developing eating disorders. Both male and female

Continued

athletes are at risk for development of an eating disorder when their activity is halted and their eating behaviors remain the same. Consulting an RD for this aspect of injury rehabilitation is essential to athletes' holistic care. This member of the sports medicine team should be included in the referral network of every athletic trainer. To find an RD in your area, visit http://www.eatright.org/iframe/findrd.aspx (connect through http://davisplus.fadavis.com).

"I Feel So Much Better Now That I Know": The Role of Education in Rehabilitation

One of the key characteristics that define injured athletes who cope well with their injuries is their apparent understanding of and knowledge about their injury and the rehabilitation process. By knowing what is going on and what is to come, athletes can alleviate a range of psychosocial responses relatively easily and also stop possible hindrances from emerging. For example, athletes who know the level of pain that is considered normal at different stages of rehabilitation are less likely to have negative thoughts associated with pain and also experience less injury- and rehabilitation-related stress and anxiety. Similarly, athletes who understand their injury and the steps required to get better again are more likely to take greater levels of ownership of their rehabilitation, and thus be more motivated and adherent to rehabilitation.

Educating athletes is paramount in ensuring successful recovery. Education is one of the key strategies that can affect injured athletes psychosocially. By increasing their understanding and knowledge, their cognitive appraisal of the situation can be altered (e.g., more accurate self-perceptions and expectations), their emotional responses can be facilitated (e.g., less frustrations and feelings of self-doubt), and their behavioral responses can be improved (e.g., better adherence to and use of psychosocial strategies to help deal with injury-related factors). Education is not only an important component; it is also an integral part of any other psychosocial strategy (see Boxes 10-1, 10-2, 10-4, and 10-5).

Educating injured athletes is important in many contexts. They need to be educated about the details of the injury, the rehabilitation process (including the different phases of rehabilitation), and how their cognitions, emotions, and behaviors can affect the overall outcome. They should also be educated regarding the different physical and psychosocial strategies they can use to facilitate healing and recovery, and how to implement these strategies successfully into practice (Box 10-6).

Implementing Psychosocial Strategies in Rehabilitation

Starting the process of implementing psychosocial strategies may be challenging for athletic trainers, and

BOX 10-6 | Issues to Consider When Implementing Education in Rehabilitation

1. Educating athletes is an important aspect of any rehabilitation. It should be done by a trusted person who is knowledgeable about the different aspects of rehabilitation.
2. One of the key characteristics of successful education is effective communication. Being able to actively listen to athletes and to discuss concepts related to the injury and rehabilitation in language that is easily understood by them is imperative for building trust and rapport, and thus effective education.
3. Educating athletes about their injury and rehabilitation is an ongoing process and should not be limited to rehabilitation. Educating athletes about how to cope with stress and anxiety can also help reduce the risk for injury or reinjury (for more details on how to minimize the risk for injury, see Chapter 3).

this may be a barrier to incorporating these strategies and skills into athletes' care. One way that the athletic trainer can introduce these strategies is to use a self-report survey to help athletes self-identify areas of psychosocial strengths and improvement areas. The Athletic Coping Skills Inventory (Smith et al, 1995) is one such instrument that can measure athletes' psychosocial skills.

The Athletic Coping Skills Inventory contains 28 items and has 7 subscales: coachability, concentration, confidence and achievement motivation, goal setting and mental preparation, peaking under pressure, coping with adversity, and freedom from worry. Athletic trainers can use this inventory in a variety of ways. During preseason, athletes can complete this inventory to help self-identify areas in which they can improve; the sports medicine team could also use this inventory to identify athletes who may be at risk for injury, thus offering prevention efforts using psychological skills training. In addition, this inventory could be used during the three phases of rehabilitation; again, athletes could self-identify areas in which they can improve or athletic trainers could identify areas in which athletes may benefit from additional training. Alternately, this inventory could identify athletes' strengths to build on during rehabilitation. For example, if athletes rate high on the peaking under pressure subscale (which measures if they are challenged or threatened by pressure situations), the athletic trainer could build on the athletes' strength by making them aware of it. The athletic trainer can point out that while rehabilitation and return to participation can be stressful, the athletes are mentally tough and capable of viewing this as a positive challenge rather than a negative threat.

Athletic trainers, however, may feel they are limited in their ability to integrate these skills before injury occurs. As such, three common barriers to athletic trainers' use of psychological skills with athletes undergoing injury rehabilitation are knowledge, time, and resources. As outlined in this chapter, entry-level athletic trainers are expected to have knowledge related to psychosocial aspects of athletic injury. Incorporating these knowledge competencies and integrating the associated clinical proficiencies into practice may help athletic trainers feel competent and confident in their abilities to holistically care for athletes. Furthermore, athletes expect the athletic trainer to be knowledgeable about psychosocial strategies that would be helpful to them in their recovery and to offer evidence-based care strategies when available.

Time, or lack thereof, is another common barrier cited by athletic trainers in incorporating psychosocial strategies into the athletic training setting. However, with practice, athletic trainers can learn to effectively teach these skills so they become a normal part of the treatment regimen. Consider how long it takes athletic training students to tape an ankle the first time; however, with practice, they are able to decrease their taping time and increase their taping effectiveness. The same can be true of teaching psychological skills to athletes; the athletic trainer can become well versed in the routine of introducing and integrating these skills with athletes. Multitasking can also often allow for time to teach and practice psychosocial skills; for example, they can introduce relaxation techniques while providing an ice-massage treatment or discuss imagery during an ultrasound treatment.

Along with having knowledge and time, finding available resources is often a roadblock to delivering holistic care. A multitude of resources are available for athletic trainers to assist with the introduction and integration of psychosocial strategies into practice. Resources available on the Internet grow more abundant every day. For example, imagery and relaxation scripts can be accessed through iTunes and other such sites, and many sporting and professional organizations provide online resources (e.g., the U.S. Olympic Committee's website is a great place to start).

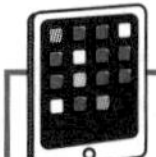

VIRTUAL FIELD TRIP

The International Olympic Committee (IOC) has several resources for athletes related to career development and time management. Specific to psychosocial strategies, time-management tools offered by the IOC may assist athletes who are involved in rehabilitation to manage their time effectively. Find a link to these resources at http://davisplus.fadavis.com.

ATHLETE INSIDER CONCLUSION

Because of the time spent educating 'A'amakua on his injuries and the rehabilitation that needed to take place, the athletic trainer convinced him to stay at school and heal his body. Only then would he be able to answer his questions about returning to play and put his mind to rest. How many times have you heard someone say, "I should have tried that; I could have done it"? The athletic trainer also suggested that 'A'amakua see another athletic trainer on campus (Hannah) who had expertise in the psychology of injury. 'A'amakua met with Hannah, and they decided to work on a few things together to improve his rehabilitation process. First, they outlined current stressors in his life and reviewed his current coping mechanisms; then, they paired these mechanisms with strategies to assist with each perceived stressor. Next, Hannah questioned 'A'amakua about things that motivate him during tough times and linked those things to iTunes Apps that would keep him on track and moving forward. Finally, Hannah educated him on how to use each skill and then set up a plan of attack for him; she outlined when he should use which skills and how often. Educating athletes about their injuries and useful strategies to improve their rehabilitation process is a key role of the athletic trainer.

Effective Psychosocial Strategies for the Athletic Trainer to Use with 'A'amakua

The psychosocial strategies listed below may prove useful when working with 'A'amakua:

1. Use goal tracker App so that he can see his daily progress and add new goals or modify current goals as needed. The key here is that not only is the athlete able to chart progress and gain motivation through that activity, but he also begins to feel in control of his progress.
2. Use an App to provide nightly relaxation reminders, which include somatic and cognitive scripts for him to use when he has trouble falling asleep. Sleep is essential to reducing stress and improving overall health.
3. Assist 'A'amakua in recording positive ***affirmations*** into an App to be played back later, when he isn't feeling so great about his recovery and life plans. It is important to provide support structures for the athlete when the athletic trainer cannot be there to remind him of his goals and that he is making worthwhile progress; these structures are a virtual "pat on the back."
4. Connect 'A'amakua to a social network page for injured athletes that the athletic trainer has experience monitoring and encourage him to read the stories of others and post his own to gather support from others. Because the athletic trainers' suggested strategies are an extension of them and their professionalism, it is important they "try out" these strategies themselves before suggesting that athletes use them to improve their well-being.
5. Create a few 5-minute focusing tasks for use before rehabilitation sessions to motivate A'amakua to get into the "frame of mind" needed to work hard that day, and put them all on an iPod for him to use during rehabilitation. Athletes are busy people, often balancing school, practice, social experiences, intimate relationships, and family. Using a focusing tool before rehabilitation sessions prompts athletes to "leave their life at the door" or to clear their mind before beginning rehabilitation. This enables them to give focus to goals set for the day and the work it will take to meet those goals.

CONCLUSION

This chapter highlighted the importance of integrating psychosocial strategies into caring for injured athletes. More specifically, the chapter introduced and provided details of various psychosocial strategies that are beneficial to athletes in the context of sport injury prevention, rehabilitation, and return to participation. This chapter also provided details for the athletic trainer on how to introduce and implement these strategies (i.e., the what, where, when, and how) with athletes and how to educate athletes regarding practice and use of these skills. This chapter also highlighted the role of athletic trainers in the psychosocial care of injured athletes. Overall, this chapter was based on the consensus that injured athletes can benefit from the use of psychosocial strategies during the three phases of rehabilitation, and that athletic trainers are in an ideal position to inform athletes and integrate these strategies into their work with them. When implementing these strategies, it is important, however, to follow five main principles: (1) strategies and interventions used need to be tailored to meet the individual athlete's needs; (2) the strategies should be used only with consent from the athlete; (3) strategies should be implemented only by a person who is appropriately trained to do so; (4) any psychosocial strategies should be implemented in such a way that athletes see them as part of treatment and rehabilitation, rather than an addition to it; and (5) if athletes display symptoms of unhealthy behaviors that could be clinical, they should be referred to appropriate mental health professionals when necessary.

REFERENCES

Andersen, M. B., & Williams, J. M. (1988). A model of stress and athletic injury: Prediction and prevention. *Journal of Sport & Exercise Psychology, 10,* 294–306.

Arvinen-Barrow, M., Clement, D., & Hemmings, B. (2013). Imagery in sport injury rehabilitation. In: M. Arvinen-Barrow & N. Walker (Eds.), *Psychology of Sport Injury and Rehabilitation.* Abingdon, Oxon, U.K.: Routledge.

Arvinen-Barrow, M., & Hemmings, B. (2013). Goal setting in sport injury rehabilitation. In: M. Arvinen-Barrow & N. Walker (Eds.), *Psychology of Sport Injury and Rehabilitation.* Abingdon, Oxon, U.K.: Routledge.

Arvinen-Barrow, M., Penny, G., Hemmings, B., & Corr, S. (2010). UK chartered physiotherapists' personal experiences in using psychological interventions with injured athletes: An interpretative phenomenological analysis. *Psychology of Sport & Exercise, 11*(1), 58–66.

Clement, D., Arvinen-Barrow, M., Hamson-Utley, J. J., et al. (2012). Injured athletes' use of psychosocial strategies during sport injury rehabilitation. Paper presented at: Association for Applied Sport Psychology Annual Conference; Atlanta, GA; October 3–6, 2012.

Clement, D., Granquist, M., & Arvinen-Barrow, M. (2013). Psychosocial aspects of athletic injuries as perceived by athletic trainers. *Journal of Athletic Training, 48*(4), 512–521.

Clement, D., Hamson-Utley, J. J., Arvinen-Barrow, M., Kamphoff, C., Zakrajsek, R. A., & Martin, S. B. (2012). College athletes' expectations about injury rehabilitation with an athletic trainer. *International Journal of Athletic Therapy & Training, 17*(4), 18–27.

Crossman, J. (2001). Managing thoughts, stress, and pain. In: J. Crossman (Ed.), *Coping with Sport Injuries: Psychological Strategies for Rehabilitation* (pp. 128–147). New York: Oxford University Press.

Dawson, M., Hamson-Utley, J. J., Hansen, R., & Olpin, M. (2014). Examining the effectiveness of psychological strategies on physiologic markers: evidence-based suggestions for holistic care of the athlete. *Journal of Athletic Training, 49*(1).

Durso-Cupal, D. (1996). The efficacy of guided imagery for recovery from anterior cruciate ligament (ACL) replacement. *Journal of Applied Sport Psychology, 8*(Suppl.), S56.

Evans, L., Hardy, L., & Fleming, S. (2000). Intervention strategies with injured athletes: An action research study. *The Sport Psychologist, 14,* 188–206.

Flint, F. (1998). *Psychology of Sport Injury: A Professional Achievement Self-Study Program Course.* Champaign, IL: Human Kinetics.

Gillet, N., Vallerand, R. J., Amoura, S., & Baldes, B. (2010). Influence of coaches' autonomy support on athletes' motivation and sport performance: A test of the hierarchical model of intrinsic and extrinsic motivation. *Psychology of Sport & Exercise, 11*(2), 155–161.

Hardy, J. (2006). Speaking clearly: A critical review of the self-talk literature. *Psychology of Sport & Exercise, 7,* 81–97.

Hush, J., Cameron, K., & Mackey, M. (2010). Patient satisfaction with musculoskeletal physical therapy care: A systematic review. *Physical Therapy, 91,* 25–36.

Ievleva, L., & Orlick, T. (1991). Mental links to enhanced healing: An exploratory study. *The Sport Psychologist, 5,* 25–40.

Jacobson, E. (1938). *Progressive Relaxation.* Chicago: University of Chicago Press.

Kolt, G. S. (2003). Psychology of injury and rehabilitation. In: G. S. Kolt & L. Snyder-Mackler (Eds.), *Physical Therapies in Sport and Exercise* (pp. 165–183). London: Churchill Livingstone.

Larson, G. A., Starkey, C., & Zaichkowsky, L. D. (1996). Psychological aspects of athletic injuries as perceived by athletic trainers. *The Sport Psychologist, 10,* 37–47.

Mageau, G. A., & Vallerand, R. J. (2003). The coach-athlete relationship: A motivational model. *Journal of Sports Sciences, 21*(11), 883–904.

Morris, T., Spittle, M., & Watt, A. P. (2005). *Imagery in Sport.* Champaign, IL: Human Kinetics.

Nathan, B. (1999). *Touch and Emotion in Manual Therapy.* London: Churchill Livingstone.

Russell, H., & Tracey, J. (2011). What do injured athletes want from their health care professionals? *International Journal of Athletic Therapy & Training, 16*(5), 18–21.

Smith, R. E., Schutz, R. W., Smoll, F. L., & Ptacek, J. T. (1995). Development and validation of a multidimensional measure of sport-specific psychological skills: The athletic coping skills inventory – 28. *Journal of Sport & Exercise Psychology, 17,* 379–398.

Taylor, A. (1995). Development of a Sports Injury Clinic Athlete Satisfaction Scale for auditing patient perceptions. *Physiotherapy Theory and Practice, 11*(4), 231–238.

Tod, D., Hardy, J., & Oliver, E. (2011). Effects of self-talk: A systematic review. *Journal of Sport & Exercise Psychology, 33*(5), 666–687.

Walsh, M. (2005). Injury rehabilitation and imagery. In: T. Morris, M. Spittle, & A. P. Watt (Eds.), *Imagery in Sport* (pp. 267–284). Champaign, IL: Human Kinetics.

Wiese-Bjornstal, D. M., Smith, A. M., Shaffer, S. M., & Morrey, M. A. (1998). An integrated model of response to sport injury: Psychological and sociological dynamics. *Journal of Applied Sport Psychology, 10,* 46–69.

Wiese, D. M., & Weiss, M. R. (1987). Psychological rehabilitation and physical injury: Implications for the sportsmedicine team. *The Sport Psychologist, 1,* 318–330.

Wiese, D. M., Weiss, M. R., & Yukelson, D. P. (1991). Sport psychology in the training room: A survey of athletic trainers. *The Sport Psychologist, 5,* 15–24.

Williams, J. M., & Andersen, M. B. (1998). Psychosocial antecedents of sport injury: Review and critique of the stress and injury model. *Journal of Applied Sport Psychology, 10*(1), 5–25.

BOARD OF CERTIFICATION STRATEGIES AND COMPETENCIES

As the Sixth Edition of the Board of Certification's Role Delineation Study outlines, athletic trainers are involved in the prevention and care of athletic injury (Domain 1). The Fifth Edition Athletic Training Educational Competencies include knowledge and skills in the content area of Psychosocial Strategies and Referral (PS), and psychosocial strategies are included within this content area. This chapter has described psychological skills (including goal setting, imagery, self-talk, and relaxation) that can be used to motivate the athlete during rehabilitation and return to participation (PS-7, PS-8). In addition, one of the Clinical Integration Proficiencies (CIP-7) aims to select and integrate appropriate ***psychosocial techniques*** (including goal setting, imagery, self-talk, etc.) into athletes' rehabilitation plans.

Board of Certification Style Questions

1. An athlete who is injured is struggling with being away from home. What are the most useful psychosocial strategies to assist this athlete? (Select all that apply.)
   a. PMR
   b. Cognitive relaxation
   c. Goal setting
   d. Positive reframing

2. Evidence-based practice in the psychology of injury suggests which of the following strategies are effective for stress management? (Select all that apply.)
   a. PMR
   b. Cognitive relaxation
   c. Goal setting
   d. Positive self-talk

3. Evidence-based practice in the psychology of injury suggests which of the following strategies are effective for motivating an injured athlete through rehabilitation? (Select all that apply.)
   a. PMR
   b. Cognitive relaxation
   c. Goal setting
   d. Positive self-talk

4. Evidence-based practice in the psychology of injury suggests which of the following strategies are effective for pain management? (Select all that apply.)
   a. PMR
   b. Cognitive relaxation
   c. Goal setting
   d. Positive reframing

END-OF-CHAPTER EXERCISES

1. Observe your athletic training room during a busy time of day. Pick a few different athletes to watch, individually, to observe their experience. What did you notice? As the Sixth Edition Role Delineation study outlines, athletic trainers are involved in the prevention and care of athletic injury (Domain 1). Did the athletes receive care quickly? Did they look lost? How were they handled? Make sure to select athletes from different sports and possibly different playing statuses (bench vs. All-Star), as they will likely be treated differently. Following your observation, what needs to be changed to provide effective care, and how do you suggest these changes be made? Complete an action plan outlining procedures/skills to implement to better your athletic training room interactions with athletes needing services.

2. Consider Table 10-2, which outlines the observable signs and symptoms of athlete distress. In the third column below, list things that the athletic trainer *could* do or implement with athletes to improve their rehabilitation or away-from-sport experience. Be prepared to discuss these activities with the class or your small group.

Stressor(s)	Resulting Athlete Behavior in ATR	Effective Responses by AT
Dealing with pain	Skipping treatments, avoiding AT, negative attitude or outlook, malingering behaviors (e.g., reporting to be ill when not ill to avoid therapy)	
Not being with team, being out of element	Looking sad, not motivated to be at treatment or to do any exercises, moving sluggishly, less eye contact, less conversation, negative attitude	
Lacking control of current situation, no longer a leader (or team captain)	Resistant to suggestions by AT, questioning of AT recommendations, uses outside resources to determine own timeline for return to play, consulting other medical professionals to ensure receiving best-practice care	
Giving up on returning to play	Not motivated by things that were once motivating, skipping treatment, atypical negative attitude, questioning every suggestion by the AT, appears depressed (lacking hygiene, no eye contact, little to no communication compared with normal behavior)	
Not invested in goals set by AT	Activity is not related to set goals, does not listen to AT recommendations, lying, communicating incorrect information to coaching staff and parents/loved ones, suiting up for practice without clearance (and other deviant behaviors)	

AT, athletic trainer; ATR, athletic training room.

3. Create a performance imagery script. Creating a performance imagery script for yourself can help you work with athletes to develop their own performance imagery script:
   a. Describe one of your *successful* plays in your sport. Write in first person, present tense.
   b. Now add in more detail. Think about what you see, feel, hear, smell, and taste. What are you feeling emotionally? What is going through your mind? What should be going through your mind? Where is your focus? Where should your focus be?
   c. Share your script with a partner to refine it.
   d. Record your script and practice!
4. Navigate the Internet to find at least five useful athlete injury education tools. These tools can vary from Apps to digital media, and you should include a link to where your instructor and classmates can find the materials. Complete the following table.

Resource Type	Purpose	Internet Resource Location
Anatomy App	To show the athlete which ligaments were damaged and how weight bearing too early can lengthen the rehabilitation/return-to-play process	https://itunes.apple.com/us/app/ankle-and-foot-pro-iii/id504805760?mt=8

5. Athletic trainers should introduce relaxation skills to the athletes with whom they work. Role-play this scenario:
   a. Introduce relaxation and educate athletes about how these skills can be used.
   b. Help athletes acquire the skills (i.e., demonstrate, run through).
   c. Help athletes identify when they will practice this skill (e.g., while heating/icing before rehabilitation, before falling asleep at night).

6. For each of the following psychological skills, describe *when* you could use this skill with an athlete and describe specifically *how* you would use it.
   a. Goal setting
   b. Imagery
   c. Positive self-talk

7. Consider the stressors faced by athletes in the rehabilitation process. Also consider the available time of the athletic trainer in meeting athletes' needs. Complete the following chart by navigating the Internet and finding prepackaged, already-made resources that would be useful in addressing those stressors.

Stressor	Psychosocial Strategy	Internet Resource Location

8. When could athletes use deep breathing? When could athletes use PMR? When could athletes use imagery for relaxation (think both preinjury and postinjury)? Compile your answers in essay format illustrating a clear strategy → goal relationship.

9. Complete the following table with common negative self-talk statements made by athletes who encounter obstacles in rehabilitation (left column) and pair them with positive, constructive statements they can use in the thought-stopping technique. Then use these with an athlete who is currently rehabilitating. You must review the thought-stopping technique in the chapter to be able to complete this exercise.

10. Navigate Facebook to find social support pages for injured athletes. What did you find? Copy and paste all links to pages into your answer. Then describe how each will be useful for injured athletes.

Negative Self-Talk Statements	Positive Replacement Statements

Chapter 11

Psychosocial Aspects of Return to Participation

Laura J. Kenow with Leslie Podlog

CHAPTER OUTLINE

CHAPTER OUTLINE *continued*

KEY TERMS

Affirmation statements Positive, action-oriented self-talk that affirms athletes' abilities.

Athletic identity The degree to which a person identifies the self as an athlete.

Autonomy A sense of choice or control over one's actions and behaviors.

Competence A sense of being capable or proficient in one's pursuits.

Functional progression A series of gradually progressive activities designed to prepare athletes for return to a specific sport.

Macrotrauma Injury resulting from a single impact or force that creates tissue damage (e.g., fracture, sprain, or dislocation).

Microtrauma Injury resulting from repeated smaller forces that gradually result in tissue damage over time (e.g., stress fracture, tendinitis).

Performance imagery The creation or re-creation of an experience in the mind from memory or quasi-experience using a combination of the five senses with the goal of improving an aspect of a performance in sport or rehabilitation.

Physiotherapists Term used for sports medicine practitioners in other countries, similar to athletic trainers in the United States.

Process goals Goals that focus on the actions an individual must engage in during performance to execute or perform well.

Reframing Changing the way one views a situation by consciously choosing to attend to different aspects of the situation.

Relatedness A sense of belonging or feeling part of a group.

Selective awareness Making a conscious choice as to what one will pay attention.

Self-efficacy Confidence in one's ability to perform a particular task in a specific situation.

Self-talk Internal and/or external statements to the self, multidimensional in nature, that have interpretive elements associated with their content; it is dynamic and serves at least two functions (instructional and motivational).

Social support Includes the feeling or sense of being supported by others, the act of supporting others, and social integration.

Tactical imagery A mental rehearsal of plays, strategies, and/or assignments.

CHAPTER OBJECTIVES

After reading this chapter, you will be able to:

1. Describe the psychological concerns injured athletes encounter as they approach their return to participation.
2. Identify sport-related concerns that injured athletes and athletic trainers need to address before returning to full participation.

3. Describe how self-determination theory applies to the return-to-participation concerns experienced by injured athletes.
4. Identify and implement psychosocial strategies to restore athletes' confidence and motivation as they return to participation.
5. Identify and implement psychosocial strategies to maintain injured athletes' relationships with their teams.
6. Identify and implement psychosocial strategies to maintain injured athletes' sense of autonomy in the return-to-participation process.

ATHLETE INSIDER

Harper arrived on campus his freshman year excited to begin his collegiate soccer career. During the first drill on the first day of preseason practice, he went to explode from a backpedal to a forward sprint and dislocated his patella. To create optimal healing, he underwent microfracture surgery along with a lateral release. His season was over before it really even began. Following off-season rehabilitation, he arrived for his second preseason camp only to fracture his big toe on the tenth day, which kept him out for 3 weeks. He returned to play in several games before sustaining a high-ankle sprain that again ended his season prematurely. In the off-season after completing rehabilitation on his ankle, Harper was playing in a pickup basketball game. He went up for a rebound, was pushed in midair, and landed awkwardly on a single straight leg. His patella dislocated again. He underwent patellar realignment surgery and arrived at preseason camp for his junior year with a good share of his rehabilitation completed, but he had yet to engage in any lateral movement activities. During functional progression exercises, Harper expressed recurring fear and apprehension about making abrupt cuts and explosive lateral movements, which had created stresses similar to those that caused his two patellar dislocations. When asked about his reluctance, he stated, "In the last two years of my life, I've spent about 6 months of it on crutches and a good chunk of the rest doing rehabilitation. I'm scared and really don't want to go back there [injured] again." He went on to state, "I know that as a junior I'm a big part of the coach's plans this year, so I need to be back soon. I just don't want to mess up my knee and miss another year."

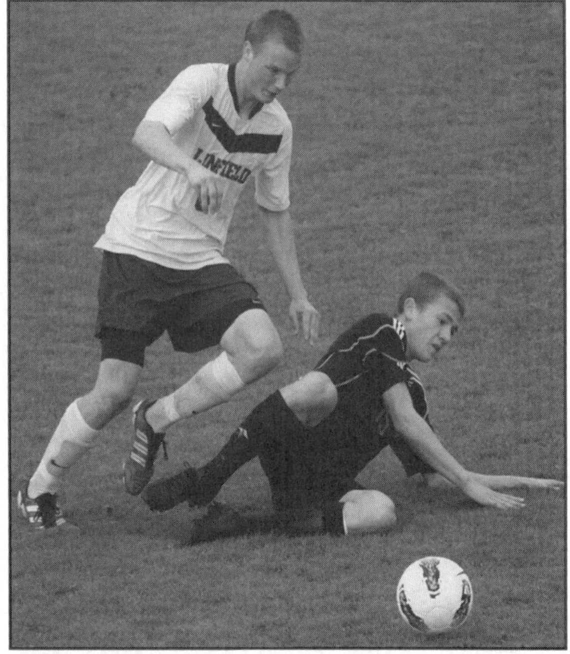

Figure 11-1 | Athlete Insider *(Courtesy of Linfield College Athletics)*

INTRODUCTION

Harper's situation is a dramatic one, yet athletes with seemingly minor injuries often express apprehension and worry about returning to participation as well. Athletes are frequently declared physically ready to compete following injury without consideration of their psychological or sport-related readiness. Ironically, athletes' overall well-being during and following return to participation after injury is impacted by a variety of psychosocial and sport-related factors. In this chapter, we review the process of return to sport participation and the athletic trainer's role related to ensuring not only physical but also psychological readiness for return. Return-to-sport confidence and anxiety over reinjury are highlighted and tied directly to current research theory. This chapter concludes with strategies that athletic trainers can use to enhance athletes' confidence, motivation, relatedness, and autonomy in the return-to-participation process.

WHAT ARE PSYCHOSOCIAL AND SPORT-RELATED CONCERNS ABOUT RETURN TO PARTICIPATION?

Following athlete injury, athletic trainers and athletes work collaboratively to rehabilitate the injured body part and maintain overall body fitness. Often, the physical aspects of recovery dominate the rehabilitation plan and are the primary measures of when an athlete is deemed ready to return to participation. However, research has shown that psychosocial and sport-related factors also play a critical role in athletes' overall readiness to return to sport following injury (Bianco, 2001; Walker, Thatcher, & Lavallee, 2010). Box 11-1 highlights the psychosocial and sport-related concerns athletes may encounter as they approach their return-to-participation date.

BOX 11-1 | Psychosocial and Sport-Related Concerns Regarding Return to Participation Following Injury

PSYCHOSOCIAL CONCERNS

Reinjury anxiety
Identity concerns
Isolation from team
Inadequate social support
Pressure to return to sport

SPORT-RELATED CONCERNS

Fitness
Role on the team
Up to speed on plays, tactics, or strategies

Psychosocial Concerns

For many injured athletes, the anticipation of a return to participation may represent an exciting opportunity. Not only does the resumption of their sport participation provide the possibility of achieving personally relevant goals, but it also signifies the chance for them to once again experience the satisfaction of sport involvement and interaction with coaches and teammates. At the same time, the prospect of returning to play may raise thoughts of doubt, uncertainty, and apprehension about what lies ahead, particularly among athletes experiencing a lengthy rehabilitation. Athletes typically have a number of common concerns as the return to participation approaches. These include, but may not be limited to, anxieties regarding reinjury, identity concerns, isolation from team camaraderie, inadequate ***social support***, and finally, pressures to return to competition. Each of these concerns is explained in more detail in the following subsections.

Reinjury Anxiety

Reinjury concerns may begin to increase as injury rehabilitation draws to a close and a return to competition draws near. In some instances, anxieties regarding reinjury may be severe enough to prevent an otherwise physically healthy athlete from returning to sport. Typically, reinjury anxieties are more common in instances where the athlete has experienced a severe injury and prolonged sport absence, heightened pain levels, setbacks throughout the rehabilitation process, and pressures to make an expedited return—an issue to which we shall return later. Box 11-2 highlights common indications that an athlete may have elevated reinjury concerns. Certainly, explicit statements regarding reinjury worries should be taken seriously and dealt with as soon as possible.

BOX 11-2 | Common Indications of Elevated Reinjury Concerns

- Malingering efforts despite positive clinical or functional indicators
- Increased negative mood states
- Hesitation to try drills or skills of which the athlete is physically capable

It is also important to consider that reinjury anxieties may increase the likelihood of actual injury. As discussed in Chapter 3, ample evidence exists demonstrating the negative consequences of stress and anxiety in increasing the likelihood of athlete injury. Typically, individuals experience stress when they perceive that the demands of a particular situation (physical, social, psychological) outweigh their ability to successfully negotiate such demands. An athlete who feels stressed may, in turn, have distracted thoughts and therefore fail to attend to task-relevant cues. An example of this would be a gymnast who focuses on the crowd or a coach's reaction rather than the technical aspects of an upcoming maneuver. Such distractions may lead to an increased risk for a fall and a greater likelihood of reinjury.

Under stress, athletes may also have a tendency to experience a narrowing of the peripheral vision, or what is commonly known as tunnel vision. In addition to the attentional consequences of stress, physiological changes in the body typically occur. For example, the football quarterback who is experiencing concentration deficits associated with stress may also experience muscle tightness, reduced timing and coordination, and increased muscular fatigue. Given the attentional and physiological deficits just outlined, it is easy to imagine how the gymnast or the quarterback might be more susceptible to falling off the beam, getting sacked, or unfortunately, sustaining a serious injury. Returning our focus to the athlete with reinjury anxiety, it becomes apparent that attentional and muscular changes may put an athlete at heightened risk for actual reinjury. From the standpoint of the athletic trainer, the need to alleviate athlete fears and anxieties becomes paramount in an effort to minimize reinjury occurrence. Specific strategies for addressing reinjury anxieties are discussed later in this chapter.

Once athletes return to competition, reinjury anxiety may adversely affect postinjury performances and athlete satisfaction regarding the return. For instance, in a study with NFL football players, performance decreased after a return to sport following a serious knee injury (Carey, Huffman, Parekh, & Sennett, 2006). Upon their return, running backs and wide receivers exhibited a 33% decline in rushing and receiving yards, as well as touchdowns. Although the researchers suggested that a loss of strength, deconditioning, and reduced proprioception were likely factors accounting for diminished performances, a possible alternate explanation may be that reinjury anxieties influenced athletes' concentration and created a sense of hesitation. It is likely that feelings of stress and uncertainty regarding the possibility of reinjury or diminished postinjury performance may have in part been responsible for the decreases in actual performance. Indeed, athletes in a range of sports such as skiing, rugby, and basketball have indicated that reinjury anxieties and diminished confidence in their ability to execute sport skills were important obstacles in their ability to regain preinjury performance levels (Bianco, 2001; Evans, Hardy, & Fleming, 2000). Once again, findings such as these highlight the need for athletic trainers to be particularly vigilant in minimizing the potentially negative consequences associated with reinjury anxiety.

Identity Concerns, Isolation From Team Camaraderie, and Inadequate Social Support

A loss of ***athletic identity*** during rehabilitation and in the initial stages of the return to sport may also be challenging for returning athletes. For many athletes, the belief that they are not a "true athlete" unless they are competing or fully involved on the field of play can influence their sense of self-worth. This idea is nicely summarized in a quote by a top-level Australian rower who experienced injury and was unable to train and compete. The rower commented:

> *"It was hard because I guess I am a rower. I define myself as a rower, and when you don't have that and you don't have those people around you, you feel worthless. It makes up a big part of your life. When you see someone you haven't seen in a while and they say 'How's the rowing going?', and you say 'Well, it's not at the moment.' When they ask 'What else are you doing?' and you say, 'Well, nothing,' there's a big void there to fill, and it's pretty hard" (Podlog & Eklund, 2006, p. 54).*

A loss of athletic identity often stems from feelings of isolation from the camaraderie of team events, being unable to experience the highs and lows of competition, and feeling unsupported by coaches, teammates, or relevant others. Feelings of detachment and isolation may occur as recovering athletes become removed from their usual training and competition venues, and spend more time in rehabilitation settings. Inadequate levels of social support may also contribute to a sense of identity loss. For example, some athletes perceive their coaches to be distant and insensitive to injury, that they provide insufficient or inadequate rehabilitation guidance, or that they lack a belief in the athlete's ability to return. Such distancing by a coach may contribute to athletes' perceptions that they are not valued members of the team and that only those who are competing are deserving or worthy of the coach's attention. Confronted with this reality, it is not surprising that athletes all too commonly feel a sense of alienation from their sport and a loss of athletic identity.

A lack of social support may not only undermine athletes' views of themselves, but may also have detrimental consequences for injury recovery progressions and knowledge about how best to proceed with the return-to-sport transition. Interestingly, athletes have reported a lack of guidance and information from coaches and ***physiotherapists*** about how to train or build up their muscles as they re-entered the competitive arena (Johnston & Carroll, 1998). Such findings contradict substantial evidence of the benefits of social support for athletes' returning to sport following injury (Bianco & Eklund, 2001). Social support from coaches, family members, and athletic trainers may be essential in assisting athletes in dealing with the demands of injury recovery and complying with the rigors of their rehabilitation regimen. Research has shown that greater compliance can increase the likelihood of enhanced clinical outcomes such as proprioception, range of motion, joint/ligament stability, muscular strength, and endurance, as well as reductions in the subsequent risk for reinjury. Techniques for enhancing social support are discussed later in this chapter.

CLINICAL TIP

Athletic trainers cannot individually meet all the social support needs of injured athletes; however, they are in a prime position to recognize these needs and serve as facilitators in mobilizing a social support network for the athletes. Athletic trainers can recruit and educate coaches, teammates, friends, family, academic advisors, and residence life staff members as key allies in providing the emotional, informational, and tangible support needed by injured athletes.

Pressures to Return to Sport

Another common injury-related challenge reported by both athletes and coaches is the issue of pressures to return to sport. Competitive athletes often face external pressures from coaches, teammates, or training partners to return to sport after an injury, in some instances, before they are physically or mentally ready.

EVIDENCE-BASED PRACTICE

Murphy, P., & Waddington, I. (2007). Are elite athletes exploited? *Sport in Society, 10,* 239–255. doi: 10.1080/17430430601147096

Description of the Study

The purpose of the study was to explore whether elite athletes are exploited in terms of their health and well-being. To address the question, the researchers focused on the case of professional English soccer and based their discussion on interviews conducted with players from the English First Division (i.e., Premier League).

Results of the Study

The researchers found that players are expected to "play hurt" and may be subjected to pressures from coaches, owners, and even sport medicine practitioners to return to play before they have fully recovered. According to the soccer players, being prepared to play while injured was, in the eyes of the coaches, a central characteristic of a "good professional." Athletes described how coaches could often exert subtle (or more explicit) pressures to encourage a return to play by making the soccer player feel that he was of "no use" to anyone unless he was contributing on the field of play. Moreover, players reported instances in which information about their injuries was deliberately withheld from them by team doctors. The doctors withheld the information so that players would not appreciate the severity of their injury and would continue to play while hurt. The researchers concluded that many sport clubs fail to meet the requirements of health and safety legislation in the United Kingdom.

Implications for Athletic Training Practice
Findings from this study suggest that, as sport becomes more commercialized, athletes' economic value to the team may be given primary importance over and above their physical and psychological health and well-being. In this environment, athletic trainers may be placed in ethically challenging situations in which the need to expedite the return to participation may be at odds with clinical indicators of readiness to return. Having ethical principles and standards (e.g., disclosure of information, comprehension of information, informed consent, beneficence) that guide decision-making processes will be essential for athletic trainers who are attempting to ensure athletes' safe and successful return to full activity.

A study with English female university athletes highlighted pressures to return to participation. In particular, athletes reported experiencing pressure to return from significant others, namely, coaches and peers (Charlesworth & Young, 2004). This pressure influenced athletes' decisions to play while in pain or to return prematurely from an injury. Although coaches and teammates may not always explicitly pressure athletes to return, their mentality, particularly at the elite level, may be such that they exert subtle or inadvertent pressures on the athlete to return. Elite coaches have conveyed instances where they felt that sports medicine physicians were too conservative in their approach to treating athletes out of fear of negligence or concern over being sued (Podlog & Eklund, 2007a). Furthermore, coaches have suggested that because some doctors lack an appreciation of the inherent risks and physical demands of elite sport, physicians may fail to be as innovative as necessary in returning the athlete to competitive play. Such a mind-set on the part of coaches may influence their interactions with athletes by encouraging them to make a quick return to competitive play. Athletic trainers need to be aware of instances in which coaches place overt or more subtle pressures on rehabilitating athletes to return to competition so that they can intervene on athletes' behalf.

CLINICAL TIP

It is essential that athletic trainers educate not only the injured athlete but also coaches and others close to the athlete about the injury and the tissue-healing process. As part of this discussion, athletic trainers should review safe parameters for rehabilitation progress and return to participation so athletes receive consistent messages about their return-to-participation timetable.

The situation is often further compounded when considering the pressure that top-level athletes face in the media. As discussed in Chapter 2, television, film, and newspaper reports regularly glorify and praise those playing through pain and injury. Recall the story of gymnast Kerri Strug, who received national fame and attention following her final vault in the 1996 Olympics, a vault that helped the U.S. women's team clinch the gold medal. On her first of two vaults, Strug under-rotated the landing, causing her to fall and damage her ankle. In the time interval between Strug's two vaults, she asked her coach Béla Károlyi, "Do we need this?" To which he replied, "Kerri, we need you to go one more time. We need you one more time for the gold. You can do it, you better do it." Strug complied, limping slightly to the runway for her second attempt. She landed the vault briefly on both feet, virtually instantly hopping onto her good foot. She then dropped to her knees and needed assistance off the landing platform. Sportscaster John Tesh commented, "Kerri Strug is hurt! She is hurt badly." Károlyi later carried Strug onto the medals podium to join her team, after which she was treated at a hospital for a third-degree lateral sprain and tendon damage. Because of her injury, Strug was unable to compete in the individual all-around competition and event finals, despite having qualified for both. Following the Olympics, Strug became a national sports hero for her final vault, visiting President Bill Clinton, appearing on numerous television talk shows, making the cover of *Sports Illustrated*, and appearing on a Wheaties cereal box with other team members. In a media environment where athletes are lauded, praised, and rewarded for their heroic ability to play with pain and injury, it is understandable that many feel obligated to return to participation. Unfortunately, athletes who return before they are mentally or physically ready may suffer performance decreases, heightened competitive anxiety, and even long-term health effects associated with recurrent or chronic injury.

VIRTUAL FIELD TRIP

For examples of media glorification of those who play through pain and injury and questioning those who don't, go to http://davisplus.fadavis.com.

Pressures to return may not only come from external sources but from athletes themselves. As discussed in Chapter 2, athletes often internalize beliefs that they must push their physical limits, relying on the principle of "no pain, no gain," and believing that training can never hurt enough. Moreover, those who exclusively identify with the athlete role, who display strong perfectionist tendencies, and who experience regular anxiety may be at greatest risk for self-induced pressures to return. It is also common for athletes to shorten their recovery because of an increasing lack of confidence in the ability to perform, concerns over losing too much fitness, or a desire to take part in an upcoming competition.

As a counterpoint, it is important to acknowledge the many coaches, managers, or athlete support systems that work to lessen such pressures and create the "culture of precaution" discussed in Chapter 2. Coaches can be instrumental in decreasing pressures to return by ensuring that athletes do not return because they are made to feel guilty or are coerced. A world-class gymnastics coach stated:

> *"We try not to bully them into feeling they should be doing it to please the coach because there can be an aspect of that if you're not careful. You can bully an athlete into doing things going 'Oh, my foot's really sore', 'Is it? OK, well, I suppose we won't be ready for Nationals, but OK; don't do anything then.' As opposed to 'My foot's really sore', 'OK, well, what do you feel you can handle? Do you feel you can do a few of these? No, not really? Well, leave that for today; we'll try it tomorrow.' That's a very different approach to making the athlete feel guilty if they've come to you and said 'I can't do it' and you go 'That's fine' or you make some snide or underhand remark, and that's very easy to do" (Podlog & Eklund, 2007a, p. 216).*

This particular gymnastics coach emphasized the importance of keeping the center of control with athletes by teaching them to make good judgments about what they were capable of doing. Although some coaches may undoubtedly exert pressures on athletes to return, others recognize the downsides of doing so. For example, the coach quoted earlier suggested that pressuring an athlete to return could ultimately result in poorer performances, an increased chance of reinjury, and the athlete questioning whether the coach really has his or her best interests at heart. Given the pressures facing athletes to return to sport, it is pivotal that athletic trainers and others act in the best interests of the athlete's health and well-being. Intervention on the athlete's behalf may be prudent (and even necessary) when it is apparent that a return to competition may result in injurious consequences or decreased performances.

CLINICAL TIP

The athletic trainer must operate as the exclusive advocate for the injured athlete's best interests. Power relations in sport can make athletes hesitant to challenge a coach's urging to return to participation following injury. Athletic trainers must be willing to step in and intervene with a coach who is pressuring an athlete to return too quickly. Educating the coach on the potential negative consequences of a premature return will be essential in these circumstances. A willingness to "take the heat" from an overzealous coach will go a long way in solidifying an athlete's trust and rapport with his or her athletic trainer. Building rapport and effective working alliances is an essential element of a successful rehabilitation.

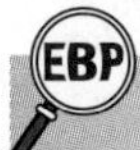

EVIDENCE-BASED PRACTICE

Creighton, D. W., Shrier, I., Shultz, R., Meeuwisse, W. H., & Matheson, G. O. (2010). Return-to-play in sport: A decision-based model. *Clinical Journal of Sport Medicine, 20*(5), 379–385.

Description of the Study

The purpose of the study was to synthesize the available literature concerning return to play (RTP) and propose a model for RTP decision making in sports medicine. The model is intended to clarify the processes clinicians use consciously and subconsciously when making RTP decisions in sport.

Results of the Study

The study proposed a three-step decision-making model that integrates and sequences the many factors associated with RTP decision-making. The model shows how these factors interact and at what point they should be considered in the RTP decision-making process. In step 1 of the model, the health status of the athlete is assessed through the evaluation of medical factors (e.g., signs/symptoms, patient demographics including age and sex, patient's medical history, laboratory tests such as x-rays or magnetic resonance imaging, severity of the injury, functional ability, and psychological state). In step 2, the clinician evaluates the risk associated with participation by assessing such variables as the type of sport played (e.g., collision, noncontact), the position played (e.g., goalie, forward), the competitive level (e.g., recreational, professional), the ability to protect (e.g., bracing, taping, padding), and the limb dominance of the patient. Step 3 in the decision-making process includes consideration of non-medical factors that can influence RTP decisions. These factors include such things as the timing in the season (e.g., playoffs), pressure from the athlete or others (e.g., coach, athlete's family), ability to mask the injury (e.g., pain medications), conflict of interest (e.g., potential financial gain or loss to the patient or clinician), and fear of litigation (e.g., if participation is restricted or permitted). Thus, the model provides a framework outlining the complex integration of components that ultimately contribute to RTP decisions.

Implications for Athletic Training Practice

Athletic trainers must appreciate that RTP decisions are not based solely on physical or medical factors. The ultimate RTP decision often involves consideration of the psychological readiness of the athlete, as well as non-medical factors such as the team's immediate need for the athlete's playing skills, the athlete's strong desire to resume athletic participation sometimes even before the injury fully heals, pressure from others to "play hurt," potential legal liability for decision outcomes, and ethical issues regarding the health risks athletes are allowed to assume. The complexity of the decision-making process highlights the wisdom of a shared-decision model that involves the athlete, the athletic trainer, the team physician, and other stakeholders in discussions regarding RTP timelines.

Sport-Related Concerns

Fitness

Concerns about overall and game-specific fitness levels may also be prevalent. During rehabilitation, losses in general fitness may affect athletes' self-esteem and can be a source of concern regarding an upcoming return to competition. For example, athletic trainers often hear injured athletes voicing concern over losing fitness during their injury rehabilitation or how they just don't "feel right" when they're not physically active. Athletes value feeling fit and may react negatively when their physical activity levels are altered or reduced.

The process of regaining match fitness may also be an arduous one, especially in cases of a severe injury or prolonged sport absence. In instances where athletes maintained their preinjury fitness through competitive play (as opposed to off-field conditioning), the challenge of regaining preinjury fitness levels may be all the more demanding. Athletes may also find that the process of achieving preinjury fitness levels is difficult even when committed to a rigorous fitness regimen that is acceptable within the confines of injury restrictions. Consider the scenario with Harper, our injured soccer player from the Athletic Insider at the beginning of this chapter. Although he and his athletic trainer implemented alternative forms of training (e.g., deep water skiing and running, strength training, cycling), throughout his rehabilitation, they often failed to match the intensity of competitive play. During his immediate post-surgical periods he was quite sedentary and gained weight, which increased the challenge of regaining his preinjury fitness levels. His athletic trainer had to remind him that attaining competitive fitness would take time, and he needed to remain patient and reasonable with his expectations.

For many athletes, a lack of game-specific fitness results in an inability to exert effort over the course of the entire game, diminished reaction times, and poorer decision-making skills. These difficulties are typically more apparent during the initial return to competition, that is, the first few weeks or month of the return. A lack of game-specific fitness and the resulting performance decrements can be a source of tremendous frustration and concern for the newly returned athlete. Athletic trainers must therefore remind athletes that the transition from rehabilitation to training and full competition will be an adjustment, and to be prepared for increased fatigue as training loads intensify and the demands of competition begin to assert themselves on athletes' minds and bodies.

Related to physical fitness concerns, returning athletes may also experience challenges associated with the physical abuse and punishment of competitive play, particularly for those in contact sports. After experiencing an absence from competition, athletes may not be used to the physicality that takes place on the field of play. As described in detail later, ensuring ***functional progressions*** in which the athlete gradually progresses from simple skills to high-intensity game-specific situations may be essential in building a tolerance to the demands of high-performance sport.

Role on the Team

Although athletic trainers may work to reduce the uncertainties of rehabilitation and a return to sport, for many athletes a number of questions nonetheless loom large. Inherent in the injury rehabilitation experience are uncertainties about how the rehabilitation will progress, what influence the injury will have on postinjury performance, and trepidations about the ability to attain preinjury levels and goals. One salient question emerging at the time of return to competition relates to the athlete's role on the team. In particular, questions about whether athletes will keep the same position, the extent to which teammates have improved and will take over a position, and what will happen to the replacement upon return may weigh heavy on athletes' minds. Undoubtedly, such questions can cause stress and anxiety, because many of these issues remain out of the athletes' control. As a result, it is essential that athletic trainers work to focus athletes' minds on factors they can influence. The strategies described later, such as goal setting, selective awareness/***reframing***, and anxiety-reduction techniques, will be instrumental in enabling athletes to focus on factors that they can modify to enhance the return experience.

Up to Speed on New Plays

Another sport-related concern of relevance during the return-to-participation transition is being up to date on new plays or strategies implemented while the athlete is out of commission. Coaches have suggested that such concerns can be alleviated by ensuring injured athletes remain involved in practice sessions and team meetings so they are on the same page as other team members. Even in instances where athletes may not be physically involved, keeping them informed about new tactical information and team plays will be important for facilitating their reintegration into the team. As suggested in the later imagery section, tactical imagery may be highly effective in enabling returning athletes to remain current with plays, assignments, and/or strategies outside of physical practice time.

Concussion-Specific Concerns

Concussion injuries present some unique considerations and challenges to athletes in the rehabilitation and return-to-participation process. These unique factors include the "invisible" nature of the concussion injury: concussions are unique injuries in that, unlike many other injuries, they tend not to have obvious external manifestations, such as limps, scars, crutches, slings, or braces. From all outward appearances, concussed athletes often look "healthy," which often results in inquiries such as "Why aren't you playing?" These inquiries can come from well-meaning fans and observers, but they can also come from uninformed teammates and coaches. Athletes may have trouble accepting the fact that an injury with no visual signs has sidelined them from active participation and feel that they should return.

Rehabilitation requires physical and cognitive rest; in the sports world, athletes have learned that hard work and persistent effort result in physical improvements and performance gains. However, this recipe for success fails them when dealing with a concussion. In rehabilitation from this injury, rest is the keyword, both physically and cognitively. "Less is better" becomes the mantra, and this runs counter to everything athletes have experienced in generating sport success. It is easy for athletes to develop a sense of helplessness and lost autonomy in the rehabilitation process. Furthermore, in most other injuries, athletes can continue to vent their energy by working out their uninjured body parts; however, this can delay healing in concussion recovery. Athletes are also discouraged from engaging in what might otherwise be useful distractions during their inactivity, such as video games, surfing the Internet, watching television, and social networking, as these cognitive activities can also exacerbate concussion symptoms. During rehabilitation from concussions, it is not uncommon for athletes to experience depressive moods, not only as a symptom of the concussion itself but also as a result of the deprivation of the psychosocial benefits that accompany physical and cognitive activity.

CLINICAL TIP

The "invisibility" of concussive injuries along with their demand for physical and cognitive rest during recovery may necessitate diligent observation of concussed athletes by athletic trainers for signs or symptoms indicating that these athletes are encountering difficulties in coping with their injury experience. It would be wise for athletic trainers to include mental health professionals as regular participants in the concussion-management protocols for all athletes (Bloom, Horton, McCrory, & Johnston, 2004; McCrory, 2011). Chapter 6 discusses how to recognize signs and symptoms of psychological distress following injury in greater detail.

RELATING RETURN-TO-PARTICIPATION CONCERNS TO CURRENT THEORY

The aforementioned concerns suggest that athletes may experience anxiety about their sense of ***competence***, ***relatedness*** (i.e., affiliation), and ***autonomy***. Figure 11-2 illustrates the relationships between the previously mentioned athlete concerns and these theoretical concepts.

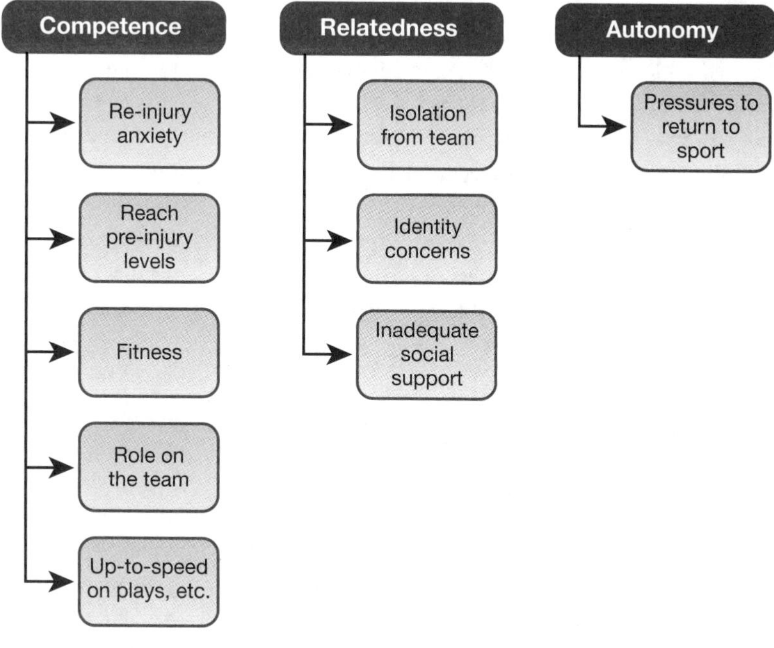

Figure 11-2 | Athlete return-to-participation concerns grouped by basic psychological needs.

Competence

Competence refers to the idea of being capable or proficient in one's pursuits and is an important psychological requirement for effective human functioning. Many of the concerns highlighted earlier relate to injured athletes' sense of competence. For example, reinjury anxieties, concerns over reaching preinjury levels, and concerns over diminished postinjury performances all relate to an athlete's desire to maintain high levels of athletic competence. Moreover, fitness concerns, worries that they may not be skilled enough to maintain their position/role on the team, or uncertainties about being up to speed on new plays all affect athletes' feelings of competence. For high-level athletes committed to the development of their physical competencies, the possibility that injury may interfere with their return performance and ultimate sporting capacities may be a daunting and unwanted outcome. In short, it is apparent that competence-related concerns may be at the forefront of athletes' minds as they re-enter the competitive arena.

Relatedness

As highlighted earlier, injured athletes experience feelings of isolation from teammates, training partners, and coaches. A lost sense of identity and questions about one's value as a person without sport involvement may impact their self-esteem and sense of worth. For many injured athletes, maintaining a sense of belonging and feeling part of the team (i.e., a sense of relatedness) may therefore be beneficial, particularly among athletes with a high athletic identity. Indeed, social support from coaches, teammates, and significant others may provide a buffer against feelings of isolation. Collectively, these findings suggest that relatedness or affiliation concerns may be important among athletes returning to sport following injury.

Autonomy

External and internal pressures to return to sport may be prevalent, thus highlighting the relevance of autonomy issues among returning athletes. The notion of autonomy refers to the idea that an individual has a sense of choice or control over his or her own actions and behaviors. Although some athletes are given autonomy to return at their own pace, others may experience pressures from coaches, teammates, and significant others to take part in certain competitions. Still other athletes may place internal pressures on themselves to meet personal standards of excellence and to be prepared for particular competitions. Thus, it is apparent that athletes may experience differing degrees of autonomy (i.e., ownership or control) regarding the circumstances of their injury recovery and return to sport.

Ties to Self-Determination Theory

Because of the focus on competence, relatedness, and autonomy issues, self-determination theory (SDT) appears to be a useful theoretical perspective for understanding and explaining athlete return-to-sport experiences and as a framework for guiding athletic trainers' intervention efforts. SDT is a motivational theory that examines the factors in the environment that influence an individual's tendency toward self-motivated behavior, psychological health and well-being, and task-related performance. According to Richard Ryan and Edward Deci (2000), the originators of the theory, all individuals have three basic psychological needs: competence, relatedness (i.e., affiliation or connection), and autonomy. When these needs are met or satisfied by the environment (e.g., athletic trainers, coaches, teammates), athletes experience better psychological health and well-being, enhanced internal motivation, and heightened performance. However, if these needs are not met, athletes may experience apathy, alienation, and elevated stress and anxiety. For example, the teammate who continually points out another's mistakes, who ostracizes an athlete from other teammates for such mistakes, or who makes pressuring or coercive statements may undermine the athlete's sense of competence, relatedness, and autonomy.

Researchers studying the relevance of SDT across various life domains (e.g., work, family, education, and sport) have found support for the beneficial effects of environments that support individuals' three basic needs. From the self-determination perspective, the extent to which injured athletes experience fulfillment of their three psychological needs will have important motivational, performance, and anxiety-related implications for their rehabilitation and return to sport.

EVIDENCE-BASED PRACTICE

Podlog, L., Lochbaum, M., & Stevens, T. (2010). Need satisfaction, well-being and perceived return-to-sport outcomes among injured athletes. *Journal of Applied Sport Psychology, 22*(2), 167–182.

Description of the Study

The purpose of the study was to explore whether satisfaction of injured athletes' psychological needs for competence, relatedness, and autonomy influenced their psychological well-being and, in turn, whether their well-being influenced their perceived return-to-sport outcomes (e.g., subjective performance evaluations, mental toughness, competitive anxiety). Subjects included 204 competitive athletes from Australia, Canada, and the United States representing a variety of sports such as wrestling, track and field, football, rugby, soccer, Australian rules football, swimming, and ice hockey. Each participant had recovered from an injury that required a minimum of 2 months of rehabilitation. Subjects completed questionnaires regarding the extent to which their psychological needs were met by relevant others (e.g., coaches and athletic trainers), their well-being (i.e., positive and negative emotions, self-esteem and feeling of vitality), and their return-to-sport outcomes.

Results of the Study

Results indicated that fulfillment of athletes' competence needs during their rehabilitation was associated with greater positive emotions and vitality (i.e., a feeling of being energized and alive), which, in turn, predicted positive return-to-sport outcomes (e.g., greater mental toughness, motivation for sport success, and an appreciation for one's sport). Furthermore, athletes whose need for relatedness was satisfied (e.g., social support from coaches) experienced reduced negative emotions and greater vitality and self-esteem that ultimately diminished return-to-sport concerns such as competitive anxiety and reinjury worries.

Implications for Athletic Training Practice

It is important to ensure injured athletes experience a sense of competence during their rehabilitation. Competence needs may be satisfied by providing functional progressions and using psychosocial strategies such as those described later (e.g., goal setting, anxiety reduction, imagery). It is also important to ensure that athletes can relate to and feel connected with their teammates and their sport through the provision of social support (e.g., emotional comfort, tangible assistance, or information about effective recovery) to offset some of the potential stressors associated with the return to full competitive activity.

It is apparent that returning athletes experience competence issues (e.g., reinjury anxieties, concerns about performing to preinjury standards), relatedness issues (e.g., feelings of social isolation and a lack of social identity), and autonomy issues (external and self-induced pressures to return to sport). SDT-based research (Podlog & Eklund, 2006, 2007b) also reveals that environments that satisfy athletes' competence, relatedness, and autonomy needs may be instrumental in reducing their anxieties and concerns regarding their return to sport. Therefore, athletic trainers, aiming to ensure athletes' holistic recovery, would be well advised to address these areas during the return-to-participation transition. The following section provides practical suggestions and strategies for addressing competence (i.e., confidence), relatedness, and autonomy needs among athletes returning to sport following injury.

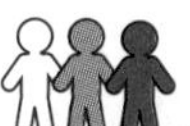

SPECIAL CONSIDERATIONS

The type of injury (i.e., acute ***macrotrauma*** vs. chronic ***microtrauma***) athletes sustain can profoundly influence their return-to-participation experience. When athletes sustain an acute macrotraumatic injury, there is

Continued

usually a single force or impact that creates the tissue damage (e.g., fracture, sprain, dislocation), resulting in a definitive mechanism of injury followed by a relatively clean and linear progression through rehabilitation and return to participation. In contrast, microtraumatic or chronic injuries (e.g., tendinitis, stress fractures) result from long periods of repeated stress with accompanying subclinical pathology until the damage summates to a point that it is recognized as injury. The rehabilitation and return-to-participation process in these cases is often less smooth and linear. Recovery from these injuries is more often characterized by repeated bouts of athletes "feeling good" and attempting return to participation only to have symptoms "flare up" and set them back in their course of healing. Despite the best efforts by athletic trainers to follow sound functional progressions, chronic injuries by their very nature tend to recur. Athletes who have endured these repeated bouts of unsuccessful return to participation or exacerbation of symptoms on return may experience frustration and greater anxieties about reinjury than athletes who are recovering from acute injuries. Although research regarding the psychological reactions to macrotraumatic versus microtraumatic injuries is lacking, athletic trainers would be wise to exercise greater vigilance for signs of reinjury anxiety, lack of confidence, self-induced pressures to return to sport, and lost identity when working with athletes preparing to return to participation following chronic injuries.

PSYCHOSOCIAL STRATEGIES

This section highlights specific psychosocial strategies that athletic trainers can use to assist athletes with the return-to-participation process. The section first addresses suggestions for assessing the psychological readiness of athletes to return to participation. The remaining strategies have been grouped into themed areas for restoring confidence, maintaining relationships, and maintaining autonomy consistent with SDT discussed earlier. In daily interactions with injured athletes, athletic trainers should be sensitive to behaviors or comments from them that may reflect one or more of these areas of concern during the rehabilitation and return-to-participation process. It is important to note that, although the strategies have been grouped under themed headings, it is highly likely that strategies will produce benefits that stretch across all three areas of concern for athletes—confidence, relatedness, and autonomy.

CLINICAL TIP

It is important for athletic trainers to be keenly aware of their scope of expertise and training when working with psychosocial aspects of the RTP process. If athletic trainers feel the situation exceeds their scope of practice, it is essential they refer athletes to other mental health professionals. Chapter 6 discusses in detail the recognition of athletes needing referral, as well as the mental health professionals to whom athletes can be referred.

Assessing Psychological Readiness

Athletic trainers receive a great deal of education on assessing injured athletes' physical readiness to return to participation; however, assuring athletes' psychological readiness to return is equally important. Sometimes this can be as easy as paying attention to athletes, observing their behaviors and moods, or having direct conversations about their readiness to return to participation. At other times, athletic trainers may want to use more formal means to evaluate athletes' psychological readiness. In these cases, inventories or surveys may be valuable. Unfortunately, the development of inventories designed to specifically address athletes' psychological readiness to return is still in its infancy. However, the following surveys may be helpful:

Injury-Psychological Readiness to Return to Sport (I-PRRS; Glazer, 2009): The I-PRRS was designed to assess athletes' ***self-efficacy*** in returning to full sport participation after athletic injury. Athletes are instructed to answer six questions on a scale from 0 to 100 (0 = little or no confidence, 50 = moderate confidence, 100 = utmost confidence). A total score for psychological readiness is calculated by summing the scores from the six individual items and dividing by 10. The maximum score is 60 and implies an athlete has the utmost confidence to return to sport at that time. A score of 40 implies moderate confidence to return, and a score of 20 implies low confidence to return. The I-PRRS can be administered within a couple of minutes and is very easy to use.

Re-Injury Anxiety Inventory (RIAI; Walker et al, 2010): One key component of psychological readiness is the extent to which athletes experience anxiety over reinjury. The RIAI was designed to assess the extent to which athletes are concerned about reinjury during rehabilitation and following a return to sport. The 28-item questionnaire takes approximately 5 minutes to complete and consists of 2 subscales (i.e., subcomponents). One subscale assesses anxieties regarding rehabilitation (RIA-R: 15 items), and the other examines anxieties regarding reinjury at return to play (RIA-RE: 13 items). Walker et al (2010) take care to differentiate fear (a flight-or-fight response to danger) from anxiety (uncertainty, worry, or concern), suggesting that anxiety more precisely captures the athletes' state of mind. In responding to the 28 items, athletes are asked to circle the appropriate number to indicate "how you feel right now, at this moment" on a scale ranging from 0 to 3 (0 = not at all; 1 = somewhat; 2 = moderately so; 3 = very much so). The RIAI is scored by computing a separate score for the two constructs by adding together the scores for the items corresponding to each construct. For the RIA-R subscale, a minimum score of 0 would indicate a complete absence of anxieties during rehabilitation, and a maximum score of 39 would indicate that the athlete had extremely high anxiety. On the RIA-RE scale, a minimum score of 0 would indicate a complete absence of any anxiety regarding reinjury at RTP, whereas a maximum score of 45 would indicate that the injured athlete had extremely high anxiety. The questionnaire is a useful tool in the identification of "at-risk" athletes and may be valuable in determining psychological readiness for a return to participation.

CLINICAL TIP

Athletes can complete the I-PRRS and the RIAI throughout the rehabilitation process. Athletic trainers can then monitor athletes' changing levels of confidence and reinjury anxiety as rehabilitation proceeds and better determine an appropriate time psychologically for injured athletes to return to participation.

Profile of Mood States (POMS) Short Form (McNair, Lorr, & Droppleman, 1992): The POMS short form can be used to assess athletes' total mood disturbance before returning to sport participation following athletic injury. The 30-item POMS short form assesses 6 mood states: Tension-Anxiety, Depression-Dejection, Anger-Hostility, Fatigue-Inertia, Confusion-Bewilderment, and Vigor-Activity. The first five mood states listed are considered negative moods, whereas the last one, vigor, is considered a positive mood. Adding the negative mood factors and then subtracting the score of the positive mood factor, vigor, calculates a total mood disturbance score. A high score implies the athlete has many negative moods with low vigor, whereas a low score means the athlete has few negative moods and high vigor. Lower scores on the POMS tend to be indicative of a more positive emotional profile and would be desirable before an athlete returns to full participation following injury.

In addition to the surveys listed earlier, the inventories highlighted in Chapter 3 to assess athletes' acute stress levels may also be helpful in evaluating an athlete's psychological readiness to return to participation. High scores on these inventories may be evidence of return-to-participation worries that need to be addressed.

Restoring Confidence

Functional Progression

As discussed earlier, restoring confidence is perhaps the foremost concern when working with injured athletes during the return-to-participation process. Fortunately, one of the easiest ways to restore confidence is through a physical intervention athletic trainers probably already use: functional progressions. Functional progressions involve a series of small incremental steps that enable athletes to safely and gradually resume progressively greater sport-specific function. From a physical standpoint, functional progressions are highly recommended because of their ability to minimize the risk for setbacks or exacerbation of injury.

As shown in Figure 11-3, functional progressions first involve the reacquisition of basic sports skills performed in isolation (e.g., jog, run, hop, cut, side slides). Next, athletes are reintroduced to progressive skill combinations through limited practice or individual work, or both. For example, athletes with a lower-extremity injury may be allowed to warm up with the team and participate in certain practice drills that require skills already achieved, but then work individually with athletic trainers or an assistant coach when practice becomes too intense for their physical status. As athletes become more proficient with their skills and their game conditioning improves, limits on their practice activities decrease. Athletes ultimately are cleared for full practice participation where they further refine their skills and fitness at game speed before reaching the final step—clearance for competition.

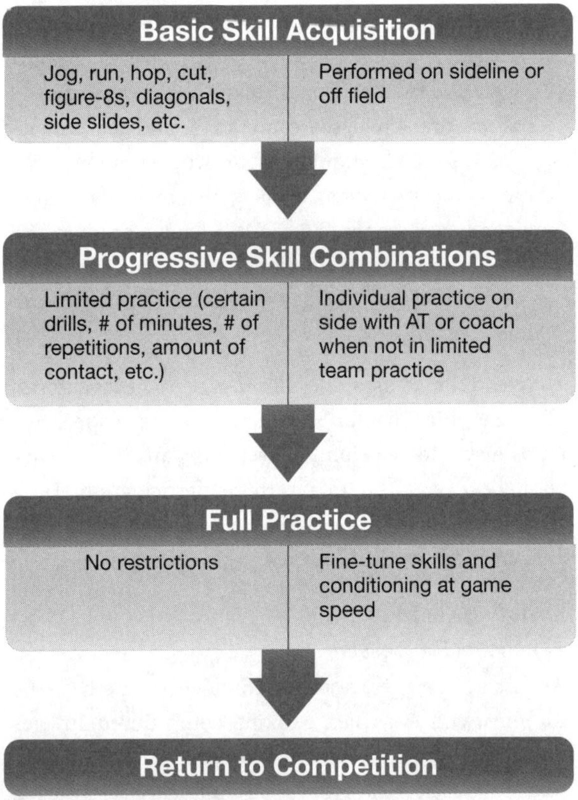

From a psychological standpoint, the small steps of the functional progression each serve as a mini-return to sport activity where athletes confirm their healing and ability to experience performance success. When monitored closely and implemented effectively, each successful completion of a step restores athletes' confidence that their injured body part is healing and can withstand sport-related demands. These small steps enable athletes to concretely see the incremental process that leads to the ultimate goal of full competitive participation. The small steps also serve to make the return-to-participation process less intimidating and daunting. Athletes gain confidence in tackling each manageable step, rather than viewing return to participation as one large leap.

For example, consider a soccer athlete recovering from an ankle sprain. Initially, he may be able to successfully run or pass in isolation; however, as he begins to combine these skills in limited practice drills, he discovers that: (1) he still is not comfortable with planting hard to fully strike a ball, (2) his accuracy in passing on the move is off, and (3) he feels "gassed" after only short bursts of practice activities. In functional progressions, he is given time to refine these technical proficiencies and game conditioning in a protected, safe environment by allowing some practice participation but still limiting the types of drills he enters, the number of minutes he actively participates in drills, and/or the amount of contact in which he engages. These limits enable him to experience continued success in his sport but discourage him from taking too large of a stride that could result in exacerbation of the injury. As his technical skills return and his fitness improves, practice limits are reduced until he is granted clearance to return to full practice without restrictions. Even at this point, it remains important to provide athletes sufficient time to restore their game fitness and test their recovered body parts at full speed before clearing them for competition. In this example, the athlete was given 2 weeks of unlimited practice before being cleared to compete. In this way, athletes can ultimately return to full competition

Basic Skill Acquisition

Jog, run, hop, cut, figure-8s, diagonals, side slides, etc.	Performed on sideline or off field

Progressive Skill Combinations

Limited practice (certain drills, # of minutes, # of repetitions, amount of contact, etc.)	Individual practice on side with AT or coach when not in limited team practice

Full Practice

No restrictions	Fine-tune skills and conditioning at game speed

Return to Competition

Figure 11-3 | Functional progression for return to participation.

against an outside opponent with confidence that has been solidified by their successful performance at unlimited practice.

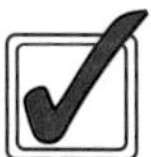

CLINICAL TIP

One advantage of functional progressions in return to participation is that they can effectively rein in potential overconforming athletes (see Chapter 2) who may think that they are immediately ready to jump back into full competition. Functional progressions can highlight athletes' abilities using their injured parts, as well as the work that may still need to be done, which may dissuade them from attempting a premature return to competition. Athletic trainers then have the opportunity to discuss realistic timelines for achieving intermediate steps that lead to a full and safe resumption of activity.

Goal Setting

The process described earlier in functional progressions is really nothing more than effectively defining the short-term and intermediate ***process goals*** that must be achieved to accomplish the desired long-term result of return to participation. Goal setting can further boost confidence by providing objective measures of improving physical health. Hopefully, throughout the rehabilitation process, the athletic trainer has recorded objective measures of physical progress (e.g., strength, power, limb girth). These can then be shared with injured athletes as their return-to-participation date nears to emphasize how far they have come and give objective feedback on the health and progress of their injured part.

For example, a female athlete had just completed her fifth month of rehabilitation following ACL reconstruction. She was voicing concerns about confidence that her knee would "hold up" in games. Her athletic trainer pulled out her rehabilitation log and pointed to the objective measures of strength (e.g., 90% of her uninjured leg as evidenced by her single-leg squat and hamstring curl comparisons) and power (e.g., preinjury and postinjury vertical jump height and 40-meter run times). The objective data that reflected her progress and physical abilities improved her confidence and ability to trust the rehabilitation work she had done. It also gave her confidence to direct her effort to achieving the objective criteria she still needed to meet before returning to full participation.

Selective Awareness/Reframing

Selective awareness refers to consciously choosing what one will focus his or her attention on. Athletes' confidence regarding return to participation can wane when they tend to focus on what they have not done or cannot yet do, rather than on what they have already accomplished and can do. It is similar to the glass is half-empty or half-full scenario. As athletes move toward full participation, they may be tempted to compare themselves with their healthy teammates regarding their fitness, speed, or technique, which causes their confidence to drop. The technique of reframing refers to helping athletes change the aspects of the situation to which they direct their attention and thereby change their perception of the situation.

CLINICAL TIP

An effective way to help athletes understand the significance of reframing is to engage them in this activity. Ask the athletes to look at the images in Figure 11-4. Although the picture itself is exactly the same in both images, the frames that surround the picture serve to change its appearance. The frames draw the athlete's attention to different aspects or colors of the picture, which ultimately changes how they see it. In injury situations, reframing does not change the fact that the athlete has been injured and may not yet be 100%; however, it does change how the athlete perceives the situation.

As discussed in the Clinical Tip box, the way one frames a picture can change its appearance. The same is true with injured athletes' perceptions of their recovery and return to participation. They need to remain focused on what they *can* do during the entire rehabilitation process, especially as they move through the functional progression to return to participation. Pessimism and doubt creep in when injured athletes frame their current status around comparisons with others and what they cannot do. In focusing on the *can*, athletes place a positive frame around their current situation that fosters confidence, optimism, and motivation.

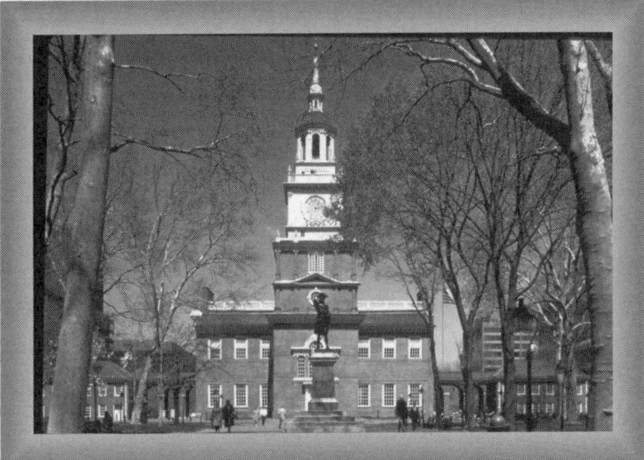

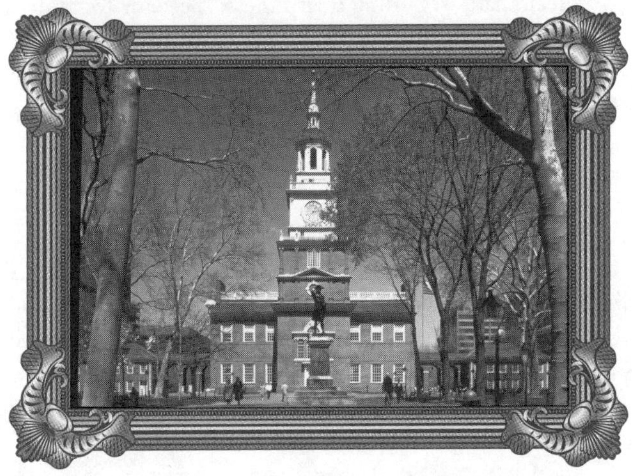

Figure 11-4 | Reframing changes perspective.

For example, look at the athlete's ***self-talk*** in Figure 11-5. In the top thought bubble, the athlete is focused on comparing his fitness with his teammates who have been practicing consistently while he has been rehabilitating from injury. He is thinking about what he *cannot* do, which results in feelings of frustration, self-doubt, and fear. However, when the athlete is challenged to reframe his current situation by focusing on what he *can* do (or what he *has been doing*), his perception of the situation changes and so do his thoughts. As a result, his emotions now include motivation to continue his rehabilitation work and confidence that he will achieve what he desires.

It is also important that, when athletic trainers communicate limits to athletes, they frame them in a positive manner. Focus should be placed on what athletes *are allowed* to do in practice, such as "I want you to run intervals at 85% of max today," versus what they should *avoid*, "I don't want you to sprint today." How limits are communicated to athletes can go a long way in directing which aspects of the situation they focus on, and ultimately how confident and motivated they feel. Another example of a selective-awareness exercise that may be useful in the athletic training setting is described in the Clinical Tip box.

CLINICAL TIP

A simple selective-awareness exercise involves constructing a "My Successes List." Athletic trainers can ask athletes to write down every success they have experienced during the last months or weeks of rehabilitation. Athletes can be encouraged to include such things as reducing the initial swelling; getting rid of crutches; returning to full weight bearing; completing range of motion, strength, and plyometric exercises; jogging; and running. Athletes should also be encouraged to include successes other than physical ones. These might include an increased understanding of the sport gained by watching practice or film during the recovery process, a new perspective on sport gained from being away from active participation, catching up on academic work, increased patience, or increased awareness of other interests besides sport. By writing a success list, athletes selectively focus on the numerous achievements they have made throughout the rehabilitation process. Focusing on the successes breeds confidence; as the list grows, so, too, does athletes' confidence in the healing process and their ability to successfully return to sport.

Affirmation Statements

Affirmation statements are positive, action-oriented statements that affirm one's abilities. Box 11-3 provides examples of affirmation statements that may be appropriate for rehabilitation settings or return-to-participation processes. The key to effectively using affirmation statements is to write them in an action-oriented, present tense beginning with "I am . . ." versus "I will . . ." This wording communicates that the event is happening and is real right now. Have athletes write down affirmation statements that enforce what they want to experience in their return-to-participation process. For example, "I am running smoothly and comfortably" or "I am strong and confident." When writing affirmation statements, athletes should be

Self-Talk
Emotions
Everyone is so fit. I've been out so long, I'll never catch up again.
Frustration, doubt, fear
I am stronger every day. I'm giving 100% in what I can do today. My fitness is returning more each day.
Confidence, motivation

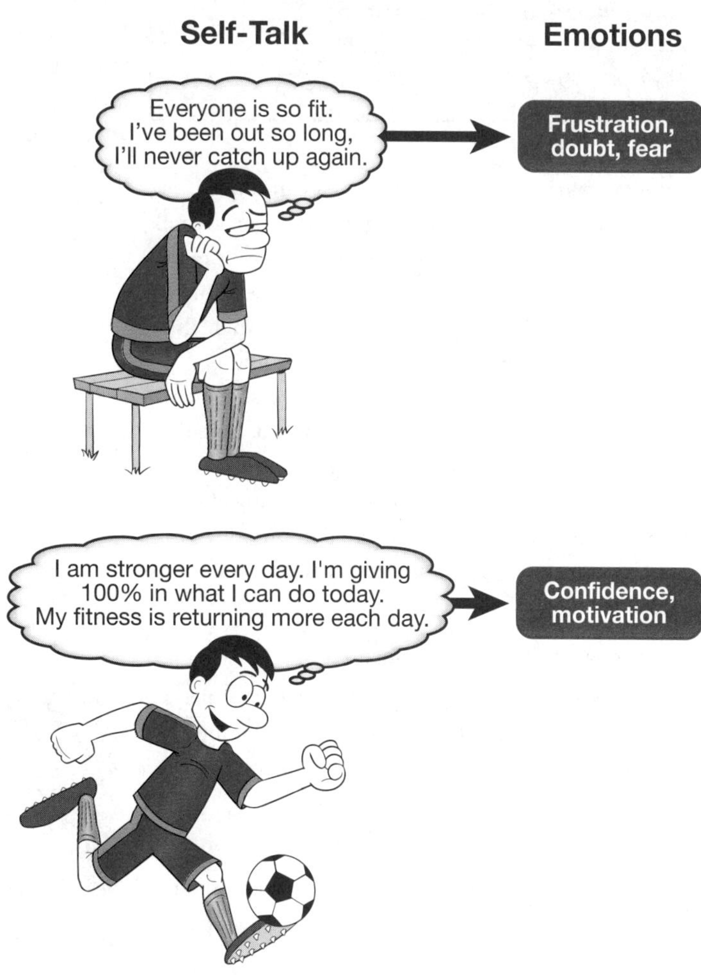

Figure 11-5 | Reframing in sport rehabilitation.

BOX 11-3 | Examples of Affirmation Statements Useful in the Return-to-Participation Process

I am stronger every day.
I am running smoothly and easily.
I am cutting with authority.
I am confident in my [insert injured body part].
I am controlling what I can in rehabilitation.
I am a skilled athlete.
I am concentrating on what's important now.
I am throwing with accuracy.
I am jumping with ease.
I am satisfied with my progress.
I trust my rehabilitation work.
I am fit.

careful to avoid using the word *not* because the brain overlooks it anyway. To confirm this, right now try *not* to think about a pink elephant. What are you seeing in your mind? Is it an elephant? The word *not* actually focuses athletes' attention on the very thing they are trying to avoid. Thus, affirmation statements must use positive wording.

Once athletes write down their affirmation statements, it is then important to increase the amount of time they spend thinking these affirmative thoughts. We all tend to believe what we hear repeatedly. Think of using affirmation statements as a bombing campaign on one's conscious awareness. To maximize the effectiveness of this campaign, follow these steps:

- Write down affirmation statements.
- Post these written statements in places where athletes will frequently encounter them (e.g., their workout bag, their locker door, their bathroom mirror, the dashboard of their car, their practice gear).
- Have athletes carry a copy in their pocket.
- Instruct athletes that, each time they encounter their affirmation statement, they need to pause and repeat it to themselves 10 times.

This bombardment with affirmative thoughts will help athletes selectively focus on the positive things that are transpiring in their rehabilitation and return-to-participation process, and can dramatically raise their confidence in their ability to achieve what they desire in their return to sport. Ultimately, the statements become a self-fulfilling prophecy.

Imagery

Athletes who lack confidence in their return to participation are often plagued by negative thinking or negative images. The earlier techniques should assist with the athletes' thinking, whereas imagery can assist with negative images. Athletes will frequently state that, when they try to use ***performance imagery*** following their injury, they tend to see the injury when they visualize the move, skill, or situation that caused their initial injury. One way to work around this is to encourage injured athletes to visualize their previous best performance. Every athlete enjoys reliving their moments of glory—it creates feelings of confidence, optimism, pride, and elation. Ask athletes to begin by enjoying the image of their best performance—recall the feelings they had, the ease of movement, the way everything clicked perfectly, the confidence and invincibility they felt in their whole body. Then ask athletes to slowly and gradually begin substituting certain parts of their best performance imagery with aspects of the current day; maybe make the opponent the same but the game a future one. Using the memories of the best performance experience mixed with some aspects of the present can help create a mental script where athletes achieve success again in the present. Many times, the confidence athletes gain from imagining their previous best performance serves as a springboard to enable them to successfully imagine their current-day performances in a positive manner.

RED FLAG

If athletes are unable to overcome flashback images of their injury or if recurring images of their injury interfere with their daily activities or sleep patterns, they need a referral to a mental health professional.

Another imagery technique that can assist in restoring confidence is to encourage athletes to use ***tactical imagery***, that is, to mentally rehearse plays, assignments, and/or strategies outside of physical practice time (Fig. 11-6). Injured athletes may lack confidence in their ability to remember plays, strategies, or assignments that they haven't physically practiced for a while, and they often feel the need to "catch up" to their teammates. Because physical repetitions may remain limited during the initial portions of the functional progression, mental repetitions can be an effective substitute to help build confidence. Although there is no substitute for physical practice, mental practice and repetitions are better than nothing. Fortunately, there are no limits on how many mental repetitions athletes can take. Mental rehearsal can make athletes feel more confident about their decision-making skills and their familiarity with plays or strategies through the knowledge of the number of mental repetitions they have experienced.

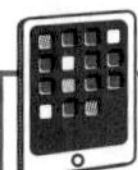

VIRTUAL FIELD TRIP

Athletic trainers can also use motivational imagery delivered through podcasts to increase confidence in the return-to-participation process. They can visit http://davisplus.fadavis.com for links to examples of motivational imagery podcasts, and learn more about how athletic trainers can make podcasts for implementation with injured athletes.

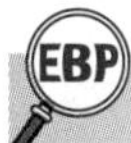

EVIDENCE-BASED PRACTICE

Evans, L., Hare, R., & Mullen, R. (2006). Imagery use during rehabilitation from injury. *Journal of Imagery Research in Sport and Physical Activity. 1*(1):Article 1. Retrieved from http://www.bepress.com/jirspa/vol1/iss1/art1.

Description of the Study

The purpose of the study was to explore the use of imagery by injured athletes during various phases of the rehabilitation process. Subjects included four athletes (two males, two females) representing the sports of hockey, pole vault, European football, and swimming at the semiprofessional or international level. Each participant had recovered from an injury that required 9 to 12 weeks of rehabilitation. Subjects were interviewed in depth regarding the type and timing of their imagery use.

Results of the Study

Participants used different types of imagery at various stages in the rehabilitation process to best meet their needs. In the early (first 3 weeks postinjury) and middle (middle 2–3 weeks of rehabilitation) phases of rehabilitation, participants made use of healing imagery, pain-management imagery, and skill-rehearsal imagery to increase their self-confidence and increase their motivation in rehabilitation and return to participation. In the late (within 2–3 weeks of return to full performance) phase of rehabilitation, participants used performance-based imagery exclusively. They focused on imagining execution of motor skills and strategy rehearsal to increase confidence, overcome fears of reinjury, and cope with their concerns about returning to play. Some variability existed in the types of imagery used and preferred across athletes.

Implications for Athletic Training Practice

It is important to assess the needs of athletes as they progress through the stages of rehabilitation and adjust the type and timing of imagery used accordingly. Performance-based imagery may be most beneficial in building confidence, overcoming fear, and coping with performance concerns as athletes near their return to full participation. It is important for athletic trainers to talk with each individual athlete about what types of imagery work best and then tailor imagery use to what each athlete finds most beneficial.

Modeling

Models, either in person or via video, can be helpful in building injured athletes' confidence regarding their return to participation. Speaking with or viewing video of

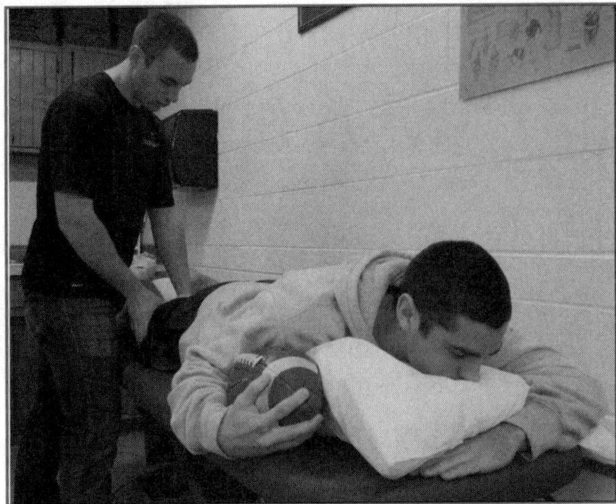

Figure 11-6 | Athlete performing tactical imagery during therapy.

athletes who have experienced similar injuries and successfully returned to sport can strengthen injured athletes' beliefs that they can also successfully return. Models allow injured athletes to vicariously experience success and affirm that successful return to participation is possible. Furthermore, models can provide comfort and reduce anxiety about potential unknowns by sharing their own experiences and challenges, as well as the strategies they used to overcome them. Injured athletes can learn from models' experiences and gain confidence in their own ability to return to participation using the suggested coping strategies. Conducting and filming interviews with injured athletes can help build a modeling resource library that can provide valuable information for injured athletes.

CLINICAL TIP

When using models, athletic trainers should encourage athletes to focus on the strategies and overall success experienced by the models rather than on the specific timeline the models' injury followed before return to participation. Athletic trainers should emphasize to athletes that every person may require different time frames in which they'll heal. Some athletes may otherwise find it discouraging if their injury is requiring more time to heal than someone else with a similar injury.

Anxiety Reduction

As indicated previously, athletes' confidence in return to participation is often compromised by anxiety. Chapters 3 and 10 discuss stress-management techniques in detail, several of which may be useful in reducing athletes' anxiety and restoring their confidence in the return-to-participation process.

Complete Breaths Ken Ravizza, a prominent sport psychology consultant, has said, "It is impossible to freak out and breathe at the same time." As mentioned in Chapter 10 with deep breathing, complete breaths are the most basic form of relaxation and can help athletes reduce their anxiety about performing a challenging skill or returning to practice. Athletic trainers can instruct athletes to use these breaths whenever they feel anxious about performing a sport skill or returning to play.

Quick Body Scan Before or during practice, athletes can use quick body scans to identify any unnecessary stress or tension and release it. They can then approach practice with a calm confidence that their body is free from unnecessary, and potentially hazardous, muscle tension.

Thought Stoppage/Thought Replacement Athletes' thinking can affect their emotions. Using thought stoppage, and then thought replacement, to change their self-talk "channel" from anxiety producing to confidence building can be helpful. The affirmation statements discussed earlier serve as good replacement thoughts for athletes to use.

Cue Words The self-talk technique of using cue words to guide attention to relevant performance cues can be applied if athletes begin to lose confidence and experience anxiety during performance. Cue words will help athletes remain performance focused and draw their attention to the relevant performance cues. Using these cue words can help restore the automaticity in athletes' performance movements that reduces the likelihood that anxiety-producing self-talk can creep in.

Normalize Reinjury Anxiety Athletic trainers can remind athletes that their anxiety about returning to play is normal considering what they have endured. Remind them that anxiety can have some adaptive value by limiting them from performing skills in which they are not fully confident or for which they are not fully prepared. Adding more steps to the functional progression or allowing more time at each progressive step can also help decrease athlete worries. Finally, athletic trainers should remind athletes that no functional step will be made unless concrete rehabilitation benchmarks indicating it is safe to proceed have been met.

RED FLAG
If athletes experience persistent or incapacitating anxiety relative to returning to sport participation, referral to a mental health professional is warranted.

Maintaining Relationships

As mentioned earlier in this chapter, when athletes become injured, their relationships and interactions with their coach and team change. Time that was once spent actively participating and interacting with their team is now replaced with rehabilitation and interactions with the athletic training staff. It is important to keep injured athletes feeling like they are still a part of the team and the social network that is so valuable to them.

Create Valued Involvement Throughout Rehabilitation

To maintain a relationship between injured athletes and the team, it is important to keep athletes involved in meaningful sport activities as much as possible throughout the rehabilitation process. This includes encouraging injured athletes to attend practices and perform as much of their rehabilitation and functional activity at the practice site as possible, so they can feel a part of the team and connect with their teammates and coaches. In support of team involvement, coaches in past research have suggested that athletes who stay involved with their team and perform rehabilitation sessions at team practices tend to be more motivated to return to sport, maintain important training routines, and are more knowledgeable about team plays and strategies on their return to sport. However, athletic trainers should exercise caution in mandating practice attendance for *all* injured athletes. Although some may benefit from being there, other athletes can perceive practice attendance as a constant reminder of what they are missing while being injured, and they could become dejected, frustrated, and disappointed. In these cases, other methods of meaningful team involvement may be beneficial.

Injured athletes can serve as player–coaches, analyze film, or scout opponents during their recovery process. These functions benefit the team but also create meaningful opportunities for injured athletes as they discover new ways to learn more about the game, develop as players, and devise strategies to successfully compete against various opponents. Through these experiences, injured athletes can gain knowledge, perspective, and insight about the sport that make them even better prepared when they return to full participation. In addition, these roles provide injured athletes with a way to contribute to and maintain relationships with the team, even if it is not in a physical capacity.

Meet with Coach to Discuss Role

Athletic trainers should encourage injured athletes to meet with their coaches to discuss their status throughout the rehabilitation process, but especially as return to participation nears. This can serve two purposes: (1) It will help maintain a sense of connection to the coach and team during rehabilitation, and (2) it can minimize athletes' anxieties regarding their place or status on the team. As injured athletes near their return to full participation, they often question their role and/or status on the team. Athletes are fully aware that someone has been playing in their place during their recovery period, and there is a great deal of uncertainty about where and how they now fit in. Frequent communication with their coach can erase many of these uncertainties. Athletic trainers should also work collaboratively with coaches and injured athletes to discuss appropriate functional progressions and expected participation goals as those athletes return to full participation.

Individual Training

As highlighted earlier in the discussion of functional progressions, injured athletes will need individual conditioning and skill practice as they work through their functional progressions. When possible, athletic trainers should have injured athletes work with assistant coaches, other injured athletes, or their healthy teammates during these activities to help maintain and enhance a sense of relationship between injured athletes, their coaches, and their team.

Mobilize Social Support Network

Throughout the rehabilitation process, it is important for athletes to feel they have a network of individuals who can support their emotional, informational, and tangible support needs. It is unrealistic and unwise for athletic trainers to assume they can fulfill all these needs. However, athletic trainers are in an ideal position to serve as facilitators in mobilizing a network of individuals who can assist in meeting these needs. Following injuries, athletic trainers can brainstorm or directly ask athletes about the types of social support (i.e., emotional, informational, and tangible) they desire. Then athletic trainers can recruit appropriate individuals to optimally meet each of those needs. For example, teammates, coaches, friends, and family members may be most effective in meeting the emotional or tangible needs of athletes, whereas members of the sports medicine team may be best suited to meet the informational support needs. It will be important to match individuals in the social support network to the needs expressed by injured athletes so as not to overwhelm athletes with support that is neither needed nor desired.

Maintaining Autonomy

Guided Choices in Rehabilitation

Injured athletes should be collaborative partners in goal setting throughout the rehabilitation process. This gives them a sense of control over their healing progression. Through creative selection of rehabilitation exercise options, athletic trainers can ensure their intended rehabilitation goals are still met. For example, if injured athletes need to work on sport-specific conditioning, athletic trainers can offer them a menu of conditioning drills from which they may choose, all of which meet the desired objectives, yet still give athletes a sense of autonomy in their rehabilitation progression.

In addition, injured athletes should be welcomed into discussions with coaches regarding limitations on drills or minutes in the return-to-participation process. Athletes will feel like they have some control if they are kept abreast of rationales for limits and at least have input into the decisions made. Although athletes' desires may not always be fulfilled, at least they know they have been heard and understand why their return-to-participation process may proceed differently than what they had hoped.

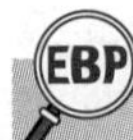

EVIDENCE-BASED PRACTICE

Podlog, L., & Eklund, R. C. (2010). Returning to competition following a serious injury: The role of self-determination. *Journal of Sports Sciences, 28,* 819–831.

Description of the Study

The purpose of the study was to experimentally examine the impact of autonomy and reinjury anxiety on professional Australian footballer appraisals (i.e., assessments) and emotions regarding a return to competition following a serious injury. Athletes were given hypothetical scenarios in which the degree of autonomy (i.e., personal control) regarding the circumstances of their return to competition and their level of reinjury anxiety was manipulated. In some scenarios, athletes were returning under conditions that were largely under their control (e.g., a return motivated by a love of the game or wanting to help the team win). In other scenarios, athletes were encouraged to think about a situation in which they were pressured to return to competition by the coach or felt guilty for not returning (i.e., lacked control over the return). Each athlete received only one scenario and was unaware that other teammates were given a different scenario, that is, one with more or less reinjury anxiety and control over the return to competition.

Results of the Study

Football players who perceived a greater sense of control over the circumstances of their return reported experiencing more positive appraisals and emotions with regard to the return to participation. Specifically, athletes with greater autonomy perceived the return-to-competition as more desirable, less threatening, less unfair, and less ego damaging than football players with less control over their return circumstances. Moreover, athletes with more control over their return to competition experienced greater happiness and lower anger and resentment than their counterparts with diminished perceptions of control.

Implications for Athletic Training Practice
Athletic trainers must ensure that athletes experience a sense of control over their return to sport. As highlighted earlier, providing athletes with options and choices (within a framework) may be invaluable in promoting a sense of control over the return-to-competition. Moreover, giving a rationale regarding the reasons behind particular exercises and encouraging intrinsic motives for a return to competition (e.g., a love of the game) may all facilitate a sense of autonomy during the return transition.

Discourage Pressure From Others

As mentioned earlier in the chapter, injured athletes may perceive pressure from numerous sources to return to participation quickly. Athletic trainers need to make concerted efforts to educate injured athletes' support networks regarding the *safe* timeline and progression for return to participation. Members in these networks most often have sincere interest in what is best for injured athletes' long-term health and well-being, and being informed of the potential consequences of premature return will help them resist pressuring injured athletes into participating before it is safe to do so.

This same support network can also be an important ally in discouraging injured athletes from trying to do too much too soon. Athletes are naturally motivated to play and want to do so as quickly as possible. An informed support network can work collaboratively with athletic trainers in sending consistent messages to athletes about being patient in the return-to-participation process so they can avoid reinjury or injury exacerbation.

Discuss Motives for Playing Sport

As athletes approach their return to participation, it is important from a psychological readiness standpoint that they are returning because it is what *they* really want versus doing it for others. Athletic trainers can informally have discussions with injured athletes about why they play their sport and why they want to return to it. Comments that raise questions regarding athletes' volition in returning to sport indicate a need for further inquiry, conversations with the coach, or encouragement for athletes to meet with a mental health professional to figure out why they are doing something they may not be internally driven to do. Also, in these conversations, it is valuable for athletic trainers to find out if the athletes agree with the timeline for return to participation. It shouldn't be surprising if athletes voice wishes to return more quickly, but if they comment that they are returning too fast, it should be considered a red flag. These athletes need to have further discussions with the athletic trainer or mental health professionals regarding their uncertainty about returning.

ATHLETE INSIDER CONCLUSION

Harper experienced an understandable lack of confidence in his injured knee and anxiety about reinjuring it while performing activities similar to the initial injury mechanisms. Harper explained that one particular drill helped him overcome much of that fear:

> *"I remember the four-cone drill that we did during individual practice as the turning point for me—the drill where I ran forward, did side slides to the next cone, backpedalled, and then did side slides back to the starting cone. As I completed those lateral movements and cutting at increasing speeds, I gained confidence that my knee would hold up, and I could do those activities again."*

The use of functional progressions that gave him time to gradually and safely discover his restored abilities provided the confidence he needed to resume full and uninhibited activity.

Effective Psychosocial Strategies for the Athletic Trainer to Use with Harper

Based on the psychosocial strategies discussed in this chapter, the following interventions would be appropriate when working with Harper.

1. Meet with Harper and normalize his hesitancy to engage in movements similar to those that caused his injuries.
2. Discuss with Harper the rehabilitation goals that have already been met and the functional progressions

designed to safely and effectively return him to full participation.

3. If necessary, create smaller steps in Harper's functional progression relative to making abrupt cuts and lateral movements so he can increase his confidence in those functional movements.
4. Administer the I-PRRS to Harper to assess his self-efficacy regarding returning to participation.
5. Assist Harper in evaluating his self-talk when he attempts to make cuts or lateral movements and point out potential areas for reframing or restructuring his self-talk.
6. Assist Harper in developing affirmation statements that he can use during functional activities that involve cutting and lateral movements.
7. Engage Harper in performance imagery of his best performances to increase his confidence in making cuts and explosive movements. Gradually incorporate current images into this process.
8. Facilitate a meeting with Harper and the coach to discuss Harper's perceived pressures to RTP quickly.

CONCLUSION

This chapter has described the psychosocial and sport-related challenges athletes face as they anticipate their return-to-sport participation following injury. Athletic trainers should bear in mind that return to participation must be based not only on physiological factors, but on physical, psychosocial, and sport-related readiness collectively. As highlighted previously, the I-PRRS questionnaire and the RIAI provide user-friendly methods for assessing athletes' confidence to resume competitive activity and the extent of reinjury worries. Given the apparent importance of confidence and reinjury anxiety to the return to participation, using the I-PRRS and RIAI will facilitate comprehensive assessment of athletes' readiness to reinitiate competitive activities. Moreover, this chapter discussed issues of competence, relatedness, and autonomy, and used them as a framework for developing and implementing intervention strategies for the return-to-participation process. Psychosocial strategies such as functional progressions, goal setting, reframing, imagery, modeling, social support, and anxiety reduction can be helpful in preparing athletes for their return to participation.

REFERENCES

Bianco, T. (2001). Social support and recovery from sport injury: Elite skiers share their experiences. *Research Quarterly for Exercise and Sport, 72,* 376–388.

Bianco, T., & Eklund, R. C. (2001). Conceptual considerations for social support research in sport and exercise settings: The case of sport injury. *Journal of Sport & Exercise Psychology, 23,* 85–107.

Bloom, G. A., Horton, A. S., McCrory, P., & Johnston, K. M. (2004). Sport psychology and concussion: New impacts to explore. *British Journal of Sports Medicine, 38,* 519–521.

Carey, J. L., Huffman, G. R., Parekh, S. G., & Sennett, B. J. (2006). Outcomes of anterior cruciate ligament injuries to running backs and wide receivers in the National Football League. *American Journal of Sports Medicine, 34,* 1911–1917.

Charlesworth, H., & Young, K. (2004). Why English female university athletes play with pain: Motivations and rationalizations. In: K. Young (Ed.), *Sporting Bodies, Damaged Selves: Sociological Studies of Sports-Related Injury* (pp. 163–180). Oxford, U.K.: Elsevier.

Creighton, D. W., Shrier, I., Shultz, R., Meeuwisse, W. H., & Matheson, G. O. (2010). Return-to-play in sport: A decision-based model. *Clinical Journal of Sport Medicine, 20*(5), 379–385.

Evans, L., Hardy, L., & Fleming, S. (2000). Intervention strategies with injured athletes: An action research study. *The Sport Psychologist, 14,* 188–206.

Evans, L., Hare, R., & Mullen, R. (2006). Imagery use during rehabilitation from injury. *Journal of Imagery Research in Sport and Physical Activity. 1*(1):Article 1. Retrieved from: http://www.bepress.com/jirspa/vol1/iss1/art1

Glazer, D. D. (2009). Development and preliminary validation of the Injury-Psychological Readiness to Return to Sport (I-PRRS) Scale. *Journal of Athletic Training, 44,* 185–189.

Johnston, L. H., & Carroll, D. (1998). The provision of social support to injured athletes: A qualitative analysis. *Journal of Sport Rehabilitation, 7,* 267–284.

McCrory, P. (2011). Future advances and areas of future focus in the treatment of sport-related concussion. *Clinics in Sports Medicine, 30*(1), 201–208.

McNair, D. M., Lorr, M., & Droppleman, L. F. (1992). *Manual for the Profile of Mood States (POMS)* (Revised ed.). San Diego, CA: Educational and Industrial Testing Services.

Murphy, P., & Waddington, I. (2007). Are elite athletes exploited? *Sport in Society, 10,* 239–255.

Podlog, L., & Eklund, R. C. (2006). A longitudinal investigation of competitive athletes' return to sport following serious injury. *Journal of Applied Sport Psychology, 18,* 44–68.

Podlog, L., & Eklund, R. C. (2007a). Professional coaches' perspectives on the return to sport following serious injury. *Journal of Applied Sport Psychology, 19,* 207–225.

Podlog, L., & Eklund, R. C. (2007b). The psychosocial aspects of a return to sport following serious injury: A review of the literature from a self-determination perspective. *Psychology of Sport and Exercise, 8,* 535–566.

Podlog, L., & Eklund, R. C. (2010). Returning to competition following a serious injury: The role of self-determination. *Journal of Sports Sciences, 28,* 819–831.

Podlog, L., Lochbaum, M., & Stevens, T. (2010). Need satisfaction, well-being and perceived return-to-sport outcomes among injured athletes. *Journal of Applied Sport Psychology, 22*(2), 167–182.

Ryan, R. M., & Deci, E. L. (2000). Self-determination theory and the facilitation of intrinsic motivation, social development, and well-being. *American Psychologist, 55,* 68–78.

Walker, N., Thatcher, J., & Lavallee, D. (2010). A preliminary development of the Re-Injury Anxiety Inventory (RIAI). *Physical Therapy in Sport, 11,* 23–29.

BOARD OF CERTIFICATION STRATEGIES AND COMPETENCIES

Several of the competencies in the psychosocial strategies and referral content area of the Fifth Edition Athletic Training Education Competencies are addressed in this chapter. This chapter has focused on the importance of psychosocial and sport-related readiness in the return-to-participation process. Issues of confidence and motivation for injured athletes in the return-to-participation process have been discussed (PS-1, PS-3). In addition, the importance of educating injured athletes' support networks regarding the psychological challenges athletes will face in the return-to-participation process have been outlined (PS-6). Finally, many psychosocial intervention strategies to improve athletes' confidence and motivation, relatedness, and autonomy in the return-to-participation process have been presented (PS-7, PS-8). Athletic training students should feel well prepared to respond to questions on the Board of Certification examination relative to these competencies.

Board of Certification Style Questions

1. Which of the following are common indications that an athlete may have elevated reinjury concerns? (Select all that apply.)
   a. Avoiding a return to sport despite positive functional indicators
   b. Increased negative mood states
   c. Hesitation in trying sport-specific skills of which an athlete is physically capable
   d. Doing more than the prescribed number of rehabilitation exercises

2. An athlete is lacking confidence in her shoulder when considering returning to participation following rehabilitation from a superior labrum anterior-posterior lesion repair. What psychosocial strategies could you use to enhance her feelings of competence? (Select all that apply.)
   a. Tactical imagery
   b. Goal setting
   c. Affirmation statements
   d. Modeling

3. Autonomy refers to the idea that an individual has
   a. social support from coaches and teammates.
   b. choice or control over his or her own actions and behaviors.
   c. external pressure placed on him or her by coaches and teammates.
   d. the skill to accomplish his or her goals.

4. Sport-related concerns frequently faced by athletes as they approach their return to participation include (Select all that apply):
   a. remaining up to speed on plays, tactics, and strategies.
   b. reinjury anxiety.
   c. identity concerns.
   d. inadequate social support.

5. Referral to a mental health professional is needed in which of the following situations? (Select all that apply.)
   a. An injured athlete is feeling isolated from his teammates
   b. An athlete is having difficulty sleeping because of "flashbacks" of her knee injury
   c. An athlete is engaging in negative self-talk following injury
   d. An athlete is concerned over whether he will have his starting position when he returns from his injury

END-OF-CHAPTER EXERCISES

1. Consider an athlete with whom you are currently working who has voiced apprehension about his or her recovering body part's ability to resume normal activity. Develop a list of progressive functional steps that will allow the athlete to move gradually from the current physical status to full activity. As you review your list, are there any steps that may seem "too big"? If so, work to break them down into even smaller pieces. Explain how you would objectively measure and record athlete successes at each of these steps to help instill even greater confidence.
2. Develop (or work with the athlete or coach to create) an imagery script that will assist an injured athlete in performing tactical imagery.
3. Describe how objective measures of rehabilitation success can influence an athlete's confidence and motivation.
4. Identify and explain the issues of competence, relatedness, and autonomy that Harper is facing (or has faced) in his injury experiences. Based on the psychosocial strategies you have just learned, identify specific ways in which you could address each of these issues.
5. Devise a list of five negative statements an athlete might make regarding a return to participation. Beside each negative statement, provide a positive statement that helps reframe the negative thought into a constructive or affirmative one.
6. As described in this chapter, athletes may experience pressure to return to participation from coaches, teammates, or training partners. Write a short script for what you might say to a coach who you are aware is pressuring an athlete to return to participation.
7. Athletes often want and need social support during the return-to-participation transition. Identify and define the three broad forms of support returning athletes may typically desire in the return-to-participation transition process and indicate who might be most qualified to provide each type of support. Then describe how you could facilitate a network of individuals to assist you in giving each of these types of support needed by the athlete.
8. Choose an injured athlete with whom you are currently working or with whom you have worked in the past. Describe different ways in which you can take his or her rehabilitation exercises (e.g., strength, power, conditioning) to the practice site so he or she can maintain greater affiliation with the team.
9. Conduct and film an interview with an athlete regarding their return-to-participation experience. Ask questions that guide the athlete to discuss his or her experiences with anxieties, feelings of isolation, or loss of control. Then encourage the athlete to discuss how he or she coped with these situations, and ask him or her to provide advice for athletes who might sustain a similar injury in the future.
10. Assume that a swimmer is recovering from shoulder impingement, and all overhead activity still produces pain. With a partner, role-play the way you'd communicate practice limits so the athlete selectively attends to what he or she *can* do versus what he or she *cannot* do.

Appendix A

Athlete Insider by Chapter

Chapter 1: Introduction to Psychosocial Aspects of Athletic Training

- Seth
- Collegiate football athlete
- Anterior cruciate ligament sprain with surgical repair

Chapter 2: Sociocultural Aspects of Injury and Injury Response

- Petra Majdic
- Olympic cross-country skier from Slovenia
- Significant pain from skiing accident

Chapter 3: Psychosocial Antecedents to Injury

- Susan
- Collegiate softball athlete
- Return to sport following successful anterior cruciate ligament rehabilitation

Chapter 4: Emotional Responses to Injury

- Maryn
- High school basketball athlete
- Anterior cruciate ligament sprain, lateral meniscal tear, osteochondral defect

Chapter 5: Communication and Athlete Education Skills for the Athletic Trainer

- Mike
- Collegiate lacrosse athlete
- Labral tear

Chapter 6: Identification of Psychosocial Distress and Referral

- Amelia
- Collegiate volleyball athlete
- Ankle sprain

Chapter 7: Introduction and Overview of Pain

- Jayda
- Collegiate soccer athlete
- Residual lower leg pain following compartment syndrome release and tibia-fibula fracture

Chapter 8: Psychosocial Aspects of Rehabilitation

- José
- High school cross-country athlete
- Iliotibial band pain

Chapter 9: Social Support and the Athletic Trainer

- Kate
- Collegiate soccer athlete
- Anterior cruciate ligament sprain

Chapter 10: Psychosocial Strategies: Effectiveness and Application

- ‘A’amakua
- Collegiate football athlete
- Multiple injuries

Chapter 11: Psychosocial Aspects of Return to Participation

- Harper
- Collegiate soccer athlete
- Multiple injuries

Appendix B

Competencies and Proficiencies by Chapter

Psychosocial Strategies and Referral Content Area From the Athletic Training Education Competencies, Fifth Edition (2011)

Knowledge and Skills	Chapter
Psychosocial Strategies and Referral (PS)	
Theoretical Background	
PS-1	3, 9, 11
PS-2	4
PS-3	2, 11
PS-4	5, 9
PS-5	5, 9
Psychosocial Strategies	
PS-6	3, 5, 9, 11
PS-7	8, 10, 11
PS-8	2, 10, 11
PS-9	2, 7
PS-10	2
Mental Health and Referral	
PS-11	6
PS-12	6
PS-13	6
PS-14	6
PS-15	6
PS-16	6
PS-17	6
PS-18	5, 6

Continued

Psychosocial Strategies and Referral Content Area From the Athletic Training Education Competencies, Fifth Edition (2011)—cont'd

Knowledge and Skills	Chapter
Clinical Integration Proficiencies (CIP)	
Psychosocial Strategies and Referral	
CIP-7	7, 8, 10
CIP-8	6

Appendix C

Evidence-Based Practice Features

Evidence-Based Practice Features by Author (Reference Chapter in Parentheses)

Boyce, D., & Brosky, J. A. (2008). Determining the minimal number of cyclic passive stretch repetitions recommended for an acute increase in an indirect measure of hamstring length. *Physiotherapy Theory and Practice, 24*(2), 113–120. doi: 10.1080/09593980701378298 (Chapter 8)

Brewer, B. W., Cornelius, A. E., Stephan, Y., et al. (2010). Self-protective changes in athletic identity following anterior cruciate ligament reconstruction. *Psychology of Sport and Exercise, 11*(1), 1–5. (Chapter 4)

Brewer, B. W., Cornelius, A. E., Van Raalte, J. L., et al. (2003). Age-related differences in predictors of adherence to rehabilitation after anterior cruciate ligament reconstruction. *Journal of Athletic Training, 38*(2), 158–162. (Chapter 8)

Burke, S., & Sabiston, C. M. (2010). The meaning of the mountain: Exploring breast cancer survivors' lived experiences of subjective well-being during a climb on Mt. Kilimanjaro. *Qualitative Research in Sport, Exercise, and Health, 2*(1), 1–16. (Chapter 4)

Clement, D., & Shannon, V. R. (2011). Injured athletes' perceptions about social support. *Journal of Sport Rehabilitation, 20,* 457–470. (Chapter 9)

Clement, D., Hamson-Utley, J., Arvinen-Barrow, M., Kamphoff, C. S., Zakrajsek, R. A., & Martin, S. B. (2012). College athletes' expectations about injury rehabilitation with an athletic trainer. *International Journal of Athletic Therapy & Training, 17*(4), 18–27. (Chapter 1)

Concannon, M., & Pringle, B. (2012). Psychology in sports injury rehabilitation. *British Journal of Nursing, 21*(8), 484–490. (Chapter 6)

Covassin, T., Elbin, 3rd, R. J., Larson, E., et al. (2012). Sex and age differences in depression and baseline sport-related concussion neurocognitive performance and symptoms. *Clinical Journal of Sports Medicine, 22*(2), 98–104. (Chapter 4)

Creighton, D. W., Shrier, I., Shultz, R., Meeuwisse, W. H., & Matheson, G. O. (2010). Return-to-play in sport: A decision-based model. *Clinical Journal of Sport Medicine, 20*(5), 379–385. (Chapter 11)

Cupal, D. D., & Brewer, B. W. (2001). Effects of relaxation and guided imagery on knee strength, reinjury anxiety, and pain following anterior cruciate ligament reconstruction. *Rehabilitation Psychology, 46*(1), 28–43. doi:10.1037/0090-5550.46.1.28 (Chapter 7)

Dawson, M., Hamson-Utley, J. J., Hansen, R., & Olpin, M. (2014). Examining the effectiveness of psychological strategies on physiologic markers: evidence-based suggestions for holistic care of the athlete. *Journal of Athletic Training, 49*(1). (Chapter 3)

Deroche, T., Woodman, T., Stephan, Y., Brewer, B. W., & Le Scanff, C. (2011). Athletes' inclination to play through pain: A coping perspective. *Anxiety, Stress & Coping, 24*(5), 579–587. (Chapter 7)

Deveugele, M., Derese, A., De Maesschalack, S., Willems, S., Van Driel, M., & De Maeseneer, J. (2005). Teaching communication skills to medical students, a challenge in the curriculum? *Patient Education and Counseling, 58*(3), 265–270. (Chapter 5)

Evans, L., Hardy, L., & Fleming, S. (2000). Intervention strategies with injured athletes: An action research study. *The Sport Psychologist, 14,* 188–206. (Chapter 10)

Evans, L., Hare, R., & Mullen, R. (2006). Imagery use during rehabilitation from injury. *Journal of Imagery Research in Sport and Physical Activity. 1*(1):Article 1. Retrieved from http://www.bepress.com/jirspa/vol1/iss1/art1. (Chapter 11)

Flint, F. A., & Weiss, M. R. (1992). Returning injured athletes to competition: A role and ethical dilemma. *Canadian Journal of Sport Sciences, 17*(1), 34–40. (Chapter 2)

Hamson-Utley, J. J., Martin, S., & Walters, J. (2008). Athletic trainers' and physical therapists' perceptions of the effectiveness of psychological skills within sport-injury rehabilitation programs. *Journal of Athletic Training, 43*(3), 258–264. (Chapter 1)

Hush, J., Cameron, K., & Mackey, M. (2010). Patient satisfaction with musculoskeletal physical therapy care: A systematic review. *Physical Therapy, 91,* 25–36. (Chapter 10)

Kenow, L. J., & Wiese-Bjornstal, D. M. (2010, October). *Risk Behavior Conformity in Sport Injury Questionnaire (RBCSI): Preliminary evidence in support of a new measure.* Paper presented at the meeting of the Association for Applied Sport Psychology; Providence, RI. (Chapter 2)

Maddison, R., & Prapavessis, H. (2005). A psychological approach to the prediction and prevention of athletic injury. *Journal of Sport & Exercise Psychology, 27,* 289–310. (Chapter 3)

Malcom, N. L. (2006). "Shaking it off" and "toughing it out": Socialization to pain and injury in girls' softball. *Journal of Contemporary Ethnography, 35*(5), 495–525. (Chapter 2)

McCrea, M., Hammeke, T., Olsen, G., Leo, P., & Guskiewicz, K. (2004). Unreported concussion in high school football players: Implications for prevention. *Clinical Journal of Sport Medicine, 4*(1), 13–16. (Chapter 9)

Murphy, P., & Waddington, I. (2007). Are elite athletes exploited? *Sport in Society, 10,* 239–255. doi: 10.1080/17430430601147096 (Chapter 11)

Newcomer, R., & Perna, F. M. (2003). Features of posttraumatic distress among adolescent athletes. *Journal of Athletic Training, 38*(2), 163. (Chapter 6)

Podlog, L., & Eklund, R. C. (2010). Returning to competition following a serious injury: The role of self-determination. *Journal of Sports Sciences, 28,* 819–831. (Chapter 11)

Podlog, L., Lochbaum, M., & Stevens, T. (2010). Need satisfaction, well-being and perceived return-to-sport outcomes among injured athletes. *Journal of Applied Sport Psychology, 22*(2), 167–182. (Chapter 11)

Russell, H., & Tracey, J. (2011). What do injured athletes want from their health care professionals? *International Journal of Athletic Therapy & Training, 16*(5), 18–21. (Chapter 10)

Scherzer, C. B., Brewer, B. W., Cornelius, A. E., et al. (2001). Psychological skills and adherence to rehabilitation after reconstruction of the anterior cruciate ligament. *Journal of Sport Rehabilitation, 10*(3), 165–172. (Chapter 8)

Stiller, J. L., & Ostrowski, J. A. (2007). Tricks of the trade: Enhancing interpersonal skills. *Athletic Therapy Today, 12*(6), 33–35. (Chapter 5)

Stiller-Ostrowski, J. L., & Ostrowski, J. A. (2009). Recently certified athletic trainers' undergraduate educational preparation in psychosocial intervention and referral. *Journal of Athletic Training, 44*(1), 67–75. (Chapters 1 & 5)

Storch, E. A., Storch, J. B., Killiany, E. M., & Roberti, J. W. (2005). Self-reported psychopathology in athletes: A comparison of intercollegiate student-athletes and non-athletes. *Journal of Sport Behavior, 28*(1), 86–97. (Chapter 6)

Taylor, A. (1995). Development of a Sports Injury Clinic Athlete Satisfaction Scale for auditing patient perceptions. *Physiotherapy Theory and Practice, 11*(4), 231–238. (Chapter 10)

Tricker, R. (2000). Painkilling drugs in collegiate athletics: Knowledge, attitudes, and use of student athletes. *Journal of Drug Education, 30*(3), 313–324. (Chapter 2)

Yang, J., Peek-Asa, C., Lowe, J. B., Heiden, E., & Foster, D. T. (2010). Social support patterns of collegiate athletes before and after injury. *Journal of Athletic Training, 45*(4), 372–379. (Chapter 9)

Glossary

A

Active listening Communication technique that requires the listener to feed back what is heard by restating or paraphrasing; to confirm what was heard and to confirm the understanding of both parties.

Acute Of short onset or duration.

Acute pain Pain of recent and sudden onset; typically high-intensity pain localized at or near the site of injury.

Adrenocorticotropic hormone A hormone secreted by the anterior pituitary gland in response to stress.

Affect A feeling or emotion.

Affirmation Statement(s) made to the self to encourage, motivate, and improve self-worth.

Affirmation statements Positive, action-oriented self-talk that affirms athletes' abilities.

Allodynia Extreme sensitivity to an innocuous stimulus (such as light touch or cold); pain from sunburn is a common example.

Antecedent A preceding event or condition, or a preexisting factor.

Anterior cingulate cortex Frontal part of cingulate cortex in the brain; plays a role in cognitive functions such as reward anticipation, decision-making, empathy, and emotion.

Arousal Psychological or physiological state of being alert.

Athlete-centered care Providing individualized care to an athlete.

Athletic identity The degree to which a person identifies the self as an athlete.

Attending skills Ability to elicit information from others and listen intently to responses.

Autonomy A sense of choice or control over one's actions and behaviors.

B

Benign pain Temporary occurrence of discomfort that is not associated with new tissue damage; characterized as dull and generalized with no swelling or localized tenderness.

Biopsychosocial perspective The view that biological, psychological (e.g., thoughts, emotions, behaviors), and social factors all play a significant role in human functioning in the context of disease or illness.

Burnout Psychological, emotional, and physical withdrawal from an activity that was previously enjoyable; a response to excessive stress and dissatisfaction with sports participation.

C

Cerebral cortex A part of the brain that plays a key role in memory, attention, perceptual awareness, thought, language, and consciousness.

Chronic Of long onset or duration.

Chronic pain Pain that persists beyond the normal time expected for healing (typically a minimum of 3–6 months).

Clinical trial Research involving tests that generate safe-use data for health interventions by comparing existing and new drugs or procedures that change a participant's health/behavior.

Cognitive appraisal Interpretation of a situation.

Cognitive relaxation A relaxation method that includes verbal and visual cues, which lead individuals to a relaxing time and place.

Cognitive rest Stopping activities that require concentration and attention; may include a temporary leave from academic/work responsibilities, reduced school day/workload, and/or additional time allowed to complete tasks or tests.

Cognitive restructuring A cognitive behavioral strategy used to identify and replace irrational or maladaptive thoughts that often occur in anxiety-provoking situations.

Competence A sense of being capable or proficient in one's pursuits.

Compliance An individual completing a required behavior.

Concussion A complex pathophysiological process that affects the brain, induced by traumatic biomechanical forces.

Coping skills Mechanisms that promote the ability to cope with a stressor or situation; built from experience or learned.

Cortisol A naturally occurring stress hormone in the human body that is associated with the fight-or-flight response.

Countering A technique used to challenge the veracity of irrational and/or maladaptive thoughts by using logical counterstatements.

D

Decoding Process of interpreting meaning from the symbolic codes used to send a message.

Demographic variables Factors that explain or provide context for data being gathered.

Depersonalization Being detached from oneself.

Derealization Feelings of unreality.

Dissociative imagery A relaxation strategy to distract the athlete from focusing on injury-related pain.

E

Emotion-focused coping Strategies aimed at reducing the negative emotional response associated with stress; may be the only realistic option when the source of stress is outside of the person's control.

Empathy Being sensitive to and vicariously experiencing the feelings, thoughts, or motives of another person.

Encoding Process of putting an intended message into symbolic code (e.g., words, gestures, facial expressions) that can be observed.

Evidence-based practice A methodology that combines clinical expertise and the best available systematic research evidence when making decisions about patient care.

Extrinsic motivation Behavior that is driven by a desire to attain a specific outcome; motivation from an outside source.

Extrovert Manifested in outgoing, talkative, energetic behavior.

F

Feedback A verbal or nonverbal response or reaction to a message received.

Functional progression A series of gradually progressive activities designed to prepare athletes for return to a specific sport.

H

Hardiness Stable personality trait composed of three components: perceived control over the situation, viewing the situation as a challenge as opposed to a threat, and commitment to changing the situation.

Healing cycle Cycle of recovery characterized by ups, downs, plateaus, and setbacks.

Healing imagery Focusing attention on a target visual stimulus to produce a specific physiological change that can promote healing.

Help-seeking Involves the willingness to ask for assistance from identified resources, such as those with whom athletes feel comfortable seeking help and advice.

Holistic Related to healing; a holistic approach includes all parts of the healing system—the mind and the body—in the healing process.

Hyperalgesia Heightened sensation response to noxious stimulus.

Hypothalamus A part of the brain responsible for certain metabolic processes and other activities of the autonomic nervous system (including body temperature, hunger, thirst, fatigue, sleep, and circadian cycles).

I

Injury pain Occurrence of pain that signals actual or potential tissue damage.

Injury severity Grading of an injury that includes the amount of deformity, disability, and lack of strength to complete daily living activities; typically includes strength, range of motion, and functional deficit.

Injury type Kind of injury; soft tissue or bony; relates to severity.

Instrumental coping Strategies that target the causes of stress in practical ways that address the stress-producing problem or situation, consequently directly reducing the stress; examples include finding out about the injury, attempting to alleviate sources of stress and discomfort, and listening to the advice of health professionals.

Intrinsic motivation Behavior that is driven by an interest or enjoyment in the task itself (e.g., personal best).

Introvert Manifested in more reserved, quiet, shy behavior.

L

Limbic system A complex set of brain structures that lies on both sides of the thalamus; supports a variety of functions including emotion, behavior, and long-term memory.

Listening Perception and understanding of auditory signals.

M

Macrotrauma Injury resulting from a single impact or force that creates tissue damage (e.g., fracture, sprain, or dislocation).

Malingering Intentionally pretending to have or exaggerating physical or psychological symptoms, especially to avoid work or a return to participation.

Matching hypothesis Involves matching the available social support to the social support needs of the athlete.

Message A thought, feeling, or idea that is conveyed to another person.

Meta-analysis A research method that takes data from a number of independent studies and integrates them using statistical analysis.

Microtrauma Injury resulting from repeated smaller forces that gradually result in tissue damage over time (e.g., stress fracture, tendinitis).

Mood Emotional state (e.g., happy, sad).

Mood state Transitory, fluctuating state of mind of the athlete.

Motivational Strategies that influence an individual's desire or drive.

Motivational orientation An individual propensity to be driven by internal or external factors.

N

Nociception The process of pain sensation by the nociceptors.

Nociceptors Sensory neurons that respond to potentially damaging stimuli by sending nerve signals to the spinal cord and brain.

Noise Internal and external barriers that prevent effective delivery or receipt of communicated messages.

Nonpharmacological pain management Strategies designed to increase an individual's perception of control over pain that he or she experiences.

Nonresponse bias A research term describing a situation in which the answers of respondents differ from the potential answers of those who did not answer.

Nonverbal communication The expression of thoughts, feelings, or ideas without the use of words.

Normative behavior Behavior that is expected by societal standards.

Noxious An actually or potentially tissue-damaging event; may be mechanical, chemical, or thermal.

O

One-way communication Communication process focused exclusively on getting messages from the sender to the receiver.

Open posture An open stance in which arms and legs are not crossed in any way.

Overconformer Athlete who unconditionally accepts the norms of the sport ethic and follows them without reservation.

P

Pain-management imagery Focusing attention on a target visual stimulus to produce specific images to promote pain-management strategies (e.g., visualizing the pain flying away or lying in a meadow free of pain).

Pain perception Conscious interpretation of nociceptive stimulus as pain.

Pain sensation Stimulus is received by the nervous system (via nociceptors).

Pain-spasm cycle Pain that causes vasoconstriction and muscle spasm, which, in turn, causes more pain, which, in turn, exacerbates the cycle; sometimes referred to as the pain-spasm-pain cycle.

Pain threshold Point at which pain begins to be felt; an entirely subjective phenomenon.

Pain tolerance The ability of the patient to withstand pain or painful stimuli for a period of time.

Paralanguage Vocal characteristics associated with communication.

Paraphrasing Process of restating what was understood in a message back to the sender.

Paresthesias Numbness or tingling sensations.

Perception The conscious interpretation of nociceptive stimulus as pain.

Performance imagery The creation or re-creation of an experience in the mind from memory or quasi-experience using a combination of the five senses with the goal of improving an aspect of a performance in sport or rehabilitation.

Periaqueductal gray A role in the descending modulation of pain.

Persistent pain Pain that meets the time frame defined as chronic but is actually a symptom of a treatable condition.

Personality A stable trait of an individual's general emotional, behavioral, and attitudinal response patterns.

Physical characteristics Factors that describe physical elements, such as strong, healthy.

Physiotherapists Term used for sports medicine practitioners in other countries, similar to athletic trainers in the United States.

Positive affirmation A positive declaration of truth; used in rehabilitation and healing to improve mind-set and to motivate.

Postconcussion syndrome (PCS) A complex disorder in which a variable combination of postconcussion symptoms (such as headache and dizziness) last for weeks and sometimes months after the concussive event.

Post-traumatic growth (PTG) A positive psychological change experienced as a result of highly challenging life events and circumstances.

Primary appraisal Initial assessment of a situation to evaluate it as a threat or challenge.

Proactively Acting in advance to deal with an expected difficulty; anticipatory.

Process goals Goals that focus on the actions an individual must engage in during performance to execute or perform well.

Progressive muscle relaxation (PMR) A technique for learning to monitor and control muscle tension.

Proxemics Communication expressed through the space between people as they interact.

Psychological skills Mental skills, techniques by which the individual can use the mind to control the body or to create an outcome.

Psychosocial Integration of psychology and sociology within injury and healing processes; interplay between the two fields best captures individual and situational factors.

Psychosocial strategies A term typically used to describe a range of psychosocial skills and techniques athletes can use to control their thoughts, emotions, and behaviors.

Psychosocial techniques Methods athletes can use to rehearse, improve, and maintain their psychological skills.

R

Rapport The harmonious or synchronous relationship of two or more people who relate well to each other.

Receiver Person to whom a sender conveys a communicated message.

Recovery status The percentage toward recovery; can be seen as varying on a continuum from 10% to 100% or reported as "not fully recovered" or "fully recovered."

Reframing Changing the way one views a situation by consciously choosing to attend to different aspects of the situation.

Rehabilitation adherence Behaviors an athlete demonstrates by pursuing a course of action that coincides with the recommendations of the athletic trainer and is aimed at recovery from injury.

Rehabilitation antecedents Biopsychosocial factors (injury characteristics, biological factors, psychological factors, sociodemographic factors, social/contextual factors) that influence rehabilitation adherence and outcomes.

Rehabilitation nonadherence The athlete working either too little (i.e., underadherence) or too much (i.e., overadherence) based on recommendations of the athletic trainer.

Rehabilitation outcomes Results of rehabilitation; examples include, but are not limited to, functional ability, strength, range of motion, readiness to return to sport, treatment satisfaction, quality of life.

Rehabilitation overadherence The athlete doing more than the rehabilitation program calls for.

Rehabilitation-process imagery Focusing attention on a target visual stimulus to produce specific images of different aspects of the rehabilitation process.

Rehabilitation underadherence The athlete doing less than the rehabilitation program calls for.

Relatedness A sense of belonging or feeling part of a group.

Relaxation Release of tension in the body; return to equilibrium.

Rumination Cyclic nature of the thought process, where thoughts that one ignores resurface more often; stable trait, linked to depression.

S

Secondary appraisal Secondary assessment of a situation, including assessment of available coping resources.

Secondary gain Favorable consequences, such as increased attention from significant others and escape from stressful situations, or medication use, that occur in conjunction with the generally undesirable injury.

Selective awareness Making a conscious choice as to what one will pay attention to.

Self-efficacy Confidence in one's ability to perform a particular task in a specific situation.

Self-talk Internal and/or external statements to the self, multidimensional in nature, that have interpretive elements associated with their content; it is dynamic and serves at least two functions (instructional and motivational).

Sender A person who wishes to convey a message to another.

Sensation Stimulus is received by the nervous system (via nociceptors).

Social support Includes the feeling or sense of being supported by others, the act of supporting others, and social integration.

Somatic Of the body; relating to the body; bodily illness.

Somatic relaxation A relaxation method that leads the participant to a relaxed state through focus on the breath and breathing patterns.

Somatosensory cortex The main sensory receptive area for the sense of touch.

Sport ethic Socially defined criteria for consideration as an athlete in competitive sports.

Sport norms Standards, beliefs, or models considered to be normal in sports settings.

Sport socioculture Social and cultural climates, contexts, and structures that surround sport and drive the way individuals act and relate to one another in the sport environment.

Stress Response of the body to any demand made on it; physiological (i.e., body, muscle tension) or psychological (i.e., overwhelming feelings that are good or bad).

Stress-induced analgesia A reduction in pain sensitivity during stress conditions.

Stressor Stress producer; may be positive (eustress) or negative (distress).

Subclinical The early stages or a very mild form of a condition.

Subjective report What athletes or patients tell the practitioner about their injury or condition.

Suicidal ideation Serious thoughts about committing suicide.

Systematic review A research method that provides a comprehensive and detailed summary of literature relevant to a research question.

T

Tactical imagery A mental rehearsal of plays, strategies, and/or assignments.

Thalamus A part of the brain that relays sensory and motor signals to the cerebral cortex and regulates consciousness, sleep, and alertness.

Thought stopping A psychological strategy that allows the athlete to gain control over the thought process, changing negative thoughts to more productive positive thoughts.

Tolerance Reaction to a drug is progressively reduced, thereby requiring an increase in concentration to achieve the desired effect.

Trait anxiety A stable personality construct of worry (includes high and low).

Two-way communication A bidirectional sharing of information between the sender and receiver.

U

Underconformer Athlete who rejects or dismisses the norms of the sport ethic.

V

Verbal communication Use of written or spoken messages to convey a thought, feeling, or idea.

W

Withdrawal Symptoms that occur due to the decrease or discontinuation in intake of drugs.

Index

Page numbers followed by "f" denote figures, "t" denote tables, and "b" denote boxes.

D

E

F

G

Q

R

T